ETHICS BY COMMITTEE

ETHICS
BY COMMITTEE

A HISTORY *of*
REASONING TOGETHER
about MEDICINE, SCIENCE,
SOCIETY, *and the* STATE

NOORTJE JACOBS

THE UNIVERSITY OF CHICAGO PRESS

Chicago and London

The University of Chicago Press, Chicago 60637
The University of Chicago Press, Ltd., London
© 2022 by The University of Chicago
All rights reserved. No part of this book may be used or reproduced
in any manner whatsoever without written permission, except in the case of
brief quotations in critical articles and reviews. For more information, contact the
University of Chicago Press, 1427 E. 60th St., Chicago, IL 60637.
Published 2022
Printed in the United States of America

31 30 29 28 27 26 25 24 23 22   1 2 3 4 5

ISBN-13: 978-0-226-81930-3 (cloth)
ISBN-13: 978-0-226-81932-7 (paper)
ISBN-13: 978-0-226-81931-0 (e-book)
DOI: https://doi.org/10.7208/chicago/9780226819310.001.0001

Library of Congress Cataloging-in-Publication Data
Names: Jacobs, Noortje, author.
Title: Ethics by committee : a history of reasoning together about medicine, science,
    society, and the state / Noortje Jacobs.
Description: Chicago : University of Chicago Press, 2022. | Includes bibliographical
    references and index.
Identifiers: LCCN 2022000988 | ISBN 9780226819303 (cloth) | ISBN 9780226819327
    (paperback) | ISBN 9780226819310 (ebook)
Subjects: LCSH: Institutional review boards (Medicine)—Netherlands—History—
    20th century. | Medical ethics committees—Netherlands—History—20th
    century. | Human experimentation in medicine—Netherlands—History—
    20th century. | Medicine—Research—Government policy—Netherlands—
    History—20th century. | Medical ethics—Netherlands—History—20th
    century. | Medicine—Research—Moral and ethical aspects.
Classification: LCC R852.5 .J33 2022 | DDC 174.209492—dc23/eng/20220124
LC record available at https://lccn.loc.gov/2022000988

VOOR MAMA EN PAPA

And we have all heard the saying, which is true as well as witty

That a camel is a horse that was designed by a committee.

ALLAN SHERMAN, "Peter and the Commissar," 1964

CONTENTS

ABBREVIATIONS

AVS	Anti-Vivisectie Stichting (Antivivisection Foundation)
CCMO	Centrale Commissie Mensgebonden Onderzoek (Central Committee on Research Involving Human Subjects)
CME	Commissie Medische Ethiek (Committee for Medical Ethics)
CMR	Committee for Medical Research
FDA	Food and Drug Administration
IRB	Institutional Review Board
KEMO	Kerncommissie Ethiek Medisch Onderzoek (Core Committee for Ethics in Medical Research)
KNAW	Koninklijke Nederlandse Akademie van Wetenschappen (Royal Netherlands Academy of Arts and Sciences)
(K)NMG	(Koninklijke) Nederlandse Maatschappij ter Bevordering van de Geneeskunst ([Royal] Dutch Society for the Advancement of Medicine)
METC	Medisch Ethische Toetsingscommissie (Medical Ethics Review Committee)
NIH	National Institutes of Health
PHS	Public Health Service
RCT	Randomized Controlled Trial
SGP	Staatkundig Gereformeerde Partij (Dutch Reformed Political Party)
TNO	Nederlandse Organisatie voor Toegepast-Natuurwetenschappelijk Onderzoek (Netherlands Organization for Applied Scientific Research)
WHO	World Health Organization
WMA	World Medical Association
WMO	Wet Medisch-Wetenschappelijk Onderzoek met Mensen (Medical Research Involving Human Subjects Act)

NOTE ON TRANSLATIONS

Unless stated otherwise, all translations are my own,

including those used in quotations. Due to space limitations,

the original Dutch texts have not been provided.

INTRODUCTION

On February 8, 1980, a short and biting letter was published in the Dutch medical weekly *Medisch Contact*. The epistle, written by a Leiden surgeon, contained no more than two hundred words and opened with an ominous warning:

> After years of silence about Him, there he is, God, the Father, with his watchful eye *also* in the Academic Hospital of Leiden. Finally in the hospital "for advanced medicine" of the Praesidium Libertatis, while the confessional universities are arduously trying to get rid of Him. His name: CME.[1]

Leiden, the oldest university in the Netherlands (1575), had adopted the motto "Bastion of Liberty"—*Libertatis praesidium*—in the nineteenth century to advertise itself as an independent university where scientific study would progress free from ideology or religious influences.[2] Yet by 1980 Leiden had also become the first Dutch university to allow a mysterious new authority passage into its hospital. Who was this "God, the Father," whose watchful eye now oversaw the activities in the hospital "for advanced medicine"? *He* was the Committee for Medical Ethics (CME), established in 1976 to advise on various issues of ethical concern, but mostly on scientific research studies involving patients. This committee was the first of its kind in the Netherlands but would soon be followed by the instalment of comparable boards throughout the country. By the close of the twentieth century, dozens of watchful eyes were active in Dutch hospitals, general practice clinics, and research institutes, to oversee the conduct of medical research with human subjects. They followed a practice that had taken hold worldwide in the second half of the twentieth century, one without historical precedent. This was the practice of ethics by committee.

Today, when a medical researcher wants to determine the efficacy of a new medicine or surgical procedure, she first has to pay a committee like the Leiden CME a visit. Although this visit is usually digital rather than physical, the idea is that the researcher goes and requests her local research ethics committee—as these boards are generically referred to—for official permission to execute her study protocol. Whether she also has to await the decision of this board depends on the country in which she is located. Nonetheless, in many countries around the world, it has become standard practice not to start a medical research study involving human subjects before a research ethics committee has granted its permission.

Plus, once our researcher tries to publish the results of her study, she will be hard pressed to find a respectable journal willing to print her paper without proof that the experiment in question was authorized by an ethics board. The same goes for grants from most funding agencies and, depending on the type of study, for regulatory agencies such as the US Food and Drug Administration (FDA) and European Medicines Agency (EMA). This is true not only for biomedical research but also for behavioral research, and is becoming increasingly common in the social sciences and humanities. Academics conducting oral history studies in the United States, for instance, will be familiar with the routine to first acquire permission for interviews from an institutional review board (IRB)—the American version of a research ethics committee. Committees like the Leiden CME, in short, have come to operate as *obligatory passage points* in the twenty-first-century infrastructure of science, i.e., as a locus of control through which scientists hoping to conduct research involving humans first have to pass before they can participate in its practice.[3]

Research ethics committees are nowadays such firmly fixed bodies in the oversight of human experimentation that it is easy to forget how novel they really are. After all, the scientific use of living human bodies is an age-old practice, going back in recorded history to at least 280 BCE, when the Greek physicians Herophilus and Erasistratus were granted permission to vivisect a condemned criminal to observe his inner workings.[4] From about the seventeenth century onward, human experiments in science became increasingly popular, and with the rise of academic hospitals and laboratory medicine in the nineteenth century, the practice positively flourished.[5] What is more, the use of humans in experiments was recognized by the early modern period to be a subject of ethical concern, and since the mid-nineteenth century, human experimentation in medicine has regularly resulted in social protest. Correspondingly, informal moral traditions have emerged encouraging researchers to seek patients' consent.[6] Yet the actual decision to go forward with a human experiment—even one expected to have few benefits for the subjects involved—remained the preserve of individual researchers until well into the twentieth century. Until at least the 1960s, hardly any formal checks or balances existed in most countries around the world for the communal oversight of medical research involving human subjects.[7]

Small wonder, then, that the Leiden surgeon in 1980 invoked the grandeur of God the Father in his aggrieved letter to *Medisch Contact*. Suddenly, within a timespan of a few decades, a practice that had existed for centuries was brought under the control of official review boards that were to decide if such studies could proceed. In the Netherlands, dozens of these committees sprang up in the 1980s, and in 1998, the Dutch parliament passed the Medical Research Involving Human Subjects Act (WMO), legislating that no medical research studies on humans can take place on Dutch soil without prior permission of a formally recognized Medical Ethics Review Committee (METC)—the Dutch term for research ethics committees. Furthermore, for certain types of studies such as cell or gene therapy, research with gametes or embryos, or nontherapeutic intervention studies with legally incapacitated individuals, only the Central Committee on Research Involving Human Subjects (CCMO) may give its permission.[8]

In the current medical research landscape, in other words, research ethics committees have acquired the hard power of the state to decide upon the permissibility of scientific research.[9] They have, as sociologist and historian Laura Stark points out, come to function as "declarative bodies." Like a priest who declares the groom and bride to be husband and wife, research ethics committees today are legally empowered "to turn a hypothetical situation (this study *may* be acceptable) into shared reality (this study *is* acceptable)," and thus bless certain ways of probing into the world and not others. "In so doing," Stark points out, "they change what is knowable."[10] Few control mechanisms in the present-day governance of science can lay claim to this sort of power.

But why did research ethics committees spring up in the 1960s and 1970s? And what sort of control mechanism were they meant to be in the governance of ethically contentious practices in medicine and science? In this book, I explore these questions to gain a better understanding of the changing relationship between medicine, science, society, and the state in the second half of the twentieth century. In this period, the professional role of physicians and medical researchers changed radically, both in the Netherlands and internationally.[11] Whereas they had up until the 1950s enjoyed a high degree of autonomy in deciding what sort of interventions were permitted in their research and practice, they were increasingly called upon in the years thereafter to justify and request permission for those interventions in formally arranged settings, as with the research ethics committee. This change in governance was not limited to the regulation of human experimentation in medicine, or even to medical science alone. In a wide variety of professional domains, the latter half of the twentieth century saw the rise of what anthropologists have termed "a culture of accountability," i.e., the instantiation of oversight regimes designed to subject the performance of professionals to regular inspection and to oblige them to account for their activities in organized settings.[12] Yet in the governance of human experimentation this shift is often argued to have been especially drastic and disruptive: a historically unprecedented aberration from the status quo.

So, how could it be, the Leiden surgeon demanded in 1980, that in times when even the Royal Dutch Medical Association professed to be no longer capable of "adopting in writing generally accepted rules of conduct," a small group of reviewers could be anointed to tell right from wrong within the walls of an academic hospital? Why was it that in an age in which traditional moral authority was withering away, a new God could be inaugurated to watch over the conduct of medical researchers? And on what grounds were reviewers deemed eligible to take part in a research ethics committee? "Are we jubilant when first a philosopher is added to the little club of moderators?" the surgeon snarled in *Medisch Contact*. "Are we then later put at ease when the philosopher turns out to be an ethicist?" Really, what sort of expertise did these scholars possess that granted them a seat at a committee table talking about medical ethics? This book answers the Leiden surgeon, by tracing how research ethics committees emerged as watchful eyes in the oversight of human experimentation in medicine, and by exploring what type of control mechanism they became in the public governance of a historically controversial scientific practice.

The Importance of Careful Historical Research

Despite the dominance of research ethics committees in the contemporary biomedical research landscape, their study has not been very popular among historians. In a 2009 issue of *Medical History*, this lack of scholarship was noted by sociologist Adam Hedgecoe.[13] As a sociologist, Hedgecoe investigates the present-day practice of ethics review: how committees assess publications, how researchers negotiate trust with reviewers, and how ethics boards function differently depending on their national context.[14] Still, what he found wanting in 2009 was "a full explanation for how these bodies developed the way they did"—a historical context for why they arose in the 1960s and 1970s. In *Medical History*, the sociologist therefore called upon historians to carry out a "nuanced, empirically detailed analysis" of the origins and development of research ethics committees.[15]

Since Hedgecoe's article, two monographs have appeared about the history of American IRBs. One is by Stark, who traces the invention of ethics review in medical research to the boardrooms of the National Institutes of

Health in the early 1950s.[16] The other is by Zachary Schrag, who investigates why federal regulations originally designed for biomedical and behavioral research also came to regulate research in the social sciences and humanities toward the end of the twentieth century.[17] Combined, these two books offer detailed insights into the origins and development of research ethics committees in the United States. For many other national contexts, however, Hedgecoe's words still apply.[18]

Of course, a gap in historical literature is not a problem in and of itself. Nor does a historical perspective automatically help one to understand the contemporary practice of ethics review. Rather, nuanced historical research is needed because history itself fulfills a central role in the present-day governance of human experimentation. Take the current *Oxford Textbook of Clinical Research Ethics*, published in 2008 to provide "useful educational materials" for researchers and members of ethics committees.[19] Of its impressive seventy-three contributions, the first ten detail case histories of human experimentation. These range from the famous yellow-fever experiments by the US army in Cuba in the early twentieth century—when the first written consent forms were supposedly used—to the gruesome experiments on prisoners in the Japanese and Nazi concentration camps during World War II. They range from the first randomized, controlled trial in 1948 to the exposé of the infamous Tuskegee syphilis study in 1972, when it was revealed that the US Public Health Service had been monitoring the progression of untreated syphilis in impoverished African American men since 1932, even though penicillin had been available as an effective cure for the disease since the 1940s and other remedies had commonly been used before then.[20] History, in this context, is used to *teach by example*: researchers and reviewers are instilled with a sense of right and wrong about the practice through historical "object lessons," in the hope of preventing unethical behavior in the future.[21] The past, in this sense, is used to encircle the present-day governance of human experimentation with a number of moral signposts that are to nudge researchers and reviewers in certain directions and steer them clear of others.[22]

In a similar manner, history is also used to *justify* the existence of strict oversight mechanisms for human experimentation. Against those who complain about the supposedly excessive bureaucratic demands that ethics review would bring with it—of which there are many—defenders of the status quo can charge that at some point no research ethics committees existed, and look what happened then: the Nazi atrocities happened, Tuskegee happened, not to mention the numerous dubious studies conducted on institutionalized groups, such as inmates or psychiatric patients, before the current review system was put in place. History, here, offers a rationalization for the often-lamented fact that human experimentation is now surrounded with an elaborate set of formal checks and balances: they are necessary because history has proven that researchers cannot simply be left to their own devices.

Thirdly, and most importantly in the context of this book, history is regularly brought to bear to *frame* the political function that research ethics committees have come to fulfill in the public oversight of science. Present-day textbooks and policy reports on the subject of research ethics governance often begin with a backstory stating that the rise of research ethics committees in the 1960s and 1970s was part of a larger cultural trend to bring the professional conduct of medical researchers and practitioners under much-needed public control. Thus, in relevant Dutch policy documents it has become commonplace since the 1990s to narrate how "since the end of the sixties the attention for the social relevance of scientific research increased significantly," resulting in "a more critical attitude with regard to the way in which research data are obtained and with the costs that are involved." "In essence," the next lines then read, "this development is a part of society-wide discernible emancipation trend. [. . .] The realization has grown that dependence obstructs a vocal attitude."[23] Review committees, the implication is, arose as part of an emancipatory movement to give research subjects a bigger voice in decision-making about scientific research and to enable them to give direction to their own lives. Put this way, history gives body to the idea that research ethics committees arose to assert democratic control over human experimentation and still exist to hold researchers publicly accountable.

The fact that history plays such an important role in the contemporary governance of human experimentation is a crucial reason why histories of this practice need to be subjected to careful scrutiny. After all, depending on the histories that are provided, different signposts, justifications, and frames will be offered for the present-day practice of ethics by committee. For this reason, historians are often wary when they encounter historical narratives in textbooks and policy reports in which the past offers a neat frame of reference for the correct interpretation of, in this case, the governing role of research ethics committees. As Thomas Kuhn famously argues in *The Structure of Scientific Revolutions*, history in textbooks functions to initiate students into the paradigm for which a given textbook is a pedagogical vehicle, and thus primarily serves to support that paradigm.[24] The same argument can easily be made for policy documents. Often, history tends to be written backward in such publications to present the policies they favor as the only logical outcome of past events. Hence, careful historical research is itself an important check on the current system of research ethics governance, to ensure that certain historical events and their political implications are not misunderstood—or, worse, misused by political actors to push through their desired policy measures.

The Changing Knit between Medicine, Science, Society, and the State

Examining the history of ethics review also helps us to gain a better understanding of the changing ways in which liberal democracies have typically sought to handle ethically controversial issues in medicine and science in the second half of the twentieth century. Research ethics committees emerged in a period during which the appropriate relationship between medicine, science, society, and the state had come into question. From roughly the 1950s onward, scientific and technological advancement brought about new questions about what was morally permissible in medicine and science and, perhaps even more importantly, who got to speak with authority on these matters. How was an open society, one that claimed to value both scientific freedom and democratic decision-making, to approach the governance of socially contentious medical (research) practices?

In 1980, the Leiden surgeon wrote his angry letter after news had broken that an internist at his university had taken blood samples from fetuses aborted in the fifth month of pregnancy to investigate fetal blood coagulation processes.[25] Due to recent developments in chemical abortion techniques, these fetuses were often left intact and sometimes still showed signs of life such as muscular movement or a heartbeat.[26] Although these signs of life did not mean the fetuses would have been able to survive outside the womb, newspapers soon reported that experiments were conducted on "live-aborted children" in the Netherlands.[27] In a radio broadcast, the Dutch chairman of the World Federation of Doctors Who Respect Human Life compared such experiments to slavery and the Nazi concentration-camp experiments: "The point is—to justify these tests, you have to assume that [fetuses] are not human [. . .] That they have no soul and feel no pain [. . .]."[28] He therefore called upon all listeners to let the government know the Dutch people would not stand for these experiments. After the broadcast, multiple families sat down to write letters of concern to the Dutch prime minister and Queen Juliana, pleading them to please bring such a terrible and ungodly practice to a halt.[29]

The chairman of the World Federation was right that a fundamental issue at stake in the experiments was the ontological and therefore moral status of the fetus: was "it" human or not? This was, as one newspaper put it poetically, a question of "To be or not to be."[30] Yet a matter of equal contention was *who* precisely got to make this decision. Was it the scientific community or the individual investigator? The women undergoing the abortions? Or was this matter something that government and parliament should decide?

In the case involving the Leiden internist, it had been the staff of the abortion clinic who had given permission for the blood tests. The women undergoing the procedure had been left out of the decision. However, it was not this failure to obtain permission that had gotten the internist in hot water. Rather, it was the failure to obtain permission from another locus of decision-making: the Leiden CME. Upon submitting his article to the *British Journal of Haematology*, the internist had received the request to procure some sort of evidence that his study had been conducted in accordance with the reigning ethical standards for clinical research in the Netherlands. To clear this hurdle, he had knocked on the doors of the Committee for Medical Ethics that had recently been established at his hospital. "A bit naïve that he did not already do so before he began [his studies]," pharmacologist Erik Noach, the chairman of the Leiden CME, reproached the internist in the media. Nonetheless, his team would take on an after-the-fact ethics review of the blood tests taken from the aborted fetuses.[31]

This admission was enough for the *British Journal of Haematology* to publish the internist's findings—and after a few more angry letters, the public unrest over this particular case died down. However, the question of who had the authority to decide upon ethically controversial practices in medicine and science proved to be more enduring. Did research ethics committees have this authority? If so, who could sit on them? And what cultural values and political norms would they use in the evaluation of scientific research? As this book will show, the answers to these questions changed radically in the second half of the twentieth century—and, consequently, so did the imagined political function that ethics review could fulfill in the public governance of medicine and science.

Histories of Outsiders and Insiders

In the existing historiography, two narratives about the rise of research ethics committees dominate. For a long time, their emergence in the 1960s and 1970s has been explained to have been part of a movement of "medical outsiders" that sought to break the monopoly of doctors on medical decisions. Historians of bioethics, for instance, often claim that institutionalized ethics review was one of the first material effects of a broad social movement that emerged in these decades in response to public concerns over the unchecked power of the medical profession. In his 1991 classic *Strangers at the Bedside*, David Rothman outlines how the traditional authority of the American physician was replaced between 1966 and 1976 by formal mechanisms of collective decision-making. After all, "when one could no longer assume that the physician shared the same set of values as the patient, it seemed vital to devise and implement new mechanisms, preferably formal or even rigid, to further patients' particular wishes."[32] The first of these new mechanisms "was an entirely new system of governance for human experimentation," i.e., federal regulations requiring IRBs.[33]

Others, such as bioethicist and historian of medical ethics Robert Baker, similarly claim that the field emerged in the United States as a result of a laissez-faire attitude toward ethical issues in the ranks of the American medical profession, particularly in the oversight of human experimentation. Thus, in his 2013 book *Before Bioethics*, Baker argues that when new medical technologies and human research scandals confronted the wider American public in the 1960s and 1970s, this "vacuum of authoritative moral leadership created a need for action in the public sphere."[34] Hence, bioethics emerged as an alternative voice of moral authority "to meet this need, to fill that space left empty by organized medicine."[35]

Ethicist Albert Jonsen, one of the founding fathers of the American bioethics movement, also argues in *The Birth of Bioethics* that the field emerged as part of the civil rights movement of the 1960s and 1970s, to rally against traditional authorities and power relations.[36] Medicine had come to be considered an institution of social control and medical ethics a tool to privilege the interests of an elite social class. Hence, the setup of a nationwide IRB system in the early 1970s was a historic moment for the bioethics field, as it meant a "transformation of the debate on the ethics of experimentation from a private argument within the world of medicine into broad, public discourse."[37] Moreover—and especially—in a democratic society, medical ethics could only be a sub-domain of a nation's moral code accessible to all citizens. As ethicist Robert Veatch puts it in his own participatory account of "the birth of bioethics":

> I suddenly saw that explicitly in the text of the [Hippocratic] Oath would-be physicians pledged they would not reveal the precepts of the profession to anyone outside the group. [. . .] Nothing could be in greater conflict with the ways of knowing morality in the secular world where reason, empirical observation, or metaphorical social contract involving all reasonable people provided a basis for knowing the moral norms.[38]

Nonetheless, despite its evident popularity, the frame proposing that bioethics and research ethics committees arose as "part of this effort to break the monopoly of doctors on medical decisions" has received a fair amount of criticism in the last few decades. Already in 1991, sociologist Charles Bosk remarked somewhat skeptically in his review of *Strangers at the Bedside* that "there is reason to believe that the changes that have taken place have done more to protect hospitals from liability than to actually change practice."[39] Likewise, historian Tina Stevens claims that the field did not win institutional legitimacy because it gave outsiders a mouthpiece, but "because it had proved far less threatening to existing social arrangements than the changes demanded by more radical, and more popular, social critics of the sixties."[40] Putting forward a somewhat different argument, sociologist John Evans maintains that bioethics could flourish in the late twentieth century because it "met the needs of the bureaucratic state" in a secularizing political climate: i.e., instead of traditionally *thick* approaches to morality in theology, bioethics offered *thin* principles of morality (autonomy, beneficence, justice) that could easily be translated into liberal policies and regulations focused on patients' rights.[41] In turn, historian Roger Cooter charges that "bioethics has a history of opportunism" because it served to secure the professional interests of "clapped-out philosophy departments" in the 1970s.[42] Public concerns over medicine became a timely source of funding for financially struggling humanities scholars, who — taking advantage of these concerns to assert their own relevance — willingly helped to devise an ethical framework to legitimize medical research and practice, thereby protecting it from social critiques that reached beyond demands for informed-consent procedures in medical decision-making.

In her 2012 book *Behind Closed Doors*, Stark applies this counter-narrative to the emergence of American IRBs. The model of group review for the evaluation of human experiments, she argues, was "invented, justified, and expanded less by 'outsiders' like bioethicists and activists than by the researchers themselves."[43] Stark traces the origin of communal ethics review to the National Institutes of Health in 1953, when a hospital opened on their premises in Bethesda, Maryland, thereby facilitating research with healthy human subjects. While scientific experiments had in the past often been conducted on institutionalized populations such as prisoners, orphans, and the mentally ill, the routine hospitalization of healthy citizens, by a government agency no less, was a new development in the 1950s.

Ethics review, Stark argues, was invented to manage this practice. Clinical directors regularly met to discuss study protocols, which allowed them to deal with issues such as study design or the interaction between researchers and subjects. In this context, communal review came to function as a new method for making moral decisions in research, but also as a technique for solving legal problems: meetings served to determine if all studies proceeded according to official guidelines, and whether any patients displayed alarming behavior that had to be dealt with before it might escalate. Moreover, when widespread public unrest followed a number of research exposés in the 1960s and 1970s, ethics review "helped researchers to manage a legal crisis that threatened their share of the federal budget and the reputation of medical researchers." In short, Stark concludes, the histories of bioethics and IRBs should be read as "two parallel stories with one common cause: medical researchers' concerns over their legal liability in clinical studies and clinical care."[44]

This shift of historical frame—from an emphasis on outsiders to one on insiders, and from much-needed public control to legal protection and political legitimization—does not limit itself to the United States. Duncan Wilson, for example, states in his 2014 book *The Making of British Bioethics* that the origins of research ethics committees in the United Kingdom have little to do with a supposed "backlash against professional society" in the 1960s, and should be disentangled from the rise of bioethics as an outsider critique on medicine.[45] Rather, they were an enduring form of "club regulation": a form of self-regulation *by* members of the medical profession *for* members of the medical profession, that ignored calls for lay involvement in the oversight of human research studies.[46] Wilson follows Adam Hedgecoe in this analysis, who likewise argues that research ethics committees did not emerge in the United Kingdom due to calls for public control, but due to changing grant policies by the US Public Health Service in 1967, requiring prior ethics review for all research to be funded. While that fact does not negate that this policy was very much developed in response to growing public concerns over human experimentation in the United States, Hedgecoe claims it would be a mistake to think of this development as expanding outsider control over medical research in the United Kingdom. Furthermore, when the British Ministry of Health became involved in the nationwide setup of research ethics committees in the late 1960s, the idea was actively preserved that ethics review was a form of self-regulation. Hence, the rise of British research ethics committees should equally be understood as a continued form of club regulation, not as a new, inclusive method for ensuring democratic control over medical science.[47]

A Cultural History of Changing Political Function

At stake in these histories is the political function of research ethics committees. According to Rothman et al., research ethics committees emerged as a tool of what I call *external control*, i.e., as an instrument to take the medical profession out of its social isolation and to subject it to "a nation's moral code," approved by all citizens. However, according to authors such as Stark and Hedgecoe, this historically unwarranted emphasis on the influence of outsiders belies the emergence of research ethics committees as a tool of what I call *internal control*, i.e., as an instrument that was primarily wielded by medical researchers, and that ultimately served "as a technique of promoting research and preventing lawsuits."[48] Which origin story is accepted as correct matters, for depending on which history of research ethics committees that is accepted as authoritative, their current political function is viewed differently as well.

Yet, despite the relatively recent emergence of research ethics committees, it would be incomplete to limit our investigation to an overview of their origins, and to present a narrative of political function frozen in time. Contemporary IRBs, Zachary Schrag rightly argues, bear a certain family resemblance to their progenitors, but in many ways "the differences are as striking as the similarities."[49] Thus, even if research ethics committees first emerged to strengthen internal control over medical science, they do not necessarily still fulfill this function today. What we need, therefore, is a better understanding of the *changing* governance functions that research ethics committees have served over the course of their existence, in order to highlight the changing relationship between medicine, science, society, and the state in the second half of the twentieth century. Such an understanding will enable us to better answer questions such as: Which problems were at different times understood to be at stake in the governance of human experimentation? Who was, in each of these periods, considered capable of passing judgement on such studies? On behalf of what and whom? And why did these configurations change over time?

Of course, this focus does not preclude attention to the role of outsiders or insiders, nor to their political interests. As sociologist Joseph Gusfield pointed out in his 1981 book *The Culture of Public Problems*, "human problems do not spring up, full-blown and announced, into the consciousness of bystanders."[50] It involves work for an issue to be recognized as a problem in need of public governance and, even then, it matters a great deal who is appointed to come up with suitable policy solutions. Why do governments allow laboratory animals to be bred for scientific research, for instance, while this practice would be considered absolutely deplorable for the animals' human counterparts? It is not that animal-rights activists have never rallied fiercely against such practices. Yet such groups have never been fully successful in convincing others, and particularly those in power, to consider the issue to be equally problematic. Instead, those in favor of animal experimentation have by and large been able to maintain that it is a scientific practice that should not only be allowed by law, but should also be advanced with streams of public funds. Likewise, this book will establish that those in favor of human experimentation have by and large been able to insulate the practice from more radical social critiques, due to their privileged seats at the policy table.

However, of primary interest is not whether lobbyists have been insiders or outsiders to the medical research establishment, but how they made sense of and gave direction to the issues at stake in the governance of human experimentation. Hence, the main goal of this book is to *re-collect* the dominant notions that once gave form to the practice of ethics by committee and to trace how these notions changed in conjunction with changing conceptions of the appropriate relationship between medicine, science, society, and the state. "At root," Roger Cooter maintains, "the history of bioethics is not about medicine and morality at all, nor about the activity of bioethicists, but rather, is a reconfiguration of what it is to be human." With this often-used expression in medical historiography, Cooter points out that historians should study how the notion of patients' rights came to be celebrated as a capstone of ethical and legal decision-making in the latter half of the twentieth century, rather than to focus on whether "the authority of doctors was displaced by the would-be authority of (laity-minded) bioethicists."[51] Hence, this book presents an approach to history that is not so much interested in that "things could be otherwise," although it certainly does not deny this fact.[52] Instead, it seeks to recover what factors configured ethics review *as it actually manifested*, and thereby to make explicit which conceptions of the appropriate societal position of medicine and science underlie the governance of human subjects research today.

Early Concerns and Delayed Action in the Netherlands

As Wilson rightly points out in *The Making of British Bioethics*, the American story of the history of bioethics — and ethics review — continues to dominate international scholarship on the topic. While both Rothman and Baker, for instance, neatly limit their work to the American history of bioethics, their account has become such a dominant trope in the literature that it often functions as a near universal explanation for the changing governance of human experimentation after the mid-twentieth century — even though new oversight mechanisms and ethics frameworks emerged at different times in different places and continue to have distinct national traditions. This view of their scholarship is problematic, as it contributes to the perception that bioethics and research ethics committees have a single origin story and concomitant political function that they fulfill to this day.

Judging from existing Dutch texts on the ethics of human experimentation, for instance, it is easy to forget that the Netherlands might have its own history of research ethics governance. Textbooks for Dutch medical students all tend to follow the same genealogy, starting with the Nazi concentration-camp experiments and the Nuremberg Code, a set of now world-famous principles for human experimentation that were promulgated as part of the Nazi doctors' trial in 1947.[53] Then, they move on to the 1964 Declaration of Helsinki by the World Medical Association (WMA), another set of principles for human subjects research that is now often called the cornerstone document of human research ethics worldwide.[54] Subsequently, the seminal 1966 article "Ethics and Clinical Research" by the American anesthesiologist Henry K. Beecher is mentioned, which listed twenty-two postwar clinical research studies that Beecher believed to be flagrantly unethical.[55] To this, the 1967 book *Human Guinea Pigs* by British physician Maurice Pappworth is added, listing numerous questionable experiments conducted on hospital patients, orphans, inmates, and other confined populations in the United Kingdom in this period.[56] The 1972 exposé of the Tuskegee study typically concludes such segments, whereafter it is concluded that, today, stringent legislation for human research studies exists worldwide.[57]

Such a placeless genealogy ignores, however, that these exposés played hardly any role in the establishment of the first research ethics committees in the Netherlands. While Dutch news did report on scandals such as Tuskegee and the exposés of "Mister Pappworth," none of these reports ever led to much government action. A placeless genealogy also neglects to acknowledge that the Netherlands itself was not free from research scandals. In the 1960s and 1970s, multiple dubious human research studies were reported on, such as experiments in a psychiatric clinic with a flu vaccine in 1966 by a prominent pharmaceutical company. But while the Dutch statespersons in office usually did issue a formal reply condemning these studies, these scandals did not lead to much government action before the early 1980s. In other words, the singular focus in historical scholarship on the United States overlooks the way in which context-specific factors shape what is taken to be ethical or problematic in different times and places. This lack of nuance may be an important cause of the at-times heated polemics over the past and present-day institutional function of bioethics: i.e., by reducing its history either to a need for action in the public sphere or to a strategy to protect the interests of scientists and physicians, one ignores that, as Wilson puts it, "bioethics is a multi-sited and interdisciplinary set of activities" which cannot be traced back to a single historical event (Tuskegee) or figure (Beecher).[58] In recent years, therefore, scholars from various disciplines have called for more-nuanced empirical studies that move away from the American story to show the varying forms and functions of bioethics and ethics review in different historical contexts.[59]

The Dutch history of research ethics committees offers an interesting case for doing so. In Anglo-American scholarship on the topic, historians have repeatedly argued that this unprecedented change in the governance of human experimentation started in the Netherlands, which is supposed to have been one of the first countries to try to install research ethics committees in the 1950s, and whose national medical society in 1952 first brought the ethics of human experimentation to the agenda of the WMA. Susan Lederer has discussed this influence in her history of the Declaration of Helsinki, and both Robert Baker and Ulrich Tröhler have pointed to the Netherlands as one of the first countries that would have recognized the principles of the Nuremberg Code by seeking to establish official ethics boards.[60] This special attention for the Netherlands fits with a broader tradition in academic scholarship on the history of medical ethics. Dutch developments are often brought to bear on the topic as a key reference culture to situate developments in other national contexts, due in large part to the unique Dutch legal history of euthanasia and physician-assisted suicide (resulting in conditional legalization in 2002).[61] Thus, in *Before Bioethics*, Baker juxtaposes the laissez-faire attitude of the American medical profession to that of the Dutch medical profession, which he claims to have retained jurisdiction over medical ethics, both in the past and the present: "The Royal Dutch Medical Association (founded in 1849) was able to negotiate physician-initiated euthanasia practices with Dutch legal authorities without involving 'bioethicists' in any major decision."[62]

In this book, I offer the first scholarly examination of these Dutch concerns to show that an early awareness of the need for more oversight of human experimentation did indeed exist in the Netherlands. I also show that this awareness was not spurred on by questionable research practices in Dutch hospitals and research clinics themselves, but by concerns over what was happening under the aegis of medical science in countries such as the United States and Great Britain. A growing group of Dutch physicians came to ask themselves in the 1950s whether some of the research published in American and British medical journals was really so different from the atrocities committed by Nazi scientists during the war.

I also argue, however, that the exemplary function fulfilled by the Netherlands in many Anglo-American histories of medical ethics has little empirical grounding, and that conclusions in these studies need revision in light of a more informed view of the Dutch context. Most importantly, this book makes clear that, contrary to widespread perception, research ethics committees in the Netherlands were at first intended just as much to advocate for as they were to curb human experimentation in medicine. If Dutch clinical science ever wanted to become as prestigious as its counterparts in the United States and Great Britain, Dutch physicians and medical researchers argued in the 1960s and 1970s, more and better experiments had to be conducted on patients. Hence, research ethics committees were imagined as what I will call *epistemic filters*, tools that would raise the quality and quantity of clinical research by taking away "undue moral concerns" among physicians and politicians, and by promoting new research methods among clinicians.

In addition, despite these early activities, it would take until the close of the twentieth century until the Dutch parliament passed a law for the regulation of human experimentation in medicine, long after many other countries had done so. This delay was not for lack of trying. From the 1950s onward, the Dutch government requested reports from official advisory bodies on numerous occasions to help decide whether legislation for human experimentation was desirable, and what such a framework should look like. In parliament, the matter was discussed at length throughout the 1980s and 1990s and politicians complained regularly that the realization of an appropriate legal system was long overdue. In the same period, both medical insiders and outsiders frequently vented frustrations about the inability of the government to enact proper legislation. "The Netherlands is becoming an international testing ground for all sorts of experimental research," commentators would write, "a *Freistaat* for experiments [. . .] which are refused elsewhere."[63]

Hence, due to a reluctant government, conversations over the ideal governance of human experimentation spanned a period of more than forty years in the Netherlands, revealing clear shifts in the conceptualization of research ethics committees and their function in the governance of medical science. Where Stark argues that ethics review in the United States had by the 1960s already become an "entrenched, routine way of doing things" that required "less justification and explanation over time," it remained an active subject of deliberation in the Netherlands until the late twentieth century, in expert advisory boards, at parliamentary hearings, and in the discussion pages of scientific journals and newspapers.[64] For years the original blueprint for ethics review was tweaked and twisted, until most parties involved deemed it ready to be cast into law. As a result, an impressive paper trail has been left behind on the shelves of the Dutch National Archive and in the proceedings of the Dutch parliament. These sources will be combined with a variety of published materials, including pamphlets, newspaper and journal articles, private correspondence, and broadcasts, to map how the idea of ethics review travelled from the first Dutch policy report on the topic in 1955 to the eventual passing of a law in 1998.

A Long and Winding Road

The following chapters make clear that this journey did not follow a straight path. Between 1955 and 1998, the original Dutch blueprint for ethics review changed substantially in conjunction with changing conceptions of the appropriate relationship between medicine, science, society, and the state. Part I of this book maps the original notion of ethics review by committee as a form of internal control over the practice of human experimentation. I show that it was developed in the 1950s and 1960s in the Netherlands as an instrument that had to be wielded by medical researchers and practitioners, that preserved the idea that the medical profession constituted a separate social class subject to its own mores and traditions, and that was intended to have systemic effects on the sort of knowledge that could pass as legitimate in modern medical science.

Chapter 1 shows how, after the Second World War, revelations of the Nazi concentration-camp experiments provoked radically different responses among social groups in the Netherlands. Leaders of the medical profession vowed to never again let the corrupting influences of political ideology and government bureaucracy take hold of medicine. Other social groups, however, including homeopaths and antivivisectionists, found definitive proof in the concentration-camp experiments of the dangers of "modern medicine" and its reductionist perspective on life. In this context, debates over human experimentation became a placeholder for larger concerns over the societal standing and epistemic authority of modern medicine. Consequently, the first proposal for a system of ethics by committee became an attempt to entice a definitive statement from the Dutch government over the rightful position of medical science in mainstream medicine and modern society.

Chapter 2 examines the first full blueprint for ethics review that was developed in the Netherlands around 1970, in response to parliamentary questions about the permissibility of a new form of human experimentation: the randomized controlled trial. The architects of this blueprint were convinced that legal measures were needed to bring this research practice under public control. However, these architects were not concerned merely with the rights and safety of human research subjects. In their eyes, clinical experimentation itself had to be protected and promoted as well, with governments having a moral responsibility to increase both the quality and quantity of human research studies.

In part II, I explain how the original notion of ethics review was adopted toward the end of the 1970s by a movement that pushed for more external control over medicine and science. In this process, research ethics committees were reimagined as instruments to take the medical profession out of its social isolation and to democratize medical research.

Chapter 3 details how, in the 1960s, a crisis emerged in the Netherlands over whether the existing medical ethics tradition was still compatible with "life in a modern society," which many commentators believed to be dominated by technological inventions, an increase in the scale of organizations, and changing societal bonds more broadly. When this crisis connected in the late 1960s to a larger rebellion against traditional authorities, multiple social groups came to argue that medicine and science required new and better democratic modes of governance. Eventually, in 1978, these arguments resulted in the establishment of a government advisory committee named Rights of the Patient, which proposed the introduction of far-reaching public control mechanisms to bring about truly participatory decision-making structures in health care.

Chapter 4 explains how, in comparison with countries such as the United States and Great Britain, unrest over unethical human experimentation initially played only a minor role in "the backlash against professional society" in the Netherlands. When such unrest did emerge more forcefully in the late 1970s, the Rights of the Patient Committee adopted the original blueprint for ethics review in an attempt to give "society representatives" an opportunity to participate in the governance of medical research. Yet I also show in chapter 4 that, just as with the original blueprint for ethics by committee, this new blueprint was likewise written with the intention to protect and promote the conduct of human subjects research. This time, however, the project of epistemic reform went hand in hand with a narrative of egalitarian decision-making in a democratic society.

Finally, I explain in part III how, in the 1980s and 1990s, against a backdrop of a rising neoliberal climate and the scaling-up and internationalization of medical science, the political function of research ethics committees was once more reimagined in the Netherlands. I also argue that this change was bound up with the international rise of a new class of professionals in this period, i.e., ethical experts.

Chapter 5 traces the emergence of Dutch health ethics in the 1970s and 1980s, a development that was modelled after the rise of the bioethics movements in the United States and Great Britain. Despite the fact that the emergence of health and bioethics is often explained as a movement that sought to democratize ethical debates and decisions on science and medicine, I argue that it is better to understand its rise as an attempt to speak with new expert authority at a time when traditional moral authority was waning. In addition, chapter 5 maps the debates that ensued in the late 1980s about the function that this field would fulfill in the public governance of medicine and science. In academic scholarship, the establishment of research ethics committees is often argued to have been the first tangible effect of the bioethics movement. However, I show that in the Netherlands the relation between these two modes of governance can best be understood the other way around: in the late twentieth century, the practice of ethics by committee, originally designed as a tool of internal control over medicine and science, became a battleground for ethicists and philosophers to flesh out *their* professional identities and political roles in a democratic society, with consequences for those who could speak with expert authority on the ethics of medicine and science in political arenas and institutional settings.

Chapter 6 examines the mushrooming of ethics review in the 1980s and 1990s, and the growing political tension between expert and democratic modes of governance that new forms of "human" experimentation, such as embryo research and gene therapy, brought along. It describes how the Dutch government, as a typical example of the Third Way politics popular in liberal democracies in the 1990s, came up with a conception of "objective ethical decision-making" that permitted politicians to kill two birds with one stone. First, it enabled the state to assert that it did not leave medical researchers to their own devices—an autonomy they had proven incapable of handling and that did not befit a democratic order anyway. Second, by suggesting that this scrutiny would proceed *objectively*, it enabled the government to assert that it did not infringe upon personal beliefs in a pluralistic society. Professional ethicists in this context were imagined as ideal fulcrums between expert and democratic modes of decision-making.

At stake in all these changing conceptions of the appropriate governance function of research ethics committees were fundamental questions about how societies are to handle morally complex issues in medicine and science, and who may legitimately speak on behalf of science and the public in deciding upon the permissibility of morally freighted research studies. By examining these complex negotiations in the context of the Netherlands, this book seeks to contribute to ongoing conversations in international scholarship about the ways in which liberal democracies in the recent past have sought to resolve concerns over charged issues in medicine and science—questions they continue to struggle with to this day.

Some Disclaimers Before We Start

Since this book focuses on policy debates, the day-to-day dealings and decisions of the more than one hundred Dutch research ethics committees that have existed since the 1970s receive only minor attention in the following pages. The emphasis lies with the language of political discourse in which their role and function have been imagined, not with their actual historical or current practices.[65] As a consequence, the question of how the development of ethics review has impacted the practice of medical science remains largely out of view. I fully acknowledge that this is a crucial question that awaits further historical research, requiring a methodology and availability of archival materials that lie outside of the scope of this book. Here, I focus predominantly on *committees thinking about committees*, i.e., on the numerous advisory bodies that have been commissioned since the 1950s by the Dutch government to write reports on the topic, and on the two "committees" ideally elected once every four years to represent the interests and concerns of Dutch citizens: the country's House of Representatives (Tweede Kamer) and Senate (Eerste Kamer).

According to sociologist Sheila Jasanoff, expert advisory committees are important resources for scholars interested in the boundary work that goes into framing contentious issues as problems in need of public action.[66] Outside the limelight that dominates parliamentary deliberations, they often establish the parameters within which subsequent policy discussions will be held. Relevant policy documents have therefore formed a central point of departure for identifying further source material. In addition, as expert advisory bodies draw on developments in scientific practice and public discourse, relevant academic journals and popular newspapers have been studied to gain a better picture of the changing cultural climate in which policy deliberations took place. All issues of the journal *Medisch Contact* (1945–present) have been studied, for instance, as have other relevant medical and academic journals. Such sources are often included in the following pages, although within limits. Discussions that hardly had an effect on the development of policies, even if they were of high concern to those involved, receive only minor attention.

The upcoming chapters also do not address the role of research ethics committees in nonmedical research contexts. Of course, depending on the definition given to concepts such as "experiment" and "research," the scope of a law regulating human subjects research may vary widely. In fact, as will become clear, a big part of the policy discussions about human experimentation was dedicated to deciding what precisely constitutes an experiment and how it differs from regular clinical interventions. As Schrag shows in his 2010 book *Ethical Imperialism*, the legal definition of research in the United States has over the years come to include most studies with human beings in the social sciences, a process that has gone hand in hand with a reconfiguration of the notion of what is considered scientific in these fields.[67] Nonetheless, Schrag also emphasizes that US federal policies for human experimentation were originally designed for the biomedical and behavioral sciences, and only later transposed to the social sciences and humanities. Likewise, in the Netherlands, policy deliberations mostly revolved exclusively around medical experimentation, and current legislation continues to speak of medical-scientific research, leaving it up to the administrative body responsible for the execution of this law to decide what types of other research studies fall within its scope.[68]

This book also does not contain a systematic comparison with historical developments in other countries. Rather, different national contexts flow in and out of consideration to highlight what is particular about the Netherlands, to show why it is worthwhile to consider the history of ethics review away from the Anglo-American narrative. I do show how developments in the Netherlands connected to broader international developments in the second half of the twentieth century, including the growing dominance of American-led transnational funding and publishing networks. Part I, for instance, details how Dutch concerns over human experimentation in the 1950s were based in large part on research done in the United States, while the desire to develop large-scale clinical research programs stemmed from attempts to catch up internationally. Part III, in turn, details how a growing dependency of Dutch medical researchers on foreign research funders and scientific journals contributed to the explosion of research ethics committees in the Netherlands in the 1980s, and also how Dutch ethicists increasingly adopted the language of American bioethics during this period. These processes of institutional isomorphism on the terrain of medical ethics are ones that historians are now beginning to consider.[69]

Finally, this book does not provide a definition of the term governance. Although it is admittedly an elusive term that cannot be translated into all languages, it is a widely recognized concept by which to consider acts of organizing, managing and ruling, by a variety of entities and actors, through formal and informal channels, in a multitude of spheres.[70] Bruno Latour refers to concepts like governance as part of a scholar's *infra*-language: "They don't designate *what* is being mapped, but *how* it is possible to map anything from such a territory. They are part of the equipment on the geographer's desk to allow him to project shapes on a sheet of paper."[71] And thus, in the upcoming pages, the term is equipped to bring into view the two fundamental shifts in the governance of human experimentation that this book wants to capture. One, the transition of the locus of ethical decision-making from individual researchers to select teams of expert reviewers. And, two, the transition from a tradition of self-governance in medical science to one of strict public control—as it occurred in the second half of the twentieth century in a small country called the Netherlands.

PART I
INTERNAL CONTROL

CHAPTER 1

A MORAL OBLIGATION

to MEDICAL PROGRESS

"Both modern medications and modern medical practice carry risk. Hippocrates' old precept can therefore in this modern day and age no longer be maintained in its entirety."[1] In 1954, Dutch internist Job Pannekoek put this conclusion on the table of the national Dutch Health Council's Committee for Tests Upon Human Beings. A few months earlier, this committee, consisting of sixteen eminent physicians, had been established to study the permissibility of human experimentation in medicine. Pannekoek and his colleagues were worried about some of the experiments conducted in Dutch hospitals and expressed deep concern about stories that reached them from countries such as the United States. Yet they also felt that traditional medical ethics no longer befitted physicians who committed themselves to the practice of modern medicine. *Primum non nocere*, the old Hippocratic precept to "first, do no harm," could no longer be maintained by physicians who had an array of tools available to actually *do good*, and who carried a responsibility to benefit as many patients as possible. Hence, a new ethical framework was needed—one that would do justice to the new role of science in medicine. Modern medicine required modern medical ethics.

This chapter explores the incentives behind the establishment of the Health Council's Committee for Tests Upon Human Beings. In 1955, its conclusions about the appropriate governance of human experimentation were published as a twelve-page policy advice report to the Dutch government, containing fourteen guidelines for medical tests involving humans and recommending the installation of a national advisory board to guide this practice.[2] According to some historians, this publication marked one of the first times that the need for institutional oversight of human experimentation was recognized in national policy circles.[3] Still, why did a national advisory body to the Dutch government formulate ethical guidelines for medical tests upon human beings in the 1950s, a decade when only few precedents existed internationally to suggest that the state rather than the medical profession should be responsible for governing this practice? Why did it decide in 1954 that the old ethical precept of *primum non nocere* in medicine had become obsolete? And what sort of oversight role did the Health Council imagine for a national advisory board in guiding human experimentation?

To answer these questions, I trace how and by whom human experimentation was turned into a matter of public concern in the Netherlands in the first decade after World War II. In this period, revelations of the Nazi concentration-camp experiments provoked radically different responses among different Dutch social groups. Leaders of the medical profession vowed to never again let the corrupting influences of political ideology and government bureaucracy take hold over medicine. Others, however, found definitive proof in the concentration-camp experiments of the dangers of "modern medicine" and its reductionist perspective on animal and human life. As a result, debates over human experimentation in the immediate postwar period came to revolve around the social standing and epistemic authority of modern medicine. Consequently, when the Dutch Health Council published its report in 1955, it attempted not just to lay the groundwork for the future governance of human experimentation in the Netherlands, but also to enforce a definitive statement about its rightful position in mainstream medicine and modern society. This chapter explores what this statement was—and who was responsible for it.

The Growing Importance of Human Experimentation

Human experimentation is an age-old practice, but it has not always been a central part of medicine. Of course, as every new medicine and surgery once had to be tried out on a human patient for the first time, it is possible to argue that human experiments are as old as medicine itself.[4] But experiments whereby an intervention on the human body is undertaken not primarily to benefit the health of the patient, but to obtain generalizable scientific insights, started to gain in popularity only during the Renaissance.[5] Many of these early experiments were conducted on the bodies of the experimenters themselves, but philosophers and physicians experimented on others as well.[6] Often, these experiments were conducted on volunteers, who participated in popular demonstrations of new machines such as the Voltaic pile or the apparatus for producing factitious airs.[7] However, medical experiments were also conducted on those who could not be considered volunteers. Londa Schiebinger describes, for instance, how English physicians in the eighteenth century experimented with cures and dosages on charity patients until they deemed these treatments ready to prescribe to paying patients. Prominent physicians in France and Germany, meanwhile, promoted submitting prisoners to extreme trials and surgeries for "the sake of humanity."[8] In general, individuals confined in closed institutions such as workhouses, orphanages, and prisons were at risk. Crammed together and dependent on the grace of others, they were often taken as "readily available material."[9]

In the nineteenth century, with the growing importance of statistical approaches in science, human experimentation in medicine intensified. In the 1830s, Parisian physician Pierre Louis famously developed the "numerical method" for medical practice, using calculus and probability theory to measure the risks and benefits of clinical procedures.[10] This numerical approach subjected individual experience to systematic comparison. Central was not whether medicines worked for one patient, but whether they produced significant effects on a population level. In addition, after the mid-nineteenth century, the growing popularity of the germ theory of disease led medical practice increasingly to model itself after scientific practice.[11] In his famous 1865 book *Introduction to the Study of Experimental Medicine*, French physiologist Claude Bernard explained: "So, among the experiments that may be tried on man, those that can only harm are forbidden, those that are innocent are permissible, and those that may do good are obligatory."[12] Under the right circumstances, human experiments were a moral obligation for physicians.[13]

This experimental tradition was facilitated by the rise of modern research hospitals. In the early nineteenth century, the idea gained prominence that hospitals were teaching and research centers as much as they were service institutes. Emphasis lay on diagnosis, not cure.[14] Based on new theoretical insights in physiology, students were trained in new diagnostic techniques to recognize which parts of the diseased body were failing. After patients passed away, autopsies served to confirm these findings. Often, these interventions served to demonstrate scientific insight and skill as much as, or even more than, they served to provide care. Patients effectively functioned as research subjects.

In this period, still, hospital patients were often from the lower classes of society. Affluent patients preferred to be taken care of in their own homes, far away from the noise and filth of hospital wards. Toward the end of the nineteenth century, however, the growing use of invasive medical technologies such as stomach tubes and x-rays ensured that well-to-do patients were increasingly taken care of in hospitals—where these technologies were more readily available. As a result, physicians' careers grew less dependent on their patients' preferences and more dependent on the approval of hospital boards and medical peers.[15] Conducting human experiments, if successful and above moral suspicion, could greatly boost a curriculum vitae.

A final, more remote, factor contributing to the intensification of human experimentation was the growing public function of medicine. In the nineteenth century, states increasingly took an interest in public health, thereby elevating the legal status of physicians.[16] In the Netherlands, the government passed legislation in 1865 that made it illegal for anyone to see patients without the right license, officially creating a "doctors' monopoly."[17] This legislation corporatized the identity of the Dutch medical profession. In 1849, the Dutch Society for the Advancement of Medicine (NMG) was created to represent the interests of all physicians in the Netherlands, a development that took place in other countries as well in the nineteenth century.[18] Such professional societies stimulated rhetoric of communal responsibility: physicians did not just carry a responsibility to individual patients; they had a duty to take care of the body politic of a nation as a whole. In the late nineteenth and twentieth centuries, this utilitarian logic served to justify human experiments. After all, if physicians were responsible for "the wellbeing of the greatest number of people," perhaps some risks could be taken with a few patients, if these risks could benefit the many.

Of course, the relevance and extent of these changes differed by country. The use of medical statistics, for instance, originated in England in the eighteenth century and was brought to fruition in Paris in the nineteenth century.[19] Similarly, in the early nineteenth century, physicians from all over Europe and the United States flocked to Paris to watch their French colleagues make rounds and use the newest instruments in their bedside diagnoses.[20] With the rise of laboratory medicine in the mid-nineteenth century, Germany took over this leading international position, whereas in the twentieth century the United States increasingly assumed international leadership in the medical sciences.[21]

In the Netherlands, the pace of change was on average slower. Throughout the nineteenth century, Dutch physicians expressed frustration at the fact that the government seemed unwilling to invest substantial sums of money in medicine.[22] These feelings of frustration lasted until well into the twentieth century. Systematic human experimentation was not possible in the Netherlands, the feeling was, as the country lacked the infrastructure to bring together the know-how of academia, the "patient material" in hospitals, and the financial means of industry. Yet, also in the Netherlands, medicine underwent substantial changes in the nineteenth century, stimulating systematic human experimentation. Around the 1850s, the statistical method grew popular, the hospital system underwent significant revisions, and diagnostic laboratories were established.[23] The idea that poor hospital patients mainly served as "research material" became a trope.[24]

Consequently, by the turn of the century, members of the Dutch parliament started to wonder if measures had to be taken to bring the practice under public control, as reports reached them, especially from countries east of the border, of all sorts of ungodly activities taking place in hospitals under the guise of science. The Dutch medical profession vehemently opposed such accusations: in the Netherlands, the NMG professed publicly, doctors knew and respected the boundaries of human experimentation. Yet, even within the ranks of the NMG, some started to argue in the early twentieth century for additional safeguards to keep the practice within bounds.

Moral Traditions and Social Concerns

Sometimes, human experimentation prior to the advent of research ethics committees is presented as a practice that was able to proceed in any shape or form without much public or professional scrutiny. Historical research has shown, however, that in the early modern period human experimentation had already attracted moral discussion. According to Erika Dyck and Larry Stewart, "trials upon the ill-informed, the desperate, and the unreliable raised clear and serious alarm in the minds of the experimenters."[25] "The point is not that this was a matter of a drastic morality," Dyck and Stewart explain, "but rather that the issue was then fairly acknowledged and well considered."[26]

In the nineteenth century, fledgling medical professions in Europe and the United States developed more pronounced moral traditions for handling the risks associated with untested remedies and surgical procedures.[27] These traditions, Sydney Halpern argues, were largely informal and uncodified. Few formal mechanisms (legislation, state inspections) existed to prevent or repress excesses by individual researchers. Nonetheless, many physicians treated these traditions as if they were self-evident, and they did not shy away from shaming colleagues whom they believed to have transgressed the boundaries of the permissible in human experimentation. Other imperatives, Halpern shows, were the practice of prior self-experimentation—the so-called golden rule—and the "logic of lesser harms," which stipulates that an intervention is justified when the benefits are likely to outweigh the risks.

Following Martin Pernick, Halpern traces this logic to the growing influence of statistical reasoning in medical practice in the nineteenth century.[28] The introduction of anesthesia in American surgical practice in 1846, for instance, was justified using "a calculus of suffering." While patients could die from this purposefully induced deep sleep, its proponents collected numer-

ical evidence to prove that surgeries without anesthetics killed a larger per-
centage of patients than surgeries with anesthetics.[29] Hence, on a population level, the calculus of suffering pointed in favor of anesthesia. According
to Halpern, this utilitarian logic was increasingly used in the early twentieth century to justify experiments without a direct benefit for participating
research subjects. Risks taken with individuals could be balanced "by the
expectation of a contribution to the greater social good."[30]

In addition to the development of moral traditions within different countries' medical professions, the nineteenth century also saw growing societal
opposition to human experiments. In conjunction with the growing popularity of experimental medicine in this period, efforts to restrict scientific
experimentation in medicine grew stronger as well. Many of these attempts
revolved around animal experimentation rather than human experimentation. Nonetheless, by the end of the nineteenth century, the use of humans
in medical research had also increasingly become a topic of concern for organizations dedicated to the prevention and abolition of animal research—
typically called antivivisectionist societies.

A fairly extensive body of literature exists that details the history of antivivisection movements in the nineteenth and twentieth century. These histories show that important differences existed among and within national
antivivisection movements. Still, on average, antivivisectionists expressed a
few typical objections to animal experimentation. First, they considered it
to be a cruel practice on par with other forms of animal violence. Many early
antivivisection societies were therefore linked to animal protection groups.
Secondly, they argued that torture inflicted on animals blunted the minds
and senses of scientists to the extent that these researchers would eventually inflict cruelty on humans as well. Thirdly, for many antivivisectionists, a
charge against vivisection included a charge against "the corrupting effects
of modern medicine." The experimental tradition, they argued, had reduced
the traditional art of healing to a cold, mechanistic science that prioritized
scientific knowledge above patient care and ignored everything not made
out of matter. The germ theory of disease, for instance, had reduced illness to
single deterministic causes that neglected the influence of the environment
and psyche. Likewise, the bewildering array of medical specialties that had
sprung up in the nineteenth century fueled a harmful, reductionist perspective on life. Such a perspective ignored that living beings were more than
the sum of their parts and could only be understood in relation to the world
around them. Felix Ortt, for instance, a founding father of the Dutch antivivisection movement, believed an inconceivable order to exist in the world

that operated on and through everything—from the electron, molecule, and cell to the organism, society, and state. Vivisectionists, he argued, cut their connection to this ordering principle and would thus never be able to produce true knowledge.[31]

Historians have often argued that the late-nineteenth-century debate over vivisection was, in fact, a debate over the cultural authority of modern science. Vivisection represented the "priorities and aspirations of science," Nicolaas Rupke argues, "and scientists defended the practice, even if they had no direct contact with it." In contrast, those who opposed the practice did so because they "saw their cultural influence waning as that of science grew."[32] Others take issue with this representation of the antivivisectionists. Susan Lederer, for instance, criticizes the equation of antivivisectionism to anti-science sentiments in the context of the United States in the early twentieth century. This dichotomy, she argues, fails to capture the multiple and fluid meanings that medical science itself embodied during this period.[33] Likewise, in her history of Dutch antivivisectionism, Amanda Kluveld points out that antivivisectionists did not denounce modern science, but rather offered an alternative integration of elements of science, religion, and philosophy to the by-then established scientific order.[34] Ortt, for one, drew on Maxwell's laws of thermodynamics in his ideas of an all-ordering principle. Still, both historians agree that antivivisectionists did *position* their perspectives as an alternative to "the evils of modern science." In turn, they were typically denounced by their opponents as a mindless group of quacks.

Human experimentation fulfilled a specific role in these tugs of war. On the one hand, for many antivivisectionists, animal and human experiments were intimately related. Not unjustly, the impression existed that vulnerable social groups were more likely to fall victim to the vivisector's knife than the well to do. Orphans, mental patients, prisoners: for antivivisectionists they were all powerless individuals in dire need of protection. As such, they were not so different from animals. A difference in degree existed, but not in kind. Yet at the same time, antivivisectionists often instrumentally drew on cases of unethical human experimentation to lobby for legislation restricting animal vivisection. In a meeting of the Dutch parliament in 1903, for instance, a member of the Anti-Revolutionary Party warned Prime Minister Abraham Kuyper against the dangers of *human* experimentation to convince him that *animal* vivisection had to be brought under legal control:

And, above all, Mister Chairman, a statutory regulation of vivisection would be necessary for the upcoming generation of professors and doctors, so that we can entrust to them with confidence the weak, the poor, amongst us. It is for the sake of them that I called vivisection a harrowing national distress.[35]

It was well known, this parliament member continued, that in "clinics abroad" the most terrible experiments were done with humans. Rumor went that even "children and chaste maidens" had deliberately been infected with syphilis for its scientific study! Hence, legislation for animal vivisection was needed now in the Netherlands, before the minds and senses of Dutch vivisectors had become so blunted that they too would be unable to refrain from conducting such godless practices on humans.

As a result of such parliamentary discussions, the Dutch medical profession started to develop more pronounced views on the governance of human experimentation around the turn of the twentieth century. In 1904, for instance, editor of the *Dutch Journal of Medicine* Hendrik Burger reacted with horror to the insinuation in the Dutch parliament that dubious human experiments might take place at the hands of Dutch doctors. Half of his reaction served to dismiss such unfounded accusations: little proof existed that Dutch physicians were equally guilty of unethical human experimentation. Half of his reaction, however, also served to remind readers of the *Dutch Journal of Medicine* that "tests upon human beings which only satisfy our medical curiosity and that do not meet the distinct medical grounds of a specific case deserve absolute disapproval."[36] Physicians who wanted to conduct human experiments could only use their own bodies for doing so.

Burger also urged his readers to be vigilant. It was the duty of every physician to speak up when he suspected another colleague to have crossed the line. To suit his actions to his words, he proceeded to scold a member of the Dutch medical profession who had recently stated that he was willing to give a homeopath access to his patients just to prove that the homeopathic doctrines were unfounded. If one was sure a therapy had no effect, Burger wrote sternly, it was deeply unethical to expose patients to such self-serving experiments. This editorial comment led to a heated dispute in the *Journal* over whether this naming and shaming was proper etiquette. Still, Burger considered it his duty as an editor to condemn unethical research studies.[37] Failure to do so, he stated, would undermine the public's trust in the medical profession.

Physicians like Burger with influential positions in the Dutch medical profession frequently used their authority to moralize the practice of medicine in the early twentieth century. They did so because they were convinced that medicine had to be governed primarily through processes of *internal control*.

Until the rise of the patients' rights movement in the 1970s, it was common in the Dutch language to refer to the doctors' collective as the *artsenstand*, i.e., "a class of physicians." Membership was allotted only to those with a license to practice, who conducted themselves in a manner that could be expected from "gentlemen": with dignity and prudence.[38] As a class, physicians were part of Dutch society, but stood apart from it at the same time. Their conduct was regulated by mores specific to the medical profession.

Ethical guidelines and peer pressure served to regulate the conduct of practitioners. While physicians were subject to the law like anyone else, ethical wisdom in medicine was understood to come with years of experience; one required the lived experience of being a physician to be able to judge what was right and wrong in medicine, and which measures had to be taken in case of misbehavior. Right or wrong depended on context and could not be fixed by hard legislation.

From this understanding, it followed that the governance of medicine was first and foremost a *professional* affair. Members of the *artsenstand* had a duty to hold each other accountable, as only they could really understand what it meant to be a physician. Conversely, the interference of "outsiders" was often treated with suspicion, as laypeople did not possess the lived experience of being a physician.

This class ideology translated itself in various safeguards of internal control. First, seasoned practitioners had a responsibility to instill a sense of right and wrong in younger generations. They led by example, at the bedside and in classes. Secondly, physicians reminded one another of the ethics of their practice via both the written and spoken word. Although it would take until 1936 before the NMG published its first booklet on medical ethics, it was common for physicians to discuss the ethics of medicine in the *Dutch Journal of Medicine* or to publish lectures on the subject.[39] Thirdly, from 1905 onward, the NMG held regular disciplinary hearings to hold physicians responsible for any misbehavior.[40] Finally, one of the most important safeguards was a physician's professional identity: the moment someone adopted this identity, he represented no longer just himself but the *artsenstand* as a whole. Since a single physician's misconduct reflected badly upon the entire profession, he carried a weighty responsibility toward his colleagues to constantly be on his best behavior. Even more, he carried this responsibility to all of society, because if patients were to lose faith in the *artsenstand* due to bad press, they would seek refuge in the arms of quacks, to their own detriment. Consequently, the duty "not to undermine trust in the medical profession" was one of the most reiterated sayings in publications such as the *Dutch Journal of Medicine* in the early twentieth century.

Human experimentation by no means figured prominently in these discussions of medical ethics. More common were themes like medical confidentiality (crucial) and commercial advertising (objectionable). From the early twentieth century onward, probably in response to growing antivivisectionist complaints, members of the Dutch medical profession did start to discuss the appropriate stance toward human experimentation more regularly, as Burger did in 1904. But such considerations did not translate into official guidelines. Even in the 1936 NMG medical ethics booklet, the topic was wholly neglected. Its chapters addressed themes like "the general demeanor towards the public," "care for the poor," and "how to pass on one's practice upon retirement," but not human experimentation.[41] This neglect held true for most countries. Explicit guidelines—let alone official regulations—are for the most part a product of the post-1945 period.[42]

Various reasons exist why formal regulations did develop in the second half of the twentieth century. One, which will be discussed in chapter 2, is the fact that World War II provided an enormous stimulus for the systematic conduct of medical experiments with humans, leading some historians to conclude that human experimentation before World War II was in comparison nothing more than a "cottage industry." Another, which will be discussed in chapters 3 and 4, is the fact that another type of societal opposition to "modern medicine" surfaced in the 1960s, which was much more successful in convincing governments that medical research and practice had to be brought under public control than the Dutch antivivisectionists had ever been. First, however, this chapter discusses the cultural impact of World War II and the Nazi concentration-camp experiments.[43] In the aftermath of the war, Dutch physicians drew on their experiences to rally against any form of state involvement with medicine. For them, the war had taught that only an *artsenstand* could safeguard the ethics of medicine. For the Dutch antivivisectionists, however, the Nazi concentration-camp experiments were definitive proof of the debilitating effects of modern medicine: this debilitation had reached its pinnacle in the horror chambers of the Third Reich. It was in the confrontation between these two groups that the Dutch government was first advised in 1955 to start governing the practice of human experimentation using communal ethics review.

The Nazi Experiments and the Dutch Medical Profession

From December 9, 1946 to August 20, 1947, twenty medical doctors and three Nazi officials were brought before the US military court in the Nuremberg Palace of Justice to stand trial for mass murder under the guise of euthanasia and for involvement in a series of experiments conducted on prisoners in the Nazi concentration camps.[44] This tribunal, which has become known as the doctors' trial, laid bare some of the gruesome atrocities committed by the Nazis in the name of medical science. Prisoners had been subjected to lethal sea-water, high-altitude, and freezing experiments; to tests measuring the effects of poisonous bullets, mustard gas, and incendiary bombs; to sterilization experiments which frequently resulted in severe debilitation; and so on. From 1945 to 1947, horrific descriptions of these studies found their way into the pages of Dutch newspapers.[45] Dutch journalists discussed them in tones of disbelief and horror. The experiments demonstrated the absolute inhumanity of the Nazi regime: how camp prisoners had been brutally tortured, maimed, and killed without so much of a hint of compassion from those responsible.

In the *Dutch Journal of Medicine*, the Nazi experiments were condemned as the work of pure evil, and a far cry removed from regular medical science. To emphasize this distance, words like "medical" and "colleagues" were bracketed in descriptions of the experiments.[46] To the same end, in discussing "regular human experiments," any connection with Nazism was emphatically denied. "We have to get rid as soon as possible of the unpleasant associations linked to experiments due to the criminal actions of many Germans," one physician wrote in the Dutch medical journal *Medisch Contact* in 1949, "as they may form a hindrance in scientific traffic."[47] Indeed, editor Joghem van Loghem of the *Dutch Journal of Medicine* stressed in 1953, "those who tackle the permissibility of tests upon humans need to dissociate the subject from its German past."[48]

Still, Dutch physicians worried that the doctors' trial had put a slur on the reputation of "scientific human experimentation." In 1953, Van Loghem lamented that "[the trial] has apparently had the result that, *more* than *before* the war, people nourish a distrust of the ethics of experimental research."[49] Not only had the revelations of the Nazi concentration-camp experiments scared people, the defense had also produced a list during the trial of international literature published in the last century—seeking thereby to prove that ethical transgressions in medicine were by no means a new phenomenon in the Third Reich. Van Loghem, who was appalled by the comparison, worried that this social unrest still had not died down almost a decade after the war.[50]

This strong dissociation does not imply that Dutch physicians expressed no concern about human experimentation in the years immediately following the war. Articles like those by Van Loghem served to remind readers of the *Dutch Journal of Medicine* of their moral responsibilities in experimenting on humans. "Every founded consideration of the subject will strengthen the awareness of our responsibility," Van Loghem wrote in 1953.[51] But the faulty association with the Nazi concentration-camp experiments was like a knife to the heart for a scientific practice that, with the right safeguards, was essential for medicine to progress.

Some Dutch physicians therefore felt that ethical concerns about medicine should not be debated in public at all. Laypeople might get the wrong impression and call for outside interference with affairs that concerned the *artsenstand* only. In 1949, for instance, editor of *Medisch Contact* Gerard Heringa wrote a stern reply to a philosophical paper published in his journal; the paper had dedicated a large segment to the question of whether therapeutic experiments with humans were permissible and, if so, under what circumstances. "Personally I regard this publication with concern," Heringa reproached, "because I fear it will cause confusion and shake trust in the *artsenstand*. I do not see much good in the public discussion which is bound to follow."[52] The paper's author was convinced that Heringa exaggerated. "Surely, the layperson intelligent enough to read our articles is capable of setting apart the mentality of a Nazi from that of a Dutch physician," he wrote in reply.[53] Heringa was adamant, however, that the subject had to be treated with the utmost care to prevent measures from being taken that could possibly shake the public's trust in the medical profession. For that reason, he persuaded another colleague that year to withdraw a submission on the ethics of clinical research. In "times of turmoil," the subject really was unfit for public discussion.[54]

That public unrest over the Nazi concentration-camp experiments might result in outside interference with the practice of medicine disturbed Dutch physicians. Partly, they framed this concern in a familiar rhetoric of the importance of protecting the *artsenstand*. But, partly, the war had also fueled a belief that medicine had to be defended against any form of political ideology or government bureaucracy.

In 1946, this feeling was articulated with passion in *Medisch Contact* by the eminent Dutch physician Jean Jacques Brutel de la Rivière. *Medisch Contact* was not just any journal and Brutel, as he was usually called, not just any physician. During the war, a number of Dutch physicians had united themselves in a resistance group called Medisch Contact (Medical Contact) which was much celebrated in later years. In May 1945, this group published its first *Announcements* and in 1946, this publication gained status as one of two official journals of the NMG—the other being the *Dutch Journal of Medicine*. Brutel had been one of the leaders of Medisch Contact and, toward the end of the war, had led the Large Advisory Committee of Illegality, established by Queen Wilhelmina to coordinate the activities of all Dutch resistance

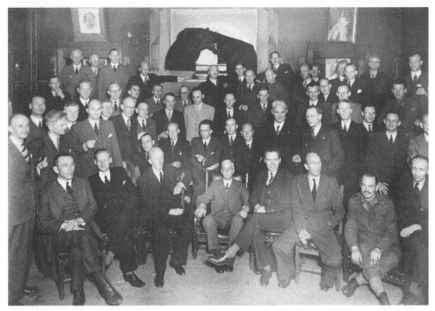

Figure 1. Jean Jacques Brutel de la Rivière, center, sitting amongst fellow members of the Dutch resistance group Medisch Contact at the organization's first national conference on June 16 and 17, 1945, shortly after the liberation of the Netherlands. Photograph by Frederik Kooij, from the personal archive of Willem Bernard Doorenbos.

groups.[55] In 1945, Brutel became president of the NMG, a position he traded in two years later for the joint presidency of the Health Council and the Central Committee for Public Health.[56] He was made an honorary member of the NMG in 1947, and was showered with other honorary titles and medals in the years thereafter, including the American Medal of Freedom, which was awarded to twenty Dutch citizens in 1953 for their war efforts.[57] Also, not entirely unimportantly, from 1953 to 1955, Brutel chaired the Health Council Committee for Tests upon Human Beings, a role in which he wrote most parts of the first-ever Dutch policy document on human experimentation.

In his 1946 essay, Brutel reflected on the societal position of the Dutch medical profession. Born in 1885, he wrote, he had witnessed the effects of urbanization, industrialization, and far-reaching *pillarization* on Dutch society (i.e., the segregation of society into groups by religion and associated political beliefs that lasted roughly from 1880 to 1960) and lived through a devastating economic crisis and two World Wars. As a result of these developments, Brutel concluded in 1946, the Netherlands had lost its internal social stability and moral anchors:

The notions of "morality" and "immorality" currently flow between anchorages lost and new ones yet unfound. Nobody knows exactly what they will mean and how they should be formulated to help us understand human behavior in an age of industry and city life. We are standing in between two worlds, one dead and the other barely born. It is our faith to live through a generation of chaos.[58]

As long as Dutch society was in flux, physicians could not trust their *milieu exterieur* to sustain them with the moral fiber needed to fulfill their professional duties. Hence, now more than ever, a strong and independent organization of the medical profession had become essential for ethical medicine.

Brutel worried, however, whether the NMG was still capable of this strength and independence. In the last half century, he wrote, the organization's professional function had watered down due to a growing influence of health insurance funds and government policies. More and more, physicians worked in employment rather than as free agents, which increasingly made them value company mores above professional traditions. Slowly but surely, this bureaucratization of medicine was eroding the moral standards held high by the *artsenstand* and replacing them with company norms that were formal and sterile, weak and capricious.

Above all, Brutel's war experiences had convinced him that medicine did not mix with state interference. Twice in his letter, he pointed out that physicians employed by the state had felt least compelled to join the resistance during the war. Twice, he referred to them as "the weakest link," individuals who lacked the professional identity and awareness of the moral duties which defined the physician.[59] "Any norms stipulated by the state or the health funds," Brutel concluded, "will inevitably carry a more formal character and will be bound to official rules and regulations. They will lose the character of living norms which have up until now kept patients safe or at least better protected than would have been possible any other way."[60]

Hence, if it was up to Brutel, the government had to stay clear from any interference with medicine. Only the *artsenstand* could cultivate a moral tradition that would guide the conduct of physicians. In 1947, therefore, the NMG announced plans under Brutel's leadership to ensure that the "spiritual unity" that had kept Dutch physicians strong during the war would not be lost. In the past, the organization admitted, it had sometimes focused too much on material gain. "The complaint, that our Society was too much of a trade union, has been voiced repeatedly, and certainly not by the least of us."[61] In 1949, when the association celebrated its centennial birthday and was awarded the "Royal" prefix (*Koninklijk*—by the addition of which it became the KNMG), Brutel ended the festivities by calling for a work to be written that would "adapt our existing medical ethics to the radical changes that have taken place in the profession of medicine and in society at large."[62] That same year, the KNMG installed a Committee for Professional Confidentiality, replaced in 1954 by a Committee for Medical Ethics, with the task (amongst others) to write a booklet on medical ethics that could be presented ceremoniously to all medical students upon receiving their degree to symbolize the moral duties they assumed as full-fledged members of the *artsenstand*.[63] The organization was confident that such initiatives would cultivate the high-standing and independent moral tradition that Brutel had in mind.

Human experimentation held a central position in this renewed attention of the *artsenstand* to its professional ethics. In 1949, the General Assembly of the KNMG debated whether to adopt the Declaration of Geneva, a document of the recently established World Medical Association (WMA) that was to provide physicians around the world with a modern-day adaptation of the Hippocratic Oath.[64] The WMA hoped that, by updating this traditional symbol of the worldwide medical profession, a global medical community could be sustained that could withstand the potentially debilitating effects of national political regimes.

The idea was that all members of affiliated national medical organizations were to take this new physician's oath. However, when the Geneva Declaration was put to vote at the KNMG in 1949, several members professed to be unimpressed by the principles set forth in it. Not only was the physician's oath phrased as a "typically sentimental American promise," it also failed to acknowledge a central element of modern medicine: human experimentation.[65] Although the General Assembly did vote in favor of the Declaration (albeit with a difference of only four votes), they urged the Board to request the WMA amend the Geneva Declaration to explicitly mention the role and responsibilities of medical researchers.[66]

In 1951, a group of Dutch physicians tried again. In a letter sent to all local departments of the KNMG, they raised the alarm about the growing number of international medical studies describing human experiments: "The mentality that speaks from the literature is an indicator that the ethical standards of doctors are in great danger."[67] Again, they urged the KNMG to persuade the WMA to issue a statement about the limits of human experimentation and to request medical journals to take these limits into consideration in their refereeing process.

The Central Board responded by asking Roel Hamburger, the most vocal member of this group, to coauthor a report on the subject that could be sent to the WMA for further consideration.[68] In 1953, this position paper was discussed by the WMA's Committee for Medical Ethics, which was the first time that the ethics of human subjects research made the agenda of an international organization.[69] In 1954, both authors were invited to present their paper to the WMA's General Assembly in Rome. Heringa, the editor of *Medisch Contact*, was also invited to give a talk on the responsibilities of medical journals in the governance of human experimentation.[70] That year in Rome, the WMA adopted its *Principles for Those in Research and Experimentation*, the predecessor of the organization's Declaration of Helsinki—a set of ethical principles for research with human subjects that was published by the WMA in 1964 and that has since acquired universal status as the cornerstone document for the ethics of medical research involving human subjects worldwide. To this day, it remains the single most influential document in the field of clinical research ethics. In *Medisch Contact* in 1955, Heringa lauded the KNMG as *the* national organization which had succeeded in bringing ethical concerns over human experimentation to the attention of an international audience of physicians.[71]

In 1955, Hamburger wrote a letter of concern to the *Journal of the American Medical Association* (JAMA) after reading in its pages about an experiment with humans testing the effects of ultraviolet radiation. "I feel we must searchingly ask ourselves," the Dutch physician penned, "if the margin between experiments such as these and those perpetrated in the German concentration camps, is so very wide."[72] Hamburger acknowledged that medicine owed much to "the splendid work done in the United States." However, this leading position was exactly why "we must expect that this country will also be one of the foremost in upholding the high ethical standards which are essential in the promotion of medical science for the benefit of mankind." In *Medisch Contact*, this letter was reprinted with a statement that it was thanks to Hamburger that the ethics of human experimentation had been, since 1954, considered internationally. The *artsenstand*, the message was, worked hard to ensure that all patients, also in other countries, remained safe in the hands of their physicians. Modern medicine presented difficult issues, but the Dutch medical profession operated at the ethical frontier of these developments. In the Netherlands, everything was done to keep medical ethics in high regard, to ensure it remained an effective mechanism of internal control for the *artsenstand*—both at home and abroad.

The Nazi Experiments and the Dutch Antivivisectionists

Not everyone in the Netherlands, however, was equally convinced that the Dutch medical profession really had such high-standing ethics when it came to human experimentation. In 1947, the Dutch *Anti-Vivisectie Stichting* (Anti-vivisection Foundation, AVS) sent an urgent letter to the minister of social affairs, to warn "[his] Excellence that the notorious experiments on human beings in the concentration camps just take up a tiny part of the countless experiments which are frequently conducted upon those of special means in normal times as well." It was of vital importance the government realized that, in the Netherlands too, "it is all which stands defenseless in life from which the scientific experimenter above all recruits his material," whether these defenseless beings were "the suckling in children's clinics, small children in orphanages, small or non-paying patients in hospitals, less wealthy women in childbed, or the tuberculosis patients and insane in sanatoriums."[73]

To substantiate these claims, the AVS presented the minister with nine Dutch research studies "of dubious ethical quality," with the apology that a much longer list could have been compiled had the Foundation's library not been destroyed in the war.[74] Most of these studies described the experimental use of invasive medical procedures, particularly on young children. A dissertation on digestion-leukopenia from 1923, for instance, recorded how a four-month-old baby—"the ill and nervous Johanna"—had been subjected to fifty-six blood tests over a period of two months.[75] Most of the studies also failed to obtain the permission of participating research subjects. Thus, one of the reports on possible exogenous causes of climate-induced asthma made mention of the fact that most "outpatient material" injected with experimental substances had been "completely unaware of what they had been injected with." The study had produced no satisfactory results, but did cause severe negative side effects in the research participants: "Once in a while a patient told us spontaneously that he had never felt this terrible in his life."[76]

Notwithstanding these accusations, the principal reason why the AVS had decided to write its letter was *not* to convince the government to bring human experimentation in the Netherlands to a halt. Instead, the organization hoped to persuade the minister of social affairs to give his consent to the establishment of a chair in vivisection-free medicine at a Dutch university. Various Dutch antivivisection groups had raised funds to subsidize an endowed chair in this area, but as professors could only be appointed at state universities by royal decree, a Dutch professorship in vivisection-free medicine could not be realized without government permission. This chair was direly needed, the AVS argued, because it allowed students who wished to pursue a medical career to decide for themselves which scientific method they believed was more convincing: one which tortured defenseless animals and neglected intuitive thinking (i.e., regular medicine) or one that appreciated the complicated nature of disease without needing to resort to abuse and murder (i.e., vivisection-free medicine). Without this option, the AVS concluded, Dutch medical education remained incomplete and dogmatic.[77]

This opinion was carried forward by more social movements in the 1940s and 1950s. The 1947 letter was cosigned by multiple organizations, including the Dutch Society for Naturopathy, the Dutch Vegetarian Society, and the Dutch Society for Homoeopathic Healers. In parliament, the Orthodox Protestant party SGP (Staatkundig Gereformeerde Partij) lobbied for a chair in vivisection-free medicine as well.[78] These parties all had their own reasons for joining the antivivisectionist cause. The Association of Homeopathic Healers made it clear, for instance, that it supported the AVS only "from a business point of view."[79] In letters to the government and the KNMG, the homoeopaths emphasized that they did not believe a true understanding of medications could be realized without animal experimentation, but that they hoped a chair in vivisection-free medicine would offer a platform at Dutch universities for the teachings of Hahnemann. The SGP supported vivisection-free medicine because it opposed state vaccination programs, which it believed to stand in direct opposition to God's providence.[80] Yet, regardless of their diverging incentives, these parties defended their cooperation on the basis of a communal anxiety over the technical nature of modern medicine, which "neglected medicine's synthetic element and treated sickness instead of the sick." All hoped that a chair in vivisection-free medicine would dilute "an understanding of medicine that is solely based on the modern sciences of nature."[81]

Even though the SGP was the only party in the Dutch parliament to support the antivivisectionist cause, the latter's political influence in the immediate postwar era should not be underestimated. Between 1945 and 1955, Dutch members of government requested the country's Health Council on no less than three occasions to investigate complaints by the antivivisectionists. In 1947, the minister of social affairs requested advice on the desirability of creating a chair in vivisection-free medicine. And in 1953, the government asked the Health Council for advice twice: once on the frequency and legality of animal vivisection in the Netherlands, and once on the legality of human vivisection. The latter resulted in the instalment of the Council Committee for Tests upon Human Beings. In each of these three instances, antivivisectionist complaints had been the cause of the government's request for advice.

The Health Council had been founded in 1902 as an independent scientific advisory board to provide the Dutch government with "objective nonpolitical advice on matters that may affect Dutch public health."[82] In 1947, Brutel had just been installed as Council president. Perhaps for this reason,

Brutel's dissertation was one of the studies which the AVS had decided to include in its letter. In 1932, the physician had successfully defended a thesis on allergic skin reactions in non-allergic persons.[83] According to the AVS, Brutel had injected a variety of substances into human subjects, including a preparation of the pneumococcus bacterium causing pneumonia and a suspension of spirochetes "which may possibly cause syphilis."[84] At first, the AVS stated, Brutel had mainly used mental patients, but a large number of positive test results had led him to question whether these subjects were suitable for his research studies. Thereafter, the physician had proceeded with patients of women's clinics, most of whom were pregnant.

No records have been preserved which suggest that Brutel was asked to step down as Health Council president after the accusations of the AVS or to refrain from chairing a committee on vivisection-free medicine. Instead, the 1947 request for advice was addressed directly to Brutel, and the physician set out to organize a committee to investigate whether animal experimentation really had a coarsening effect on vivisectors and whether "vivisection-free medicine" was able to develop treatments that were on par with the prophylactics and therapeutics that had been realized via established experimental methods.[85]

Brutel asked two antivivisectionists to participate in the committee: a homoeopath and an osteopath who had been proposed by the AVS as suitable representatives of the vivisection-free cause. The majority of seats, however, were taken up by physicians who were convinced that vivisection was indispensable for medicine to progress. Not surprisingly, this committee makeup had the effect that, while the two antivivisectionists did try to convince their fellow committee members of the value of vivisection-free medicine, the outcome of the deliberations was set in advance: in 1949, the majority of the committee advised the Dutch government against the establishment of a chair in vivisection-free medicine.

Despite this position of power, however, the organized Dutch medical profession was far from confident that the government would not decide to act against the "solemn scientific advice" of the Health Council. This concern was not without reason. In 1949, when the Health Council advice on vivisection-free medicine was debated in the Dutch parliament, the SGP demanded an explanation from the government. How was it possible that the establishment of a single professorship was actively obstructed in a country that supposedly stood for freedom of education?[86] At first, the responsible minister of education replied that the request could not be honored because he had realized in conversations with the AVS that the organization did not just wish to add to the existing Dutch medical curricula, but to realize an entirely different system of education. This goal, the minister stated, was "practically unrealizable for the time being."[87] After some debate, however, he agreed that an academic climate should be open to multiple philosophies and promised once more to take the request for a professorial chair in vivisection-free medicine into consideration.[88]

This commitment caused considerable commotion among the ranks of the KNMG. In *Medisch Contact*, physicians cried out that antivivisectionists simply denounced all of modern medical science and thus had no right to take part in academic life. Heringa was sure that the realization of a chair in vivisection-free medicine was "an experiment of massive gruesomeness that far surpassed any human or animal vivisection imaginable."[89] The KNMG president posted concerned letters to the prime minister; the minister of social affairs; the state secretary of public health; and the minister of education, arts, and sciences to warn them that such a chair would not only endanger the general level of scholarship in the Netherlands, but would also cause substantial damage to public health by instilling young, impressionable students with grossly flawed doctrines.[90] Really, they had to understand that the antivivisectionist stance posed a threat to the entire nation. As a result of this lobby, the minister of social affairs convinced the minister of education that, in the interest of public health, it was best to leave the matter alone.[91]

Throughout the 1950s, Dutch groups kept pushing for an alternative to "an understanding of medicine based solely on the modern sciences of nature" in academia. Every other year, the government received a request for a chair in vivisection-free medicine or homoeopathy. In the *Dutch Journal of Medicine* and *Medisch Contact*, proponents of experimental medicine kept on eyeing such requests with concern.

At stake in these heated debates over a single professorial chair was the ideological embedding of modern medicine in the Dutch state. For the proponents of vivisection-free medicine, the experimental tradition in medicine was based on a flawed conception of health and healing. It was a dangerous practice, which meant the government had a duty to intervene in the organization of medicine, open up universities to other ways of knowing, and, ideally, prohibit all forms of animal and human vivisection. In contrast, those in favor of the experimental tradition argued that such experiments were an intrinsic part of the modern health care state. Without vivisection there would be no medical progress and hence no potential for realizing better futures for citizens. The government therefore had a duty to support medical experiments and to protect experimenters from undue attacks. As Brutel wrote in a letter accompanying the presentation of the 1954 Health Council advice on animal vivisection:

> We have considered adding a passage about the actions that the Government could take to protect those who work in the field of vivisection […] Although such recommendations lie outside the mandate of this committee, I would like to point out that the Government has the possibility to critically investigate the defamatory methods used by the AVS.[92]

This type of reminder, the essays in medical journals denouncing vivisection-free medicine, the letters by the KNMG: they all indicate that the organized Dutch medical profession was by no means certain in the mid-twentieth century that "modern medicine" was ingrained enough in society to withstand the accusations which its critics brought forward. Hence, when the Health Council received a request in 1953 to explore the conduct of human experimentation in the Netherlands, the physicians that gathered to consider its permissibility were highly aware of the possible political consequences of their findings. They had to develop a report that suggested how human experiments could be kept within bounds, without exposing modern medicine as such to fundamental questions about its legitimate societal position.

A Modern Approach to Medical Ethics

The affair over vivisection-free medicine in the late 1940s did not end wholly without success for the antivivisection movement. In 1949, the minister of social affairs decided to have his civil servants chart how often and under what circumstances animal experiments were conducted in the Netherlands. This report was presented to the Health Council in 1953, with the request that the Council determine whether any further legal measures were needed to keep this practice under control. That same year, the Health Council was also asked to investigate whether the Dutch government needed to take any action in the governance of human experimentation.[93] The government made this request after newspapers reported on a lecture night by the AVS at which an experiment in the Academic Hospital of Leiden on the etiology of nettle rash had been discussed. To test whether the disease was caused by a virus, the researcher in question had dripped "sterile urine and feces filtrates" into the noses of babies admitted to the hospital.[94] "Serious accusation against Leiden hospital," one headline read the next day. "Babies and lunatics used for experiments?"[95] Were these accusations true, the government wished to know from the Health Council, and if so, did measures have to be taken to prevent such actions in future?

The then-Council president decided to answer these questions by installing the Committee for Tests upon Human Beings, this latter phrase being the common terminology for human experimentation in the Netherlands until the 1970s. This committee seated prominent members of the *artsenstand*. First, there was Brutel, who acted as chairman for most of the two years it took the committee to produce its final report. Then, there was internist Cornelis Douwe de Langen, a highly honored member of the Dutch medical profession and the other coauthor of the report on human experimentation that had been sent to the WMA in 1952.[96] There was internist Job Pannekoek, another previous leader of the Dutch medical resistance.[97] Pharmacologist Samuel de Jongh, soon-to-be rector of Leiden University, participated.[98] Willem Karel Dicke, director of the Juliana Children's Hospital, took part.[99] Willem Paul Plate, gynecologist to the royal family, held a seat.[100] And so on and so on.[101] No antivivisectionists were invited. No "medical outsiders" were asked to hold a seat. Apparently, in the 1950s, the governance of human experimentation was still a subject which, in the eyes of the Council president, should be considered by the *artsenstand* alone.

These participants were furthermore expected to consider the subject under investigation *solely* from their perspectives as physicians. As the Council president proclaimed in his introductory speech during the first committee meeting:

> I have the hope that the significantly different sources from which we derive our ethical principles, like religion, philosophy or conscience, will not be brought to the fore during our discussions. What this circle of physicians has in common is medical ethics. While nuances are also possible in this area, I am confident that it is this commonality which will allow us to formulate one definitive advice.[102]

In other words, even though the participating physicians might in their personal lives be members of different religious congregations or have different political tendencies, in the Committee for Tests upon Human Beings such differences were considered background noise. Professional ethics were expected to trump personal viewpoints.

Indeed, the professional identities of the committee members proved crucial for the way in which they approached the question of whether additional safeguards should be required for human experimentation. For one thing, they shared many of the concerns that had led physicians like Hamburger to address the international medical community in the 1950s. All felt that, judg-

INTERNAL CONTROL

ing from research studies that recently had been published in medical journals, it was high time that international guidelines were formulated to keep this practice in check. Certainly in countries like the United States, the committee members argued behind closed doors, medical researchers seemed to have little hesitation to subject "prisoners, negroes, and orphans" to all sort of risky procedures that hardly had any benefit for the participating research subjects.[103] And in the Netherlands too it seemed as if every new generation felt it could go a bit further in experimenting on patients.[104] The *artsenstand*, all felt, had to put a lid on things before they really got out of hand.

At the same time, however, the committee was very aware of the immediate cause behind its congregation and sought to use its position to *protect* the experimental tradition. De Langen, an outspoken conservative in allowing human experimentation, drummed it into the committee that it had to think long and hard about which ethical provisions it was willing to defend in public and which should remain absolutely confidential.[105] Its final advice should not provide grist to the mill of the antivivisectionist cause.

This tension between the desire for internal control and fear of undue outside interference dominated the committee meetings. Its members attempted to formulate safeguards that would prevent unethical behavior among medical researchers while reaffirming to those in power that human experimentation as such was beyond moral suspicion.

It was a balancing act that took various forms. First of all, the committee spent much time on the exact wording of its report. It would recommend that additional measures be taken to safeguard human experimentation, but with words that would reassure the government that no reasons existed for drastic action. Thus, words like *many* [dangerous experiments] were changed into *some*, terms like *often* into *sometimes*.[106] Likewise, the sentence "If the doctor uses a patient for a different goal [than the recovery of his health], the doctor violates his position of trust" was deleted when the committee recalled why the government had asked the Health Council for advice.[107] Instead, the report included reassuring segments stating that "comments that patients are used as guinea pigs" in Dutch hospitals were "false depictions" that needlessly caused anxiety.[108]

Second, the committee sought to disarm any antivivisectionist claims about the "corrupting effects of modern medicine" by dismissing outright that they had any bearing on the topic whatsoever:

This committee wishes to stress that the scientific methods [...] have proven their value for science and humanity. They need no defense and the Committee only has to ascertain if their application has in exceptional cases led to irresponsible acts, and in those cases outline the means to combat these excesses.[109]

By stressing that medical experiments need "no defense," the committee took pains to emphasize that neither the epistemic status nor the social worth of human experimentation was at stake in its governance. The Health Council only needed to formulate safeguards against a few excesses.

Third, and most importantly, because the practice as such needed no defense, the committee proposed a new ethics framework for regulating it. Antivivisectionists frequently argued that all human experiments in medicine violated traditional medical ethics, as the ancient Hippocratic precept *primum non nocere* prescribed that physicians above all had a duty to abstain from causing harm.[110] Thus, in the Council committee on vivisection-free medicine, the two antivivisectionists had argued that the "the official science of healing has come to wander from its original goal," as "physicians have a duty to help not harm."[111] In response to this, the Health Council concluded that the problem was not the experimental tradition in medicine, but traditional medical ethics. "Both modern medications and modern medical practice carry risks," the internist Job Pannekoek stated firmly, "Hippocrates' old precept can therefore in this modern day and age no longer be maintained in its entirety."[112] Instead, physicians had to balance the risks of an intervention against its benefits, as they did when using narcotics or vaccinating healthy patients.[113]

The cardinal question was, of course, whether such a "calculus of suffering" also held up when risks were taken by some individuals to benefit others. Some committee members seemed to think it did. Pediatrician Dicke, for instance, brushed aside the issue by stating that modern life itself, with its high-tech goods such as cars, detergents, and insecticides, was full of risk: "We live in technical times and we simply need to adapt to them. The existence of risk is not a medical problem. It is a problem of society at large."[114] Others argued that life in modern society had simply become more "group-minded" than "individual-minded."[115] While no one stated it outright, some seemed to think it was justifiable to expose a few individuals to more-than-average risk if doing so could possibly benefit a great many others. Others disagreed. De Langen, for one, stated that a crucial difference existed between the conscious decision to drive a car and unconsciously being experimented upon as a hospital patient. The doctor-patient relationship always had been of an individual nature and had to remain so. Brutel, also, had his doubts. He felt strongly, at least, that *if* the committee decided that medicine was to become more group-minded than individual-minded, it had to inform the general public of this shift. Patients had a right to know if "the old principle that was once the position of trust between patient and physician has been forsaken."[116]

Eventually, the committee decided that the solution was not to formulate ethical imperatives that held up under all circumstances—e.g., "first, do no harm" or "the greatest benefit for the greatest number of people"—but to propose safeguards that made it possible to decide on a case-by-case basis whether risks were worth taking. "When experimenting on humans is absolutely necessary," Brutel concluded (and the committee strongly felt it was), "we need to create conditions that keep each risk as small as possible."[117] The goal was not to avoid all risk, but to minimize those risks that simply had to be taken. Modern medicine required a modern approach to risk governance.

What were these safeguards, then? The first was formulating guidelines for tests on humans that "carry some risk, extraordinary discomfort or pain with them." These guidelines were strict. They emphasized patients' consent and made clear that, even then, "the responsibility of the researcher and not the willingness of the subject is primary." They forbade experimental tests on children, prisoners, or "lunatics," and prohibited group investigations with more-than-average risk in homes of children or the elderly. Tests on dying people were forbidden under all circumstances. The guidelines also advised against tests on patients who suffered from incurable diseases and disapproved of tests that carried substantial risk, as such tests were "not in harmony with the nature and goal of medical science." Furthermore, all tests immediately had to be brought to a halt if patients asked for it or if unforeseen danger arose. Finally, researchers were not allowed to bother patients with "unnecessary tests"—and, the committee added, "it goes without saying that any not strictly unavoidable physical or mental suffering and danger have to be prevented."[118]

At the same time, however, the committee made sure equally to emphasize that human experimentation really was a crucial component of modern medical science. Thus, the 1955 report also stated that:

> The Committee feels obliged to point out that hospital patients profit significantly from experiences that physicians have gained from past patients. The public knows that hospitals do not only exist to nurse and treat the sick, but also to increase scientific knowledge.[119]

And also, despite the emphasis on consent in the guidelines:

> The position of trust between physician and patient is not violated if the physician, without actually asking permission, performs actions

that serve to increase knowledge or his own experience, as long as these actions do not do any damage or delay recovery.[120]

According to the committee, participating in experiments that did not seriously harm them or delay their recovery was a moral duty of patients. Dicke even felt that patients were morally indebted to the medical profession, as it had brought so much relief to modern society. Others, however, remarked that a term like moral debt should not be used in a public report.[121] Still, the committee felt, it could not hurt to remind people that hospitals did not just exist to heal the sick, but also to further medical progress.

Lastly, the report recommended that physicians who wanted to conduct experiments on patients currently in treatment had to "mobilize an advisory committee" before they could proceed.[122] In addition, the government would do well to install a national advisory board with "persons who are familiar with the subject of tests upon human beings" that researchers could turn to for advice.[123] Too often, the Health Council argued, experiments in medicine were either redundant or invalid because researchers had not kept abreast of current developments in their field or had failed to pick the right research design. Hence, it made sense, both ethically *and* methodologically, to pool expertise in order to prevent bad science and promote good science. The 1955 Health Council advice concluded, therefore, with the sort of poetic statement that only policy documents can muster: "For this goal, the Committee proposes to bring a Committee into being."[124] Together with the suggestion for advisory committees at the local level, it was the first-ever proposal for the governance of human experimentation in the Netherlands through a system of ethics by committee.

Officially, the Council's advice regarding tests upon human beings was directed to the Dutch government. In practice, however, its recommendations were directed at the organization heading the Dutch medical profession: the KNMG. To make sure that the medical community would take notice of the guidelines, the Health Council proposed that the government ask the KNMG to "push the thoughts contained in the advice on its members" through whatever measures the organization saw fit. Furthermore, the government had to request that the KNMG exert its influence on medical journals to make sure that article submissions "in conflict with medical ethics" would be refused.[125] Finally, the government was to ask the KNMG to incorporate the most important elements of the Health Council report in the booklet on medical ethics it was currently preparing.

These were the recommendations of a group of physicians who believed strongly that a practice such as human experimentation was best governed by an *artsenstand*. The safeguards the Health Council proposed were all meant as measures of internal control: *by* members of the medical profession *for* members of the medical profession. All the government had to do was to protect experimental medicine from undue attacks by the antivivisectionists.

In the 1960s and 1970s, in a remarkably short period of time, this belief that an autonomous *artsenstand* was best capable to govern the conduct of physicians started to show cracks that many believed were beyond repair. In a period of only a decade, the ideals of men like Brutel gave way to a sense of crisis about the *artsenstand*. The existing code of medical ethics, even when modernized, came to be considered outmoded, while a cadre of medical out-siders united to rally against the *artsenstand* in ways that were much more successful than the antivivisectionists had ever been. Medicine in modern society, the argument became, did not require internal but external control.

However, before moving on to this call for more external control, I first take up another proposal for more internal control over human experimen-tation, one that was proposed by elite members of the Dutch medical pro-fession in the late 1960s. By then, the antivivisectionist threat had largely retreated into the background. Instead, the most vocal advocates of the experimental tradition in medicine had started eyeing their own medical col-leagues with concern. Most practitioners, it turned out, did not keep abreast of new developments in the field, nor did they show much interest in things such as research design. Hence, the reform of medicine was direly needed, these reformers came to argue, perhaps even with use of government force. After all, internal control over medicine could only be realized if the average practitioner was actually made to listen to what the profession's experts had to say.

CHAPTER 2

A MORAL NEED *for*
EPISTEMIC FILTERS

In 1962, the *Dutch Journal of Medicine* published an op-ed about the need for clinical trials. "The resistance a physician feels against experimenting on his patients is understandable," the author started off.[1] After all, every patient deserved the best treatments currently available. Yet, due to the recent boom in pharmaceuticals, it had become increasingly difficult for physicians to decide which treatments really were best. Even worse, as "products of the pharmaceutical industry generally find their way into practice before a sound judgement has been obtained about their value and risks," it was very well possible for physicians to prescribe ineffective or unsafe drugs to their patients. "Peripheral doctors" especially, the author complained, constantly felt pressured by patients and industrial firms to prescribe the newest wonder drugs available. "In this new situation, thousands of physicians are constantly experimenting," often with high risk and little reward, as it was usually hardly possible to speak of sound scientific research. "One can thus state without reservation," the author concluded, "that the conduct of good experimental research is ethically more responsible than the usually ineffective evaluations in practice." It was high time for reform. A moral need existed in the Netherlands for *proper* human experimentation.

This chapter examines two more policy reports that were written by the Dutch Health Council between 1968 and 1981. In this period, an awareness grew among Dutch politicians that the rights of research subjects in human experimentation needed additional protection, resulting in various requests for advice to the Health Council on whether public policy in this area was desirable. In 1971, the advisory body delivered the first of these reports, which contained the first fully developed Dutch blueprint for research ethics committees.

Who participated in these two Council committees? Why did they diverge from their 1955 predecessors, who had shied away from any state involvement in the oversight of medicine? And, once more, what role did these advisory bodies imagine for research ethics committees in the oversight of human experimentation? This chapter traces the development of these two reports and argues that they have to be viewed in light of a larger international reform movement in the twentieth century that sought to make medicine more rational by submitting therapeutic interventions to systematic clinical experimentation.

The members of the two Health Council committees were concerned over the rights and safety of human research subjects. Yet, just like their predecessors in 1955, they were equally motivated to strengthen the epistemic authority of medical science. Even more, while in 1955 the Health Council had still primarily sought to *protect* human experimentation from outside attacks, sixteen years later it actively came to *promote* such experimentation, in the hope of rationalizing Dutch therapeutic practice. This chapter makes clear that research ethics committees were imagined to fulfill a specific function in these attempts at reform.

Therapeutic Reform and Clinical Experimentation

I borrow the term therapeutic reform from Harry Marks, who introduced it in his 1997 book *The Progress of Experiment* to identify "individuals who sought to use the science of controlled experiments to direct medical practice."[2] This movement first emerged in the United States in the early twentieth century in concern over the growing range of pharmaceutical products put on the market by the nascent drug industry. The precise composition, safety, and efficacy of these products was often unclear, while drug firms heavily targeted both patients and clinicians with promises of medical breakthroughs or attractive discounts.[3] According to Marks, the American medical profession's scientific elite had little faith in the capacities of the average physician to handle these challenges: "Among therapeutic reformers, the gullible physician soon vied with the ignorant layman as a symbol of the corrupt state of therapeutics."[4] With true reformist zeal, therefore, they set out to enlighten "the peripheral physician" in particular of the importance of an intellectual program they called rational therapeutics.

In this program, therapeutic agents were only considered rational if their mechanism of action had been established scientifically. In addition, physicians could only use these agents to treat ailments for which they scientifically had been proven effective. Yet what was considered "scientific" in medicine was changing in the early twentieth century. Drawing on the ideas of the nineteenth-century French physician Pierre Louis, therapeutic reformers in this period came to argue that the efficacy of therapies could only be established by systematically comparing the effects of different treatments on groups of patients suffering from the same disease—i.e., by conducting clinical trials.

In practice, however, such trials were difficult to organize. Unless enough comparable cases were available on the same hospital ward, clinicians in different institutions had to agree to follow the same agreed-upon treatment plan and to keep note of their findings in such a way as to permit comparison. Hardly any money or infrastructure was available for this practice in the first half of the twentieth century, and it proved notoriously difficult to get clinicians to accept the limits these trials imposed on their professional autonomy.[5]

According to Marks, this state of affairs changed during World War II. In 1941, the US government created the Office of Scientific Research and Development (OSRD), which was given almost unlimited funding and resources to coordinate scientific research for military purposes.[6] This office included a Committee for Medical Research (CMR), which received about twenty-five million dollars between 1941 and 1947 to plan and oversee medical research—an unparalleled amount of money at the time.[7] Its management was put in the hands of prominent academics who adhered to the ideals of rational therapeutics, offering these scholars an opportunity to put their notions of reform into practice. The centralized and militaristic organization of the CMR, combined with its available funds, greatly favored the conduct of controlled clinical trials. After the war, this infrastructure was maintained. In 1945, the US Congress decided to reorganize the National Institutes of Health (NIH) along the lines of the CMR, resulting in its unparalleled expansion in the postwar decades. Whereas the NIH had still received about $700,000 a year for medical research in 1945, this number had increased to almost $437 million by 1965. In 1970, this had become $1.5 billion.[8]

This development was augmented by a new method for conducting clinical trials in the immediate postwar period: the randomized controlled trial (RCT). In 1948, the *British Medical Journal* published the outcome of a clinical study on the effects of the antibiotic drug streptomycin on pulmonary tuberculosis.[9] Modelled after statistical theories developed earlier in the century, the experiment allocated patients randomly between a treatment group and a control group receiving bed rest. All other variables had been kept as constant as possible to determine if the variable under investigation—the administration of streptomycin—produced a statistically significant effect. Patients in neither group had been informed about which treatment they received, nor did the specialists grading the monthly X-rays or the bacteriologists examining patients' sputum know. To eliminate any potential bias all parties had been kept as ignorant as possible. The trial was, as it is now called, double-blind. Within a decade, the RCT was described internationally as the "gold standard" for therapeutic evaluation.[10] Soon, regulatory agencies such as the American Food and Drug Administration (FDA) also started to demand that medicinal products only be made eligible for market authorization if their efficacy had been proven via controlled clinical trials.[11] If therapeutics was ever to become fully rational, the dominant adage became, *more* and *better* clinical research was necessary.

Historians have at times expressed their surprise (and dismay) about the fact that there appears to have been little consideration of the ethics of human experimentation in this crucial period in its history. Rothman, for instance, remarks that while the first two decades after World War II "witnessed an extraordinary expansion of human experimentation in medical research," they were marked at the same time by a remarkable neglect of the rights of research subjects. In a period when the Nazi concentration-camp experiments should have been fresh on the minds of clinical researchers, "utilitarian justifications that had flourished under conditions of combat and conscription persisted, and principles of consent and voluntary participation were often disregarded." In the media, the Nuremberg Code received only sporadic attention, while in government "the thrust of public policy was not to check the discretion of the experimenter but to free up the resources that would expand the scope and opportunity for research."[12] In this Gilded Age of clinical research, Rothman concludes, an astonishingly laissez-faire attitude persisted among medical researchers and practitioners with regards to the ethics of this practice.[13]

Rothman is right that fairly little attention was given to the rights of research subjects in the immediate postwar decades. Only from the mid-1960s onward did the language of patients' rights start to take center stage in international discussions over human experimentation. However, that does not mean that the ethics of human experimentation—and of clinical research in particular—was not discussed in the 1940s and 1950s. "Historians [who] have puzzled over the relative absence of ethical discussions over medical research in the first twenty years after World War II," Marks remarks delicately in response to Rothman's claims, "have been looking in the wrong place." Debates over clinical research in this period *were* highly ethically charged, even if contributors did not typically emphasize the importance of patient autonomy. "The ethics in question," Marks writes, "was the traditional ethics of therapeutic reformers, who tried to persuade physicians that their beliefs about therapy were unjustified."[14]

By the early 1950s, many new drugs were coming onto the market each year, including a stream of antibiotics, hormones, and antipsychotics—all potent drugs with a capacity to cause great harm.[15] These developments caused a new generation of therapeutic reformers to rally with ever-greater intent for the need for controlled trials to evaluate the uses and effects of new and existing medicines. Clinicians who still prescribed "unproven cures," these reformers maintained, were the ones who played with human lives, who experimented without any hope of trustworthy results, and who ultimately conducted themselves unethically. "In treating patients with unproven remedies we are, whether we like it or not, experimenting on human beings," statistician and "father of the RCT" Austin Bradford Hill wrote in 1954, "and a good experiment well reported may be more ethical and entail less shirking of duty than a poor one."[16] In the world of therapeutic reformers, controlled clinical trials were ethically more justifiable than no systematic experimentation at all.

Indeed, in the 1960s and 1970s, the time period during which discussions of human experimentation came to be dominated in the United States by concerns over the rights of research subjects, parallel discussions in the Netherlands were influenced just as much by concerns over the apparently dismal state in which Dutch therapeutics found itself—at least according to a group of pharmacologists who hoped to reorganize clinical research in the Netherlands after the American model. More controlled trials had to be conducted in the Netherlands, this group of scholars claimed, if Dutch therapeutics ever was to become fully rational. A moral need existed for therapeutic reform.

Dutch Attempts at Therapeutic Reform

In the mid-1950s, when the Health Council was asked by the government to write a report on "tests upon human beings," there were arguably not that many Dutch clinical researchers in need of ethical constraint. Better put, there were not that many Dutch clinical researchers at all, although antivivisectionists might have countered that all of modern medicine was one big experiment that put innocent creatures in harm's way. Unlike the United States, where medical research became a national industry during World War II, the occupied Netherlands did not develop centrally coordinated clinical research programs, nor were significant sums of money made available in the aftermath of the war. Physicians who did manage to conduct research in this period were lauded in later years for their work, which they had "performed under difficult circumstances during the war."[17]

In this period, a number of Dutch physicians did start to *lobby* for more-systematic clinical trials. This group consisted of researchers and practitioners from a variety of backgrounds. Some had been trained as internists, others as statisticians. However, the leading Dutch spokespersons for this movement in the mid-twentieth century were pharmacologists. Pharmacology, the study of drug action, had flourished in the Netherlands in the first half of the twentieth century, due to financial investments by the Rockefeller Institute and the Dutch pharmaceutical industry.[18] Yet, as in most countries, Dutch pharmacological research had mostly proceeded in this period through animal experiments. Although large-scale clinical trials did at times take place, clinical tests usually occurred in the form of sending out samples to clinicians who were asked to report back their findings in case reports, usually with only a handful of patients.[19]

By the early 1950s, Dutch pharmacologists increasingly evaluated this practice as unsatisfactory. Inspired by the recent developments in the United States and Great Britain, they started to advocate the need for systematic clinical experimentation to determine the efficacy of medications. Without comprehensive knowledge of the physiological responses of drugs in actual human patients, they argued, the study of drug action remained incomplete. A new branch therefore had to be added to medicine, i.e., the branch of *clinical* pharmacology.

An early and prominent advocate of this view was the pharmacologist and rector of Leiden University Samuel de Jongh. De Jongh, a physician, had begun his scientific career in 1923 at the Amsterdam pharmacological-therapeutic laboratory of Ernst Laqueur, the famous German-Dutch scientist who had co-founded the pharmaceutical company Organon in that same year and who spearheaded the industrial production of insulin in Europe.[20] In 1935, at the age of thirty-seven, de Jongh was appointed as professor in pharmacology at Leiden University, and in 1952 he was promoted to dean of the medical faculty. De Jongh was an adviser to organizations such as Organon (by that time a thriving international business), the Medical Service of the Dutch army, and the State's Defense Force of the Netherlands Organization of Applied Scientific Research (TNO). In 1958, he was made both acting president of the Dutch Health Council and the rector of his university.[21]

In that capacity, at the yearly birthday celebration of Leiden University in 1958, De Jongh decided to use the occasion to make a passionate plea for the need for more controlled clinical trials in medicine. Pharmacotherapy, the rector told his audience, found itself in the midst of "tempestuous times."[22] Although more diseases could now be cured or prevented with pills, sera, and vaccines than ever before, clinical practice was increasingly flooded with products whose safety and effectiveness remained unclear. The only way out of this predicament, De Jongh argued, was more controlled clinical experimentation. Some clinicians, he continued, objected to such trials because they withheld possibly effective therapies to patients in need. But these clinicians were wrong. "The unjust, although well-intended, omission of a control group in the past has had the result that the effectiveness of currently established therapies is strictly still unproven."[23]

For De Jongh, a previous member of the Health Council Committee for Tests upon Human Beings, this was a distinctly *ethical* argument. Unless the introduction of new medicines was categorically forbidden, he argued, every new drug at some point had to be tried out on patients for the first time: "It does not do to obscure the affair with fine words, the first application in man has the character of an experiment."[24] In other words, unless no new drugs were ever to be introduced into clinical practice anymore, De Jongh considered it more ethical to subject patients to well-designed experiments than to just keep on handing out medicines to patients that could very well be worthless, or—worse—dangerous.

In the late 1950s and 1960s, a new generation of Dutch medical researchers repeatedly started to use this line of argumentation to promote controlled clinical trials. In 1956, pharmacologist Frans Nelemans, the first Dutch *privatdozent* in clinical pharmacology, declared in his inaugural lecture that "a clinical trial is only called reliable these days if the results can be treated statistically."[25] Hence, controlled trials were the only clinical research method that could be defended morally: the risks that human experiments brought with them could only ever be justified if they had possible yields as well. In 1958, pharmacologist Chris Rümke, the first Dutch *privatdozent* in medical statistics, stated in *his* inaugural lecture that it was an "ethical necessity" that "efficient use be made of the data obtained from experiments on human beings."[26] The only method capable of doing this, Rümke maintained, was the double-blind RCT.

Nelemans, De Jongh, and Rümke were therapeutic reformers: they were convinced that more controlled clinical experimentation would ensure better knowledge about clinical drug use, which would in turn contribute to better therapeutic practice. They were also—at times—frustrated elitists. They felt they understood better than the average practitioner which courses of action should be considered rational, but they had few means at their disposal, other than the power of persuasion, to make their medical colleagues comply with their epistemic convictions. In other words, they desired *internal control* to realize their ideals of rational therapeutics, but lacked hard political and economic power to bring these ideals to fruition. In his 1958 lecture, De Jongh lamented the fact that no "communal apparatus" existed in the Netherlands to direct the experimental investigation of new pharmaceutical products. A group consisting of "chemists and physicians, scholars and manufacturers, laboratory workers, and clinicians" did cooperate occasionally in the attempt to determine the clinical safety and efficacy of new drugs, but this situation was "far from ideal."[27]

One Dutch research organization was trying to organize such a system for the conduct of coordinated clinical trials in the mid-1950s. This was the Netherlands Organization of Applied Scientific Research (TNO), an independent research organization established in 1932 by the Dutch government to conduct applied scientific research studies "in service of the public interest." The organization received government funds, but—as an independent body—made its own decisions about what type of research it would fund. By the mid-twentieth century, TNO had become the largest Dutch research organization for applied science.[28]

In December 1951, Dutch pharmacologist Johan Gaarenstroom, a previous pupil of De Jongh and a former supervisor of Rümke, had just finished a memo for TNO on "the possibilities of coordinated research on pharmaceuticals" in the Netherlands.[29] In this memo, Gaarenstroom concluded that Dutch scientists were "at their wits' end" due to a lack of any infrastructure for clinically testing the safety and efficacy of drugs. Sometimes, researchers knew "a friendly clinical relation willing to try out a new substance," but this option was scarce. With the help of TNO, therefore, Gaarenstroom hoped to organize systematic clinical trials in the Netherlands after the American model.[30]

Despite its central position in the Dutch scientific research landscape, TNO was initially skeptical of Gaarenstroom's plans. When his memo was discussed by the organization's Health Department, most board members doubted whether "any willingness can be found in the Netherlands for the systematic conduct of clinical research," since "a complete lack of interest" existed for these matters in the country.[31] From others in academia and industry, Gaarenstroom received similar replies. Most were unconvinced that cooperative clinical studies had much chance of success in the Netherlands.[32]

Another difficulty that Gaarenstroom's respondents foresaw was the professional ethos of Dutch clinicians. According to a board member of TNO, the reigning Dutch medical ethics made physicians reluctant to participate in clinical trials.[33] Another contact (probably from industry) replied: "I would have thought you knew the Dutch clinician well enough to know that this proposal in its current form does not have much chance of success." Sure, in the United States, where "the *big bosses* have access to much more patient material," "agreements exist between industrial firms and certain clinicians that oblige clinicians to test everything for these companies in exchange for significant sums of money":

> Do you deem this possible in the Netherlands? I don't. The entangle-ment of research with teaching, the overburdening of clinicians, the small size of this country, the specialization of interests—they make that I have little hope of radical change. Also here, industry will have to find her own way.[34]

Despite these objections, TNO did install a Committee for Clinical Drug Research in 1952 to "fill the existing void of clinical research in the Neth-erlands."[35] It included prominent Dutch physicians and medical scientists, including Rümke, Gaarenstroom, and Nelemans—who was appointed as its chairman in 1956.[36] But this committee had limited funds at its disposal, which made it difficult to set up large trials and "to acquire representative data."[37]

Other attempts at reform were made as well. In 1961, Nelemans co-edited a Dutch handbook on pharmacotherapy, in which he emphasized the impor-tance of controlled clinical experimentation: "Even though tests with the double-blind technique cannot always be conducted on patients because of ethical concerns, relatively few cases are known in which a study without the double-blind method has led to sound judgements."[38] And both Nelemans and De Jongh gave lectures for the Dutch pharmaceutical industry in the 1960s to convince drug manufacturers to engage in systematic clinical exper-imentation.[39] In newspapers, these talks were reported on with headlines such as "New Medicines Demand Experiments on Humans," "The Neces-sity of the Clinical Experiment," and, in one newspaper with a bit of flair for drama, "Humans are the Best Laboratory Animals."[40]

It all seemed to have little effect. As time went on, the Dutch call for therapeutic reform grew considerably more sour. In 1970, Nelemans coau-thored another booklet on clinical drug research. With it, he wrote bitterly in the preface, he hoped "to ask attention for one of the most stepmotherly endowed branches of science" and to point out "the pitfalls [. . .] that are responsible for the fact that an intolerable number of therapeutic studies go wrong." "As difficult as it must be for many physicians to process," he car-ried on in the introduction, "conclusions about the therapeutic value of a medicine based on observations of the patient who is 'only treated' are almost always useless and misleading." The two authors sorely hoped, there-fore, "that with the publication of this booklet *more* physicians than is cur-rently the case will delve into the problems that play a role in [clinical drug research]."[41]

In spite of their renewed attempt, the two seemed to have little faith in their ability to convince their colleagues of the importance of clinical exper-imentation. In the future, they supposed, the Dutch government would likely come to play a more dominant role in *enforcing* the cooperation of physicians and patients with clinical trials:

> On the one hand, it will become acceptable to demand that every prac-ticing physician, when an appeal is made on him, cooperate with stud-ies that serve to determine the value of medicines and to spend part of his working hours [...] in this vein. On the other, society may expect and perhaps even demand from her patient-members that they make themselves available for the type of studies discussed here.[42]

Reform would be realized in the end not with the soft power of academic persuasion but with the hard power of state force. Nelemans was careful to present this possibility as an *external force*: a government intervention on which he and other therapeutic reformers really had little influence. "We leave open whether this development is desirable, we just signal its likeli-hood."[43] In reality, however, reformers like Nelemans actively lobbied the government in the 1960s and 1970s to enforce their ideals of rational ther-apeutics. If Dutch clinicians would not cooperate willingly, they had to be made to walk the line using state force. In 1971, one of these lobbying attempts contained the first fully developed Dutch blueprint for the gover-nance of human experimentation using research ethics committees.

State-Imposed Epistemic Reform

In August 1967, the Dutch parliament for the first time discussed the public governance of controlled clinical experimentation. The debate was requested by liberal-conservative parliament member Henk Vonhoff, in reaction to an RCT that had recently been conducted, under Nelemans' leadership, on the effects of oral anticoagulants on coronary afflictions. While this trial was con-sidered a success from a scientific point of view, Vonhoff wished to know whether the government had been aware that such experiments were con-ducted in the Netherlands, and whether it was true that patients participating in these trials usually were not asked for their permission. Also, was it true that Dutch law encouraged the conduct of RCTs and did this method truly have such great advantages that it should be accepted as an integral part of Dutch society? Finally, if so, did the state not carry a responsibility to monitor how these studies were conducted?[44]

With his question about Dutch law, Vonhoff referred to the 1958 Medicines Supply Act, which demanded that a yet-to-be-established regulatory agency would in the future only register packaged medicines in the Netherlands "of which it may reasonably be expected that they possess the advertised effect."[45] Although this article was subject to interpretation, the Medicines Evaluation Board (MEB) established in 1963 decided early on that "possession of the advertised effect" could only be measured via "clinical trials with truly double-blind investigations from which real evidence can be obtained to establish a significant difference between a group that is treated with a certain drug and a group that is not."[46]

The two pharmacologists responsible for this decision, Poppe Siderius and Willem Lammers, in later years commemorated this move under the banner "A Law is Just a Law."[47] The MEB was established just after the infamous thalidomide disaster of 1961, when it became clear that the over-the-counter drug thalidomide, which had been sold since the late 1950s as a low-risk medicine against nausea and morning sickness, had in a few years' time caused more than ten thousand infants to be born worldwide with severe teratogenic deformities.[48] Marketed in the Netherlands under the brand name Softenon, thalidomide had also been prescribed to pregnant Dutch women, although much less frequently than in other countries.[49] Nonetheless, the disaster caused a big scare in the Netherlands. Newspapers reported that such disasters could easily occur again, not least because the government was hardly prepared to prevent them.[50]

Because of this scare, the board members of the MEB were given much leeway by the government to develop a regulatory system capable of preventing something like the thalidomide disaster from ever happening again. For the government, this injunction meant that the MEB was to push down hard on the *safety* of medicinal products, but Siderius and Lammers decided early on that the MEB would also make specific demands about the *efficacy* of products.[51] The government had put the MEB in the position to regulate the Dutch drug market, and the board would use the opportunity to demand that manufacturers prove drug efficacy with evidence gathered from RCTs.

At the time, not everyone in Dutch academia was enthusiastic about this coup. In meetings of the TNO Committee for Clinical Drug Research, the famous Dutch pharmacologist Ulbe Bijlsma—a representative of an older generation—stated that this epistemic "tunnel vision" made him feel uneasy. For one thing, it would turn many patients into "nothing more than lab rats."

For another, it was questionable whether such a singularity of epistemic norms should be enforced by the state. "In former times, without statistical research," Bijlsma remarked sharply, "medicines were also developed." Indeed, another Committee member added, all clinics had their own methods. The forced standardization of these practices was problematic, as it took away physicians' autonomy. However, Chairman Nelemans had been adamant that the Medicines Supply Act offered an opportunity for improving clinical drug research in the Netherlands: "If these methods would be standardized, and if only those medicines that have been tried and tested according to these methods would be accepted, much would have been accomplished already."[52]

In the Dutch parliament in 1967, the state secretary of health responsible for answering Vonhoff's questions took a similar line. In response to the question of whether the RCT had to be accepted as an integral part of Dutch society, the state secretary—himself a physician—replied confidently that "leading experts from around the world agree that double-blind trials as a rule should be regarded as inevitable."[53] Hence, the Medicines Supply Act could indeed be interpreted to encourage RCTs. It was not true, however, that such studies were usually carried out without patients' consent. While they were not allowed to choose if they preferred the treatment or the control group, patients were "usually informed that an experimental investigation was taking place," leaving them free to withdraw from the study at any time they wanted.[54]

Vonhoff was not convinced. Armed with newspaper snippets, he confronted the state secretary with the fact that research leader "Dr. Nelemans" had said on multiple occasions that the requirement of informed consent did not apply for clinical trials. Only recently, Nelemans had been quoted as saying that research subjects could only truly provide informed consent if they were fully aware of all risks and that, if this information were available, no need would exist to conduct the experiment. In addition, the pharmacologist had stated that since written consent forms often served only to absolve researchers in case experiments went south, the emphasis on informed consent could also be considered unethical.[55] Vonhoff suspected a different reason underlay the reluctance to obtain consent: "In *Medisch Contact*, I at one point find the statement that the manner and persuasion in which a physician prescribes a recipe to his patient has important effects on the healing process and that this placebo-effect needs to be eliminated to get objective results." In other words, omitting to inform patients that an experiment was being conducted was not primarily in the interest of those patients, but in meeting "the requirements of an ideal trial."[56]

Other members of parliament voiced concerns as well. A member of the Labor Party—also a physician—agreed with the state secretary that double-blind investigations were needed, but had heard that such experiments were usually only conducted with publicly insured patients; i.e., those patients who depended on health funds provided by the state because their income was too low for them to afford private health insurance. Again, the state secretary offered a reassuring reply: "In my experiences in academic hospitals, class patients are also included in these types of research studies."[57] Nonetheless, he promised to investigate the concerns voiced in parliament. In particular, he would seek advice about one of the last questions posted by Vonhoff: whether the state had a responsibility to monitor the conduct of double-blind pharmacological studies in the Netherlands. To this end, the state secretary submitted a request for advice to the Health Council: was legislation for clinical drug research needed in the Netherlands and, if so, what should such regulations look like?[58] To answer these questions, four internists, two pharmacologists, a general practitioner, and a pharmacist met up thirteen times between 1969 and 1971 to write a report on the regulation of clinical drug research.[59] One of the two pharmacologists was Frans Nelemans.

Research Ethics Committees as Epistemic Filters

Appointed as the chairman of the Council Committee for Clinical Drug Research was the Leiden pharmacologist Erik Noach, a former student of Samuel de Jongh who had taken over the latter's professorial chair in 1963.[60] At Leiden University, he had been experimenting with the communal review of clinical research studies since 1965, which made him an excellent candidate to chair a committee on the regulation of clinical drug research. During his career, Noach would make various important contributions to the organization of medical science in the Netherlands. He was one of the architects of a new curriculum for the biomedical sciences at Leiden University, for instance, and was considered an authority on the appropriate regulation of alternative medicines and animal experiments. First and foremost, however, Noach is remembered for his contributions to the Dutch governance of human subjects research. In many ways, as will become clear, he may be considered the founding father of Dutch research ethics committees.

In 1968, Noach advised the Health Council president to compose the committee of three types of experts: practitioners of the clinical and pre-clinical sciences, stakeholders of the pharmaceutical industry, and representatives of civil service. Finally, if the Council president found it desirable to seek advice from a "non-medical expert in ethical issues," Noach recommended he invite Leiden Professor in the Philosophy of Religion and Ethics

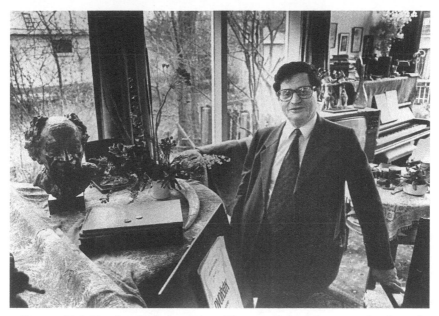

Figure 2. Erik Noach in his home in 1984. Photograph from the personal archive of Arthur and Stella Noach, children of Erik Noach.

Herman Heering.[61] No records have been preserved to indicate that Heering, who would go on to become a prolific author on medical ethics in the 1970s, was invited to join the committee. Instead, the Council president invited seven physicians and a pharmacist, all established disciplinary insiders to the Dutch field of medicine and health. Around 1970, apparently, the ethics of human experimentation could still be considered solely by members of the medical profession.

The men were each appointed in a personal capacity, yet each of them did represent an organization relevant to the practice and politics of clinical drug research. The industrial pharmacist worked for Brocades & Stheeman, one of the largest Dutch pharmaceutical companies at the time.[62] The first internist sat on the board of the National Specialists Association, the second was employed as a public health officer, the third was a highly esteemed academic, and the fourth, internist Louis Stuyt, headed a department of internal medicine at a large hospital (and would go on to become minister of public health and environmental hygiene in 1971). The general practitioner, in turn, sat on the board of the College for General Practitioners. Finally, there was Frans Nelemans, longtime leader of TNO's Committee for Clinical Drug Research, a known advocate of the controlled clinical trial, and, as it happened, the direct reason why the state secretary of public health had requested that the Health Council develop a policy report.

In a memorandum prepared by Noach for the first committee meeting, the pharmacologist laid down a framework for its deliberations that contained a clear rhetoric of therapeutic reform. All committee members had to accept, for instance, that "human experimentation to determine the useful, undesirable, and toxic effects of medicines is of the utmost importance" and "to a certain extent mandatory by law." Also, they had to agree that researchers needed to follow "rigorous scientific methods" to ensure that their studies "yield[ed] optimal information with minimal risks":

> The committee needs to develop a description of clinical drug research in such a way that it will encourage the conduct of experimental tests—which are scientifically and ethically correct—as being in the interest of public health and therefore necessary, while scientifically flawed tests—which on this ground are already ethically deplorable—will be hindered as much as possible.[63]

Noach, in short, made it clear from the start that any regulation for clinical drug research would have to both accept and promote its conduct. In addition, he envisioned any form of state oversight to function as what I call an *epistemic filter*: a porous device that would sift out good clinical experiments from bad clinical experiments—*good* here meaning simultaneously "methodologically sound" and "ethically just"—and, as such, improve the quality of clinical research and practice in the Netherlands.

In the Council report submitted in 1971, this intricate link between sound research and moral conduct figured prominently. Its opening pages, for instance, quoted a 1968 World Health Organization (WHO) report on clinical drug evaluation, drawn up under the leadership of Austin Bradford Hill, which emphasized that "for the investigation of drugs, planned scientific studies in man are always necessary. It is not always recognized that it is unethical to introduce into general use a drug that has been inadequately tested." (The WHO report continued: "The ethical problem is not solely one of human experimentation; it is also one of refraining from human experimentation.")[64] In addition, the Council report added, since clinical research increased medical knowledge and had a positive pedagogical effect on students and physicians, the government had every reason to support and promote it.[65] This fact did not mean, the Health Council emphasized, that principles of medical ethics did not have to be taken into account.[66] However, the report *literally* underscored multiple times, the conduct of clinical research itself was *necessary* and *inevitable*.[67] Hence, like the Council Committee for

Tests upon Human Beings before it, the Council Committee for Clinical Drug Research maintained in 1971 that all it could sensibly do was propose measures that minimized risks of human experimentation and ensure that no fundamental ethical lines were crossed in the process.

The question of what these policy measures should look like formed the core of the thirteen committee meetings that took place between 1969 and 1971. Its eight members eventually agreed on four general guidelines. First, conducting clinical drug research was only permitted for physicians and dentists. Second, while no group of research subjects should a priori be excluded from clinical research, strong caution had to be exercised in experimenting with special groups such as children or mentally ill patients. Third, as testing drug samples on individual patients "as a rule misses any scientific value," that practice should only be allowed with registered pharmaceuticals with a known composition. Finally, following the 1964 Declaration of Helsinki, the report stated that "in general" the informed consent of research subjects was required. Notably, however, the committee made a distinction between the consent of healthy research subjects and those participating in a clinical trial. In the case of the first group, informed consent was always necessary. Yet, in case of the second group, the Health Council recommended that the government demand only that permission should be acquired "as is common in normal medical treatments."[68] Thus, clinical researchers had to be permitted to take the consent of patients for a clinical *procedure* as sufficient information that they were also willing to take part in a clinical *trial*. Whether a researcher was obliged to inform patients that they might possibly receive a placebo was left unspecified.

In his 1970 booklet, which appeared in the midst of the committee deliberations, Nelemans defended this rule by invoking the 1964 Declaration of Helsinki. This declaration, he argued, was of crucial importance for clinical trials, but researchers really had to interpret it "to the spirit of the letter." Its passage on informed consent, for instance, "really has to be understood to mean that no research may ever be conducted if the patient would not have given his permission had he been informed of all available data."[69] Otherwise, pretty much all clinical experimentation would become impossible, which "certainly cannot have been the intention of the Declaration." "It makes more sense," Nelemans and his coauthor concluded, "to automatically assume the cooperation of a patient, unless there is clear evidence to the contrary."[70]

To be sure, Nelemans did emphasize the need for strict ethical guidelines in clinical experimentation. Such experiments could only be permitted "if they satisf[ied] medical ethics, perhaps most easily described in practice

as that the physician would not hesitate to let himself or his family participate [in the trial]."[71] They also had to—at least potentially—yield important new insights, and existing pharmacotherapies needed to have objections
held against them that could "be overcome completely or partially by the
new medicine." In addition, Nelemans made very clear that "a scientifically
sound trial, *no matter how important it is,* may *never* be executed if it sins
against medical ethics."[72] The pharmacologist was simply unconvinced that
the requirement of informed consent added much to these rules. Instead,
the medical community had to invest in its professional ethics and institutional safeguards.[73]

The Committee for Clinical Drug Research followed Nelemans in this
logic. Instead of giving suggestions for how best to ensure the freely given informed consent of patients, it advised the government to develop a system of
oversight "that should better guarantee the safety and wellbeing of research
subjects."[74] This system worked as follows: a physician or dentist who wanted
to conduct a clinical drug trial would have to make a report about his plans
to the Dutch Medical Inspection. He could then commence his study. However, if the Inspection suspected something to be wrong, it was entitled to
bring this study to a halt. If a researcher failed to report his study and was
found out, legal steps could be taken and penal measures imposed.

The committee formulated two main tasks for the Medical Inspection.
The first was that "in the interest of science only technically correct investigations, in which a warrant of optimal information acquisition is present, may
be conducted." Thus, one of the main things the Dutch Medical Inspection
had to assess was whether reported clinical studies were methodologically
sound. The second was that "on ethical grounds, it is necessary to establish
impartially if the objectives and execution of the study weigh out against the
risks taken by research subjects."[75] If a clinical trial simply duplicated another
study, for instance, no new scientific insights would be gained—a state of
affairs the committee deemed to be a wasteful use of resources. Or, if a hospital did not have the right research facilities to properly execute a clinical trial,
no valid results could be obtained and participants could be put in danger,
which would be another reason to bring a clinical study to a halt.

To assist the Medical Inspection in this task, Noach et al. proposed to set
up local review committees in the main Dutch research centers, including
medical faculties and academic hospitals. Experts in the field of clinical drug
research would sit on these committees to evaluate "the scientific merits of
a proposed study as well as its closely related ethical aspects."[76] The Health
Council compared the functioning of these committees to the practice of

refereeing that had long been popular with academic journals and, somewhat more recently, with grant organizations.[77] Thus, the committees would be asked primarily to assess the scientific quality of proposals and the availability of appropriate research facilities. If all were in order, the study could proceed. If not, suggestions for improvement would be made. Hence, as the MEB was imagined to operate as an epistemic filter at the end of the clinical drug research pipeline, ethics boards were imagined to operate at the beginning of it. As the 1968 WHO report stated, "investigators should discuss their plans of investigation with other physicians and experienced medical research workers before embarking on the initial investigation of a new drug [...] best done by a local medical or scientific committee rather than by an official control organization."[78] The more epistemic filters in place, the better the system functioned.

Noach et al. were confident that this type of oversight would benefit the *quality* of Dutch clinical drug research. "Consultation of this nature is a powerful tool to raise the level of science," the 1971 report stated, "which is in the long haul also in the interests of the participants in the study."[79] In addition, they hoped it would increase the *quantity* of such research as well. A main reason why it remained difficult to conduct controlled trials in the Netherlands was that many clinicians did not want their patients to receive a placebo drug. But physicians who felt this way did not truly understand clinical science: "The committee cannot shake the impression," the 1971 report read, "that these restraints are often more founded on emotion than on reason."[80] Noach et al. envisioned ethics boards, therefore, to reach out to physicians to explain the logic of clinical research and to take away unnecessary ethical doubts. In addition, they could offer "moral backing" if critics unjustly accused researchers of unethical conduct.[81] This way, researchers would no longer stand alone when attempting to bring about medical progress, a development that would surely help to "contribute to the intensification of clinical drug research in the Netherlands, which has been developed insufficiently in part because of hesitations of physicians on ethical grounds."[82]

Finally, Noach et al. recommended that the government enforce this system by law. In theory, they stated in 1971, the voluntary cooperation of researchers was possible. Equivalent to the general practitioner who had grown accustomed to consulting specialists, a researcher could be conditioned to consult experts in clinical drug research. Sadly, however, these experts remained a scarce good: "As long as no specialized training in clinical drug research exists [...] the danger remains that voluntary oversight will lead to unacceptable risks, for instance because a necessary correction is not made because of the misplaced self-confidence of a researcher."[83] Thus, as long as clinical research was not up to par in the Netherlands, state force was needed to direct the professional conduct of Dutch researchers.

Still, the precise involvement of the state had to be carefully orchestrated. "A straitjacket that is too narrow," the report read, "will reduce the enthusiasm for conducting clinical drug research [...] which certainly cannot be in the interest of public health."[84] After all, "a Government generally exercises more caution than is strictly necessary on ethical or scientific grounds, as she is vulnerable to public opinion, even if the latter is predominantly based on emotional grounds."[85] The role of the state, therefore, had to be strictly limited to authorizing the conglomerate of review boards to keep watch over clinical research and to demand that researchers report all clinical research studies to these bodies. The actual review of these studies had to remain the prerogative of the medical profession itself. Or, more precisely, it had to become the prerogative of specific elite members of the medical profession, who would use the hard power of the state to control those peripheral researchers who did not always know what they were doing. Only in this way would therapeutic reform finally be realized in the Netherlands.

In 1971, Noach et al. did not yet refer to the review boards they envisioned as research ethics committees. In the 1970s and 1980s, however, their ideas for the oversight of human experimentation became the main blueprint for Dutch policy debates on human experimentation, and Noach became widely considered as the national authority on research ethics governance. Research ethics committees, in this original conception, were *expert* committees, intended to promote more and better clinical experimentation. Noach et al. acknowledged that methodologically good science did not necessarily equate to ethically good science. However, they were convinced that methodologically bad science did equate to ethically bad science. Hence, they imagined review committees to function first and foremost as epistemic filters, which they believed to be an absolute moral requirement for the conduct of all forms of clinical — and other types of human — experimentation.

A Lack of Proper Expertise and More Policy Reports

After the Health Council sent a confidential version of its report to the government in December 1971, nothing happened for almost two years. Only in May 1973 did the Health Council receive a reply, with the remark that the government agreed that "national legislation for the protection of those involved in clinical research is desirable," but that questions still existed about the oversight system proposed by the Health Council. First, was the Council absolutely certain that it would not "put a halt to clinical investigations, which are necessary"? Second, given the scarcity of relevant expertise in the Netherlands, which experts precisely would take up seats in local review committees? Before the government would undertake any further steps, therefore, it first wanted the Health Council to think further about the implications that these measures could have for the development of clinical drug research.[86] Evidently, in the early 1970s, the Dutch government was not in any hurry to realize additional oversight for human experimentation.

In response to this request, the Council president duly brought another committee into existence, which started its deliberations in 1974. Noach this time served as a regular committee member, as did eight other physicians, a pharmacist, and a legal scholar. Again, this committee set out to write a report on the regulation of clinical drug research, to make sure it *absolutely* would not "put a halt to clinical investigations," and to make policy suggestions about how enough national expertise could be cultivated to effectively take on the oversight of clinical experiments.[87] Its final report was published in 1981, fourteen years after Vonhoff had first asked the government whether the state was not responsible to monitor the conduct of RCTs.[88]

There were various reasons why it took the Health Council this long to finish a report that was only meant to provide some additional reflections. The main reason was that now that the committee members, all enthusiasts of clinical pharmacology, had the ear of the Ministry, they used the opportunity to develop elaborate plans for the expansion of their discipline.[89] In this process, the realization of research ethics committees increasingly took a backseat. By the late 1970s, some committee members even remarked that it would be a waste if their plans for the growth of clinical pharmacology went unrealized simply because their report also contained chapters on the regulation of clinical experimentation.

One committee member did continue to care intensely about the sections on ethics review. This was Erik Noach. In an early stage of the deliberations, the majority of the Committee for Clinical Pharmacology had decided to resolve the problem of the lack of relevant expertise by advising the government to install a single, national Council for Clinical Research that would evaluate all patient-related research in the Netherlands. Researchers would still be obliged to report all studies to this council, and the council would still inform the Medical Inspection if it suspected any wrongdoings, but the committee now argued that "this Council is not supposed to act as a scientific advisory body for clinical researchers."[90] Noach disagreed. The centralization of review procedures, he warned, "will greatly stall the much-needed growth of clinical research in the Netherlands."[91] Given that researchers would likely await the verdict of the central Council before starting their studies, undesirable delays in the conduct of clinical trials could be expected. In addition, Noach felt that ethics committees did have to evaluate the scientific quality of research protocols. By the late 1970s, in fact, he had come to argue that clinical trials should only be permitted in the Netherlands *after* "a review committee has notified a researcher in writing that no scientific or ethical objections exist against the research study."[92]

Noach could not convince the other committee members. The majority maintained that a single Council for Clinical Research was the most practical solution for the problem of insufficient expertise and that, moreover, "the installation of the Council and the duty to report research studies is only meant to stimulate sound research, not to make scientific research dependent on the medical insights of the Council."[93] Noach decided, therefore, to invoke his right as a Council member to write a minority report in which he set out alternative plans for the governance of clinical experimentation by means of local review committees, which he now explicitly referred to as ethics committees. In his alternative system—which resembled much of the system that the Council had proposed in 1971—one national Council would function as a coordination and supervision office, but local ethics boards would form the backbone of the oversight of clinical research. What was more, the ethical evaluation of research protocols would very much include an evaluation of their scientific quality.

Noach's diverging opinion slowed down and further weakened a policy report that had already for quite some time started to look like a failure. When the definitive version of the report was sent to the government in November 1981, political winds had changed. By then, ethical discussions over the rights of research subjects, which had dominated public discourse in the United States and Great Britain since the late 1960s, had finally reached the Netherlands. All of a sudden, a report from a scientific advisory body that emphasized the need for more clinical experimentation and increased power for elite members of the medical profession appeared incredibly outdated. So much so, in fact, that the Dutch government had decided a few years earlier, in 1978, to request *another* policy report on the governance of human experimentation. Only this time, it sent this request not to the Health Council—an expert advisory body—but to the Central Council for Public Health, an advisory body that seated representatives of various political and civil organizations.

Since 1975, this Council had been tasked with developing policy reports for the realization of patients' rights in the Netherlands. In 1982, this Council also published a report recommending the oversight of human experimentation by local ethics committees. In contrast to the Health Council reports, however, this report did not advocate the need for therapeutic reform or more internal control. Instead, it emphasized the rights of research subjects and the need for additional democratic oversight mechanisms: i.e., research ethics committees were now argued to provide more *external control* over human experimentation. Still, one member of the Central Council for Public Health, the one who in fact wrote most of its 1982 report on the governance of human experimentation, was a familiar face. This Council member was Leiden pharmacologist Erik Noach.

PART II
EXTERNAL CONTROL

CHAPTER 3

MEDICAL ETHICS *in a*

MODERN SOCIETY

In August 1969, the social-democratic newspaper *Het Vrije Volk* ran a full-page interview with psychiatrist Rudi van den Hoofdakker, better known as poet Rutger Kopland.[1] A photograph accompanied the piece. Sitting on a camping chair without any shirt on, legs crossed, he was vigorously arguing a case. Addressing someone outside of the frame, his brows were furrowing, his hands gesticulating. "Artsenstand," the headline read, "a drift anchor that inhibits progress."[2] According to Van den Hoofdakker, the *artsenstand* resembled a "stronghold of know-it-alls."[3] The moment students started medical school, they learned to don themselves in age-old cloaks of medical ethics, hanging nicely ironed next to their white coats, just waiting to be put on. They did not have to decide themselves what was morally right or wrong; they just had to act as members of the *artsenstand* would. This conservatism, the psychiatrist felt, inhibited social progress. Physicians and patients had to break free from the chains of medical paternalism, in which the child constantly expected the father to solve all problems, while the father was afraid to violate the trust the child put in him. Physicians had to learn to "talk, talk, talk" and make decisions with patients instead of for them. What was needed was an "ethics against ethics": a close examination of why doctors held the moral beliefs they did.[4] For, like many others around 1970, Van den Hoofdakker had come to believe that a modern society required modern medical ethics.

In the following two chapters, I explore the growing call for *external control* over Dutch medicine in the 1960s and 1970s, and the encapsulation of research ethics committees by this movement in the early 1980s. In 1982, the country's Central Council for Public Health published a report stating that communal ethics review was needed to secure the rights of human research subjects in medical experiments. After all, in a modern democratic society "seclusion and mystery have to make way for openness and transparency."[5]

The specific events that led the Dutch government to request this report from the Central Council for Public Health will be examined further in chapter 4. First, this chapter details the rise of the Dutch patients' rights movement in the 1960s and 1970s. According to Robert Baker, the Dutch medical profession in this period held on to its jurisdiction over medical ethics, which made it less necessary for others—i.e., "medical outsiders"—to step in and "fill the space left empty by organized medicine."[6] In this chapter I show, however, that even though the KNMG announced after World War II that it would make significant investments in its medical ethics tradition to ensure that the professional identity that had kept Dutch physicians strong in times of war would not wither away, this optimism crumbled in the decades thereafter. By 1970, the *Dutch Journal of Medicine* and *Medisch Contact* were filled with concerns over a crisis of medical ethics that had descended upon medicine. In parliament, politicians began to call for "medical ethics that better fitted a modern, open society," and an amalgam of social movements started to advocate the need to elevate the position of the patient in health care. Instead of "vertical relations of dependence and subordination," the new mantra became, the government had to realize "horizontal relations of consultation and participation." Eventually, toward the end of the 1970s, research ethics committees became part of this discourse.

The Dutch Crisis of Medical Ethics

In the first decade after World War II, medical ethics had been an important area of focus in the Dutch medical community. In 1947, the (K)NMG announced plans to establish medical ethics departments. In 1949, *primus inter pares* Brutel called for a work "that adapts our existing medical ethics to the radical changes that have taken place in the profession of medicine and in society at large." And in 1954, the KNMG established a Committee for Medical Ethics that would write a new ethics booklet.

In the 1950s, the Dutch medical community took pride in this renewed attention to medical ethics. *Medisch Contact*, for instance, regularly kept its readers updated of the excellent progress made by the Committee for Medical Ethics. Between 1954 and 1958, the journal frequently printed draft versions of chapters of the committee's new ethics booklet, with the request for readers to send in comments and questions. This collective effort, the idea was, would result in robust ethics guidelines that carried the seal of approval of the majority of the Dutch *artsenstand*.[7] Similarly, in the mid-1950s, the KNMG relished the fact that the Dutch had brought the ethics of human experimentation to the attention of the international medical community. In the Netherlands, its message was, everything was done to keep medical ethics in high regard, to make sure it remained an effective mechanism of internal control.

At the start of the 1960s, this positive image continued to reign supreme. In 1959, the KNMG had finished its new ethics booklet.[8] Titled *Medische ethiek en gedragsleer* (Medical ethics and behavioral rules), it covered all sorts of subjects, such as the importance of medical confidentiality, the rights and responsibilities of practitioners when handing over their practice to colleagues, the appropriate attitude toward the pharmaceutical industry and general press, the position of physicians vis-à-vis health care funds, etcetera.[9] The plan was that all members of the KNMG would be sent a copy of the ethics booklet, and that all medical students would be presented with a copy upon graduating to remind them of the moral duties that this rite of passage bestowed upon them. The Committee for Medical Ethics, in the meanwhile, would be reinstated by the KNMG as a permanent advisory board for all matters concerning medical ethics.[10]

In their discussion of the booklet in 1960, the editors of *Medisch Contact* expressed their excitement over the realization of a new medical ethics. In the past, the editors explained, Dutch physicians had at times mistakenly spoken of *ethics*—which was a "heavy word," suggesting deep moral reflection—when they had really meant to talk of *etiquette*: the customary mores of polite conduct among colleagues. The new booklet therefore strictly distinguished the two, "so that it is clear that also in the leading circles of [our] medical society this distinction is appreciated."[11] Given the wealth of material that each chapter contained, the editors were convinced the booklet offered physicians solid handles for the sometimes-difficult ethical decisions that awaited them in their practice.[12]

That same year, the Protestant internist Gerrit Arie Lindeboom published another booklet on medical ethics, *Opstellen over medische ethiek* (Essays on medical ethics), which contained chapters on subjects such as medical confidentiality and vivisection, but also on subjects such as artificial insemination and euthanasia.[13] In the *Dutch Journal of Medicine*, Lindeboom's booklet was recommended as a learned and thoughtful publication.[14] Various newspapers also reviewed the booklet positively.[15] One, which printed a joint review of Lindeboom's essays and the KNMG booklet, commented enthusiastically on "the curious fact that, as much as their belief systems may differ, physicians have ever since Hippocrates displayed a profound agreement on medical ethics." The publication of these two ethics booklets was only further proof of the "fortunate fact that physicians in difficult circumstances can rely on a common opinion."[16]

Over the course of the 1960s, however, this image changed radically. In a period of just ten years, the perception in Dutch medical circles of its ethics tradition took a sharp downturn. In 1970, a physician declared in *Medisch Contact* that Dutch medical ethics was "in full crisis."[17] Anyone denying this crisis just had to reread a recent policy report by the KNMG. There, tucked away between a few policy decisions, a paragraph titled "Serious Problems" contained the admission that the Committee for Medical Ethics had been unable to write an updated version of *Medische ethiek en gedragsleer*.[18] The committee could, if desired, create another edition containing behavioral rules for physicians, but it had "given up hope of composing another *Medische ethiek*."[19] The physician felt this failure stood testimony to a deep crisis in moral medical authority that had "become manifest around 1960" and that had brought about a "degeneration in medical thinking."[20] Within a single decade, the medical society had lost its once easy connection to that "heavy word": ethics.

What happened to Dutch medical ethics in the 1960s? On March 24, 1961, *Medisch Contact* printed a review by Utrecht theology and ethics professor Johannes de Graaf of the KNMG ethics booklet and of Lindeboom's *Opstellen* that was much less enthusiastic about both booklets than other reviews had been. While both publications had clearly been written with good intentions, De Graaf wrote, neither could exactly be called *modern*: "One senses a certain longing for the good old days of personal relations [...] as if physicians still feel helpless in the industrialized mass society of today."[21] Both booklets, he felt, envisioned the doctor-patient relationship to be a special bond of trust between two individuals who knew one another intimately. Yet, like most of "modern society," the health care system was now organized through collective social structures (hospitals, health insurance plans) and a far-reaching division of labor (specialization, teamwork). In effect, doctors and patients had often become strangers to one another and their interactions had become functional and fleeting.[22] That relational shift did not mean medical ethics no longer mattered in a modern society, De Graaf continued. Quite the opposite: In a world with weak social ties, clear moral guidelines had become more important than ever. Still, the ethics professor argued, the medical profession had to find a new way of relating to patients, and to "tune in the ethos of the physician to the modern wavelength."[23]

De Graaf was wary, for instance, of the recurring appeal to the conscience of physicians in the KNMG booklet: "As if we may just trust this conscience as long as the physician acts in the spirit of the professional ethics formulated in this book." In ethics, the professor argued, scholars had since long stopped using the conscience as a normative authority: it served to recognize feelings of guilt and remorse, but did not provide an index of moral guidelines. In fact, De Graaf continued, for a work with the words "medical ethics" in its title, the KNMG booklet had surprisingly few moral guidelines to offer for medical practice. That is, it dealt in detail with a specific subset of ethical problems—those "on which consensus long since exists"—like the need for professional confidentiality or the (im)permissibility of commercial advertising. But subjects that most people now associated with medical ethics, such as the permissibility of birth control, artificial insemination, or lobotomy, were mentioned only in the chapter "The physician and religion," and only with the comment that physicians should respect patients' personal viewpoints. Perhaps such an elusive approach was inevitable for any association hoping to represent all physicians in a single country, De Graaf remarked delicately, but it did mean the KNMG had little to offer for physicians struggling with truly difficult ethical questions.[24]

A year later, in April 1962, the editors of *Medisch Contact* responded to De Graaf's critiques with a leading article entitled "Ethical problems for the physician." Given the editors' enthusiastic reaction to the new KNMG booklet only two years earlier, their reply demonstrated a surprisingly pliable attitude. While physicians could rest on a longstanding tradition of moral contemplation, they wrote, it was true this tradition increasingly seemed to fall short. The main cause of such failure, the editors asserted, was the "dizzying speed in which 'the new sciences' [had] penetrated the terrain of the physician" in the last century. In recent years, for instance, the medical profession had tried to come to grips with the implications of new respiration and resuscitation technologies that fundamentally altered the possibilities of a physician to *preserve* life. But before a moral consensus had been reached on this topic, "a new wave of technical skill" was already "poured out onto humanity" in the form of artificial insemination, which now offered physicians the possibility to *conceive* life as well. The editors agreed that such developments demanded more reflection than was currently the case, but they understood why this reflection often did not happen:

> The consequences of these technical possibilities are so far reaching, that some are hardly willing to think further about them. [...] People want to be undisturbed and live their old lives as much as possible, not just because these new possibilities are incalculable and frightening, but because they do not know how to cope with the type of ethical concerns that these [technologies] bring.[25]

Nonetheless, the editors did feel the KNMG had a leading role to fulfill in this regard, and they emphasized that debates about these new developments could also be held in the pages of their own journal: "The more use is made out of this [...] the more seriously we can strive to stay faithful to the tradition that physicians can draw support from their professional ethos in determining their point of view."[26]

This call for more communal reflection was certainly put into effect in the 1960s. In 1962, the KNMG issued a reflection paper on the ethics of artificial insemination and organized a live debate at its General Assembly.[27] Over the next few years, *Medisch Contact* published essays on the ethical implications of new medical technologies almost every other week. The most frequently asked question was whether the old adage in medical ethics—to sustain life as much as possible—still held true in an era when the possibilities for doing so seemed to grow ever more endless. In 1965, a two-day conference was held on the theme "Ethics or Etiquette," with talks like "The inadequacy of our existing medical ethics" and "What should the norm of our practice be?"[28] In 1966, the KNMG considered whether it should start to study medical ethics "scientifically," and in 1967, it decided that its Committee for Medical Ethics was in serious need of rejuvenation. Among other things, the committee had to critically scrutinize the contents of the KNMG ethics booklet—only eight years old at the time—and, if necessary, completely rewrite them.[29] In 1968, the KNMG approached all Dutch medical faculties with the request that they pay more attention in their curricula to medical ethics.[30]

This increase of communal reflection, however, did not quite have the desired effect. The more frequently journals like *Medisch Contact* discussed the ethical implications of new technologies, the more it became clear that doctors often could *not* "rely on a common opinion in difficult circumstances." Sure, separate factions had existed for a long time in the *artsenstand* that were aligned to the (in)famous "pillars" in Dutch society (i.e., the Catholic, Protestant, socialist, and liberal pillars).[31] Yet until the 1960s, the elite of the Dutch medical profession had often confidently maintained that "personal viewpoints" did not conflict with the professional ethos of physicians, which they derived from being members of the *artsenstand*. But when the Dutch medical profession started increasingly in the 1960s to discuss ethical issues other than the importance of medical confidentiality or the problem of commercial advertising, it became clear that physicians often did not agree on the morally right or wrong thing to do in difficult circumstances. On closer inspection, it turned out, the unitary ethos of the Dutch *artsenstand* was much less solid than had often proudly been assumed.

The Rise of the Modern Patient

These first dents in the professional identity of the *artsenstand* were further exacerbated in the mid-1960s by a growing recognition that patients, also, seemed increasingly to question the moral authority of the physician. In 1966, psychiatrist Jan Marlet—an oft-cited contributor to Dutch debates on medical ethics at the time—coauthored a book with his two brothers (one a jurist, the other a theologian) to examine why, despite a lack of much evidence of medical malpractice among Dutch physicians, Dutch patients increasingly seemed dissatisfied with their doctors.[32] An important psychological reason for this shift, the psychiatrist Marlet asserted, was the growth of medical power in recent years. It had made patients continuously expect more and better care, ironically leaving them less satisfied than when physicians had only been able to offer pastoral care.[33] A cultural reason, the jurist Marlet stated, was the strong levelling of social classes in the Netherlands in recent decades. In the year 1966, the doctor was no longer revered as a true "authority figure." Instead, patients' "sense of self-worth" had increased: if they did not like their physicians, they no longer hesitated to simply choose different ones.[34] A key economic reason, the jurist added, was the fact that since the 1940s many more people had acquired health insurance in the Netherlands. This change had caused waiting rooms to flood, leaving much less time for the average physician to spend per patient, who felt neglected because of it. The doctor-patient relationship, the psychiatrist Marlet concluded with some sadness, was likely to turn into an ordinary business arrangement in the Netherlands with two parties—a supplier and a consumer—constantly in search of "best value for money."[35]

Around the same time, authors in *Medisch Contact* also started to comment on the changing attitude of the patient. The modern patient, the expression went, had become *mondig* ("mouthy," assertive, mature): he no longer just accepted the authority of his physician, but made demands as to the type of treatments he wished to undergo.[36] Doctors were no longer respected as "magi," as members of a priestly caste who could ease suffering with a touch of their hands, but were taken to be mere technical engineers.[37] In 1967, the liberal newspaper *Algemeen Handelsblad* caused a stir under the headline "The doctor is not God."[38] Medical malpractice *did* occur in the Netherlands, the article stated, but the general public was often willfully kept ignorant of misbehavior or mistakes in Dutch medical practice:

> The *artsenstand* uses the term "trust" as a sacred token necessary for a proper medical treatment. In principle, that is true. The danger exists, however, that it also uses the same term as a shield to keep issues that hurt the medical treatment and therefore the general interest out of the public eye.[39]

The KNMG tried to account for such complaints. Already in 1958, its board had proposed to include a legal counsel in its disciplinary courts. At first, this proposal had given rise to fierce opposition among members. "Outsiders" had no place there, the argument ran, as collegial justice was administered according to "the principles of medical ethics which only slowly mature in each physician through his education, experience, and insights."[40] In 1964, however, the KNMG did install a committee with five physicians and three jurists for the modernization of its justice system; the committee strongly advised openness in the association's juridical proceedings. Verdicts had to be made public, including the identity of the accused, *even* if complaints had been ruled unfounded. Moreover, jurists most certainly had to take up seats in the disciplinary courts. These measures were needed, both to allow for a more open dialogue with the Dutch public and to ensure the KNMG "ke[pt] pace with social life."[41]

Yet such measures did not take away a growing unrest about the uneven dynamic of the doctor-patient relationship. In 1968, jurists organized a conference on "the physician and the law." Physicians often failed to realize, speakers complained, that they were bound to the same laws as everyone else.[42] According to one speaker, it was just typical how "in the familiar ethics booklet of the KNMG [...] the personal bond of trust between physician and patient is repeatedly emphasized," while their legal relation was, if referenced at all, interpreted mostly as an impoverishment of the vocation.[43] This attitude, wherein physicians kept on thinking of their profession as an ordained ministry akin to priesthood, agitated people. For society to keep its trust in the medical profession, it was essential that physicians start to recognize the patient as a "legally equal contract partner" and to resist the temptations of paternalism. This idea that doctors were like fathers to their patients simply did not fit life in a modern society anymore.

This surging criticism of the doctor-patient relationship did not hamper the enthusiastic production of new works of medical ethics in the late 1960s. In 1968, a long-running editorial series published the title *Recent medisch ethisch denken I* (Recent medical ethical thinking I) to do justice to "the evolution, one might even say revolution, that is unfolding itself in thinking about medical ethics."[44] The chapters were mostly written by physicians, but one was by Remonstrant theologian Herman Heering and one by legal scholar Jaap Rang, both of whom would go on to become leading public authorities in Dutch debates over medical ethics in the 1970s. Its contents, moreover, were starkly different from the KNMG booklet that had been published a decade earlier, with chapters taking on topics such as euthanasia, artificial insemination, and contraception. In 1970, another edition with topics such as sterilization and sexuality was added to the series.[45] In 1969, a journalist published the booklet *Medische ethiek vandaag* (Medical ethics today), which featured interviews of "sixteen prominent physicians who are confronted day-in-day-out with the most strange and complex new questions of ethics and religion."[46] That same year, a conference was held on "medical ethics between science and society," Herman Heering brought out a book on (medical) ethics titled *Ethiek der voorlopigheid* (Provisional ethics), and Catholic theologian Paul Sporken—who would go on to become the first Dutch professor of medical ethics in 1974—published a book titled *Voorlopige diagnose* (Provisional diagnosis).[47]

Heering and Sporken were popular among Dutch physicians. Both men were regularly invited to publish in *Medisch Contact*, asked to give lectures, and nominated to participate in advisory bodies like the Health Council. Their works helped to ensure that the Dutch discourse on medical ethics was livelier and richer by the end of the 1960s than it had been for a long time. Still, at the close of the decade, a feeling that something was sorely amiss with the existing Dutch medical ethics tradition dominated public debate. If change and temporality dictated ethical thinking, the worry was, and if patients' voices had to be included as well, it was next to impossible to formulate moral guidelines that would transcend the here and now. The idea of a longstanding tradition of medical ethics shared by all members of the *artsenstand* was evaporating into thin air.

In April 1970, the KNMG held its biannual General Assembly. At the meeting, the president announced that the standing Committee for Medical Ethics would be dissolved.[48] "The acceleration in the evolution of science and society," the president explained, demanded a more "modern approach" to medical ethics.[49] In the past, the medical community had often thought that only the opinions of physicians mattered in the moral reflection on medicine, but it now recognized that two groups could be distinguished as having claim to this terrain: "physicians and others."[50] Hence, while the KNMG did feel that "the circle of physicians" had its own unique perspective on what was morally right and wrong in medicine, the association would start to "give room to representatives of the non-medical population" in the formulation of new medical ethics. "If this does not happen," the president warned, "the danger exists that the ethos of physicians will be alienated from the ethical feelings in the population [. . .] to the detriment of its trust in the class of physicians."[51]

The KNMG would therefore establish a new committee with "representatives from the Roman-Catholic medical community, Protestant-Christian medical organization, Remonstrant medical association, and humanistic group *Socrates*" that would be tasked with modernizing the behavioral rules for physicians — strictly keeping in mind that social structures had changed radically in recent years and that patients were now increasingly *mondig*.[52] In addition, the association would start to publish loose-leaf essays on pressing ethical issues, preferably written by experts from the fields of law, sociology, psychology, and theology. These essays would have to take a "pluralistic approach" and include literature suggestions for further self-study. This way, the KNMG hoped to kill two birds with one stone: (1) to ensure that "the ethical aspects of the rapid developments on medical-scientific and technological terrain are brought to the attention of physicians and medical students in a timely manner," and (2) to provide a solution for the growing dissatisfaction in the Netherlands with the social functioning of physicians. "The times have passed," the KNMG president declared solemnly in conclusion to his speech, "that we could pretend medical ethics to be a secret doctrine belonging to the professional secrets kept by physicians."[53] In modern society, everyone had something to say about medical ethics.

The First Steps of Political Interference

In 1970, the KNMG still believed that all it needed to do to defuse this crisis was to invest even more in the formulation of new medical ethics — this time with the input of a whole range of "outsiders." Yet, around the same time that the KNMG president held his speech for the General Assembly, the Dutch parliament started to interfere in discussions over Dutch medical ethics as well. On Tuesday, February 3, 1970, to be exact, during a debate in parliament over the annual budget of the Department of Social Affairs and Public Health, the leader of the Protestant Christian-Democratic Party, Arnold Tilanus, used his allotted speaking time to address "the position of the physician in modern society."[54] According to Tilanus, a growing discomfort could be detected in the Netherlands about this position. Trade unions regularly complained that medical fees were too high; consumer organizations accused medical specialists of treating publicly insured patients less carefully than — the more lucrative — privately insured patients; frequent complaints were made that doctors and nurses refused to work night and weekend shifts; and concerns could be heard about the growing unwillingness of general practitioners to make house calls. All in all, Tilanus concluded cautiously, the societal functioning of physicians "has become a public phenomenon, about which this House can and should speak."[55]

The examples given by Tilanus were all of a socioeconomic nature. Nonetheless, the Protestant politician continued, whilst turning to the Labor Party across the aisle, it would be a mistake to solely attribute the growing popular discomfort about the Dutch medical profession to economic inequalities in Dutch health care. No, Tilanus stated, "the causes of the existing discontent between physician and patient lie much deeper."[56] To make his case, the politician invoked the booklet *Medische macht en medische ethiek* (Medical power and medical ethics) published a year earlier by Dutch *zenuwarts* (neuropsychiatrist) Jan Hendrik van den Berg.[57] In this publication, Van den Berg had, like many others in the late 1960s, argued that new medical ethics had to be developed to account for the growing technical powers of physicians. Unlike many others, however, Van den Berg had written his booklet for a lay public and had included multiple confronting images of suffering patients who were alive only because they had been "saved" by medical technology: a man whose lower body had been surgically removed, a baby with a split spine and hydrocephalus (also called "water on the brain"), etcetera. In "the era of medical power," the psychiatrist had concluded, the once "holy rule" of medical ethics to preserve life at all costs had to be replaced by a new rule stating the physician only "preserves, spares, and lengthens human life when this makes sense."[58]

Medische macht en medische ethiek was, in short, a plea for passive and sometimes even active euthanasia. As such, it caused great uproar in the Netherlands. The booklet was widely read and stayed on Dutch bestseller lists until the spring of 1970.[59] It was not the first Dutch essay to make this plea, but it was the first to actively seek out a nonacademic audience and to provoke great debate in the mainstream media.[60] Some commentators expressed sympathy for Van den Berg's ideas. Sporken, for instance, stated that he could "follow most parts of the road that Van den Berg is travelling with him."[61] Others, however, voiced deep concerns. In Reformed circles, the booklet was referred to as a "Godless book" and its author a "competitor of God."[62] And in left-wing intellectual circles, Van den Berg's ideas were compared to Nazi doctrines. "Even people with few taboos will shudder when reading this," one author wrote, "and wonder where it is that we are going and whether physicians really have any competence in making this type of decision."[63]

In the Dutch parliament, Tilanus drew on Van den Berg in support of his claim that the growing unrest over the medical profession went much deeper than annoyances over the working hours of doctors. The growth of medical power, the politician stated, had brought about new "fundamental questions about the beginning and end of life." And while he did not "want to go as far as Professor Van den Berg in his booklet," Tilanus agreed that "new medical power perhaps requires new medical ethics." Thus, he had an official request for the government: to ask the KNMG to bring together "a group of physicians and ethicists to study the problem of medical power and ethics and to submit a report about this."[64]

The responsible state secretary reacted positively to Tilanus's request. He agreed that the societal functioning of physicians had been subject to much debate in recent years—a fact *he* had been reminded of when reading an article by psychiatrist Rudi van den Hoofdakker, who had criticized the inability of physicians to properly communicate with their patients. Across the world, the societal functioning of physicians was changing due to the rapid transformations of societies: "Questions that hardly used to be questions, now bring unrest and demand constant attention from the government."[65] Hence, the state secretary agreed that medical ethics had turned into something about which politicians could and *should* speak, which was why he planned to request that the Health Council develop a report on the societal position of physicians, and the role fulfilled therein by medical ethics.

Tilanus was pleased with this promise from the state secretary, although he was a bit confused about the sort of policy document that would be written and by whom. He had understood the state secretary to say that he would request the Central Council for Public Health to write a policy report, a choice that Tilanus found unfortunate. The Central Council had been installed in 1958 as a complementary body to the Health Council; it advised the Dutch government on the *organization* of health care. Relevant stakeholders held seats on the Central Council: government representatives, health inspectors, health insurance agents, the KNMG, etcetera.[66] But the council's makeup was exactly the reason for Tilanus's confusion. Rethinking the societal position of physicians and Dutch medical ethics, the politician put forward, required "qualified scholarship" of "professors of medicine, ethics, and possibly social psychology." Such scholarship was not the terrain of the Central Council.[67] Sure, the state secretary replied, which was why he would contact the *Health* Council. "I find," he concluded, "this belongs much more with a specific *expert* committee than with the Central Council."[68]

The Emergence of the Patients' Rights Frame

In response to this request, the Health Council brought together a Committee for Medical Ethics in 1971 that was "to position the physician and patient within the social order [. . .] according to the insights that exist and are developed within society, so that the government can found policy on this."[69] It would inform the government of the circumstances under which physicians were "ethically allowed to put to use the available medical-technical possibilities" and whether any additional steps had to be taken to codify these moral precepts into criminal law.[70] The committee seated eight physicians, five legal scholars, a judge, a nurse, a sociologist, and a moral theologian. In 1973, theologians Heering and Sporken, along with a philosopher, joined the committee deliberations as well, to "reinforce the representation from the side of ethics."[71]

Although the committee was supposed to be an expert group, some members did question whether the group's composition befitted a topic like medical ethics. During the first meeting, for instance, one of the physicians brought up the question of whether, say, patients were not underrepresented.[72] Similarly, when the committee prepared to discuss euthanasia in newborn babies, Heering asked whether mothers should not be included in the deliberations, as they were "most closely involved with the issue."[73] Other members, however, strongly objected to such suggestions. Their work was "of a scientific nature" and therefore did not include the perspective of "interest groups."[74] Plus, one of the physicians remarked, while the committee did not "represent the Dutch cultural pattern in every detail," it also did not "deviate that much from it." Hence, it should be able to formulate "a *communis opinio* that will serve as a benchmark for the Minister to base his policy upon."[75]

In reality, however, this benchmarking quickly proved to be more difficult than expected. In its first report of 1972, on the topic of euthanasia, the committee admitted it had been "difficult, yes, even virtually impossible" to formulate ethical norms that would be acceptable to the majority of Dutch people.[76] Pointing to recent public upheavals over the permissibility of abortions, the committee explained that the Netherlands had become a pluralist society in recent years. "It used to be possible to speak of a *communis opinio* among the majority of physicians and other groups of the population on this topic," the report read, "but now this same measure provokes contradictory and often strong reactions among various social groups and among doctors themselves."[77] Hence, even though the government had asked the Health Council to formulate ethical norms that could be codified into criminal law, the committee felt it would be wrong for any government advisory body to stipulate normative rules as long as a plurality of opinions in Dutch society continued to exist. Any state had to avoid acting as "a master of morality," the report concluded, as "the boundaries between democratic and dictatorial governance are, after all, fluid."[78]

The committee did, however, have a different proposal. In recent years, the report read, a societal trend had been noticeable in which the longstanding authority of paternal figures—like "the government, Church, or scientifically formed expert"—had come under attack: "The conviction is gaining ground that every individual has enough self-knowledge to decide for himself what is in his own best interest."[79] Thus, instead of codifying potentially oppressive *norms* of moral behavior into criminal law, the government could better stipulate "what a patient is entitled to demand from a physician" and "to what extent a physician is entitled to meet such demands."[80] Modern medical ethics should take its starting point in the *rights* of patients and physicians.

In 1972, the Health Council was the first-ever Dutch advisory body to propose a rights frame as a suitable alternative to a more-traditional conception of the doctor-patient relationship. At the time, the term patients' rights was not new. Back in 1953, Dutch Senator Arie Querido had coauthored a Declaration of the Rights of the Patient, which was presented that year in Amsterdam to the World Health Organization (WHO).[81] The code had ten principles, such as the right to be seen as a person instead of a complex of organs and symptoms, the right to all possible help in overcoming concerns and anxieties, and the right to full attention to one's sociocultural background and moral and religious attitudes. However, the WHO had not accepted this declaration in 1953, and neither had patients' rights gained much traction in Dutch political circles in the 1950s and 1960s.

Why the patients' rights frame did gain political currency in the 1970s is a question that cannot easily be answered by pointing to a single cause. An important context, of course, is the fact that the 1960s had also in the Netherlands been a decade of social turbulence. As in other countries, the Dutch counterculture of the sixties had included a rebellion against traditional modes of authority.[82] The medical profession was not exempt from these attacks. In the late 1960s and early 1970s, numerous conflicts erupted in Dutch care facilities over their "paternalistic set-up"—at times resulting in the occupation of buildings by activists (and, in one instance, in widely broadcasted police raids).[83] Occupiers typically protested the hierarchical organization of these facilities and demanded that residents be empowered to influence their own living conditions and treatment plans. In a democratic society, the argument was, everyone should be able to take charge of their own lives. Similarly, in 1970, a group of Dutch physicians began the "kritiese artsen" (critical doctors) movement, which identified repressive social structures as the main cause of disease in civilized society.[84]

Yet, that the discourse of patients' rights would emerge victorious from this period is not as self-evident as it is sometimes taken to be. In the Netherlands, at least, the most vocal social criticism over the organization of health care was predominantly a socialist critique: a conviction that skewed

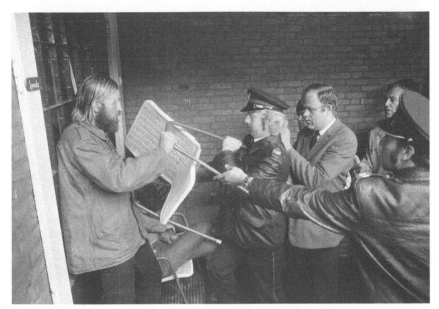

Figure 3. On July 3, 1974, Dutch police cleared the care facility Dennendal by force, after years of conflict over the appropriate treatment of the facility's mentally disabled patients. The occupants propagated the ideals of an "anti-authoritative organizational structure" and believed that all traditional power structures in medicine should be dissolved. Photograph from the National Archive, The Hague.

socioeconomic structures and institutional hierarchies were to blame for the suffering of patients. Hence, grand plans to right these injustices were not geared so much toward the codification of rights for individual patients—a liberal ideal—but toward the realization of alternative social structures and a better economic position for historically disenfranchised groups. In the Dutch parliament, by contrast, the initial response to the crisis of medical ethics had been predominantly conservative. When Tilanus called in 1970 for a reconsideration of medical ethics, he emphasized that he wanted the *artsenstand* to get its house in order before growing public unrest forced the government to step in. For the Protestant politician, the governance of medicine had mostly to be left to the field itself—as it had been in the past. As he stated in support of his request:

> The physician has to integrate in modern society and make himself familiar with the modern thinking of the people. When he fails to do so and when he keeps on resisting modern thinking men and the mod-

ern and open society, this society will try to encapsulate him because it cannot miss [the physician]. By isolating himself, he provokes socialization. I would regret that. I am an opponent of that.[85]

Of course, the perception that patients increasingly seemed dissatisfied with mainstream medical practice did play a central role in the emergence of the Dutch crisis of medical ethics in the 1960s. Still, only few commentators on this crisis in the late 1960s had proposed a patients' rights frame as the new foundation for medical practice in a modern society. Sporken, for instance, who probably stressed the inclusion of patients' perspectives most strongly out of all commentators in that period, did not write much about patients' rights. His approach was more discursive. The conception of "what it means to be human" in modern medicine, the theologian frequently stated, had come to differ too much from what it had always meant in social life. Medical ethics, Sporken maintained, was therefore in essence cultural criticism.[86] Similarly, Van den Hoofdakker had proclaimed his mantra of "talk, talk, talk" to encourage patients and doctors to express their insecurities and doubts — not for patients to start using their newfound voices to claim their rights. Only Van den Berg, really, stated outright in the late 1960s that new medical ethics had to be formulated which should revolve primarily around patients' rights to decide their own lives.[87] Yet Van den Berg's work was also most controversial in the early 1970s.

In the Committee for Medical Ethics, however, the patients' rights frame had already been proposed during the first committee meeting. According to chairman Jan de Vreeze — a legal scholar — "the relation between the rights and duties of the physician and rights of the patient will be an important point for this Committee." Not all members had immediately agreed with this statement. The participating theologian, for instance, had proposed that the committee take a broader approach: medical ethics was an application of "the general ethics" of society, which the committee had to study first to determine what could be considered morally right and wrong in medicine. Likewise, physician Gerard Dekker, the previous secretary of the KNMG, had remarked that the existing medical ethics did not deny patients' rights and that the KNMG these days made it a point to develop moral guidelines together with medical outsiders. So why would new medical ethics have to revolve around the notion of patients' rights? Because, De Vreeze had replied, medical ethics could simply no longer be "medico-centric." "In practice," another jurist added, "the ethical viewpoints of physicians sometimes deviate strongly from patients' wishes."[88] Modern medical ethics had to take these wishes as their starting point.

The influence of the five participating legal scholars on the Committee for Medical Ethics was considerable. They prepared discussion papers for committee meetings, participated actively, and often reminded the other members that the reports they were preparing would likely form the basis for government policy. Their findings therefore had to be translatable into administrative and legislative measures. The majority of the committee accepted this approach. Their first report stated, for instance, that an intimate connection existed between the domains of medical ethics and law. The first domain was an application of general moral principles, while the second derived its precepts from basic human rights, but both could be traced back to generally accepted norms for human interaction. This shared origin was why ethical principles, the report read, were over time often encoded in laws and treaties.[89] Medical ethics, in short, could be debated with a predominantly juridical approach.

After Sporken and Heering joined the committee in 1973, this juridical approach came to be questioned more frequently. However, in Dutch policy circles in the early 1970s, the input of legal scholars was weighted more strongly than that of ethicists. In part, legal scholars were invited to participate more often because their legal expertise was considered a sine qua non for formulating public policy. Yet, in part, they were also invited more often because they were better organized and better politically connected than ethicists in this period.[90] All jurists participating on the Committee of Medical Ethics, for instance, were members of the Dutch Society for Health Law, which had been established in 1968 by upcoming legal scholar Henk Leenen.[91] Health law, Leenen argued, had to be understood as a subcategory of law, not medicine—and health jurists had to use "the definitions and categories of the law," which required legal training. Hence, while Leenen considered it valuable that medical students took notice of the field, it had to be clear that the topic could only be studied in the faculty of law. Jurists were the experts and health law was *their* terrain, even if they would cooperate closely with "experts in the field of executive health care."[92]

In 1973, legal scholar Jaap Rang was appointed as the first Dutch professor in the field of health law. The title of his inaugural lecture was "Patient Law."[93] According to Rang, it was "undeniable that the patient is a key figure in both the ethics and morality of medical practice, but when it comes to the translation of this [precept] in terms of legislation, the patient appears to have been lost."[94] It did not matter whether one checked the first (1929) or last (1972) Dutch handbook on "the physician and the law"—in neither volume did the patient even make it as an index entry.[95] Hence, the freshly appointed professor stated, it was high time the government took action and started integrating the rights of patients into its health laws.[96] Solid health laws were to be synonymous with patients' rights.[97]

Both Leenen and Rang participated on the Committee for Medical Ethics and took up seats in multiple government advisory bodies in the 1970s and 1980s concerned with the revision of Dutch health care.[98] They were academics, but they were also practitioners: both men actively wished to influence government policy. And in their role as policy advisers, both of them emphasized again and again that the most crucial change that had to be brought about in the Netherlands was the overthrow of the traditional, hierarchical doctor-patient relationship by the codification of patients' rights.

In May 1973, another government took office in the Netherlands: the Den Uyl cabinet, a coalition of five political parties that is often remembered as the most left-wing government the Netherlands has ever had. An important goal of this administration was to replace "vertical relations of dependence and subordination" in public institutions with "horizontal relations of consultation and participation."[99] The underlying ideology of this ideal was the notion of the *mondige burger* (assertive citizen) who sought to make his voice heard in Dutch society, but who lacked institutional outlets for doing so. By then, the term *mondige patient* had also become a commonplace in the Dutch media.[100]

Initially, the term "patients' rights" did not form a big part of this discourse. Solutions were sought *not* in the legal codification of individual rights but in the realization of alternative social structures: citizens had to be made *mondig* through a levelling of social classes and a public school system.[101] In May 1975, however, during a debate on the reform of Dutch health care, member of parliament Dick Dees—a representative of the Conservative-Liberal Party—complained that the government paid hardly any attention to the codification of patients' rights, even though "the call for a better description of the rights and duties of the patient, the call for better legal protection is getting louder."[102] In support of this statement, Dees pointed to the recent development of health law as a "new scientific discipline," the establishment of multiple patient associations in the early 1970s, and the growing body of "excellent publications," especially those of "Leiden professor of health law, Prof. Rang." Dees filed a motion, therefore, requesting that the government conduct a study on the "recalibration of patient law."[103] His request would find overwhelming support. On May 13, 1975, the "motion-Dees" was adopted unanimously by the Dutch House of Representatives. As a member of the Labor Party, then the biggest political party, put it: it was crucial for patients' rights to be codified "in the shortest time possible."[104]

"The shortest time possible" quickly proved to be an elastic concept in Dutch policy circles. Only in 1977 did the Central Council of Public Health receive a request to study the subject of patients' rights; it took the council another year and a half to install a Committee for the Rights of the Patient. Henk Leenen served as chairman; the vice-chairman was Wim van der Mijn, a legal scholar and then-secretary-jurist of the KNMG, who had been a vocal advocate of a rights approach to medical ethics since the early 1970s.[105] Together, they were responsible for gathering a versatile committee with "adequate representation from the side of the patient/client or, put differently, the *consumer* of health care."[106]

In their first plans, however, of a total of nine committee members, only two patient representatives were included, with one of these two representing the Dutch Consumer Association.[107] The other members were mostly legal scholars or health professionals. The Central Council's Committee of Delegates—which had to approve these plans—was the first to express dissatisfaction over this distribution. One delegate felt that a member of the Diabetes Association should be elected, another that someone from the National Council for Social Welfare should participate as well. Also, would it not be a good idea to invite someone from "the circles of women's associations"? And perhaps someone from "the group of homophiles" should be included too, given the delicate subject matter of the committee.

Van der Mijn, who was also a delegate, protested. The upcoming study concerned the rights of *patients*, he argued, not "the rights of citizens in general."[108] Still, he was willing to concede that patients were perhaps somewhat underrepresented in the current proposal and that a representative from the women's associations and the National Council of Social Welfare could be invited (the Association for Housewives eventually made the final cut). However, when this amended proposal was discussed by the Central Council itself, additional protests could be heard that still too-few seats were reserved for patient representatives. The council member representing the Society for Outpatient Mental Health Care even argued that the committee should consist solely of patient representatives, as "in the circles of patient/client-organizations a widespread belief exists that nothing will change if patients' rights are approached from the perspective of caregivers."[109]

Again, Van der Mijn—who was *also* a council member—protested. Such complaints really exaggerated the situation and "in no way [did] justice to the serious aim [...] to give sufficient voice to all those who clearly represent the interests of the patient." In addition, "the slightest need" existed "for a report in which the rights of the patient are proclaimed for the umpteenth time, as [...] no one benefits from rights when they cannot be realized in practice."[110] Most council members agreed and gave Leenen and Van der Mijn permission to proceed with the installation of the committee.

In the months thereafter, however, the Central Council kept on receiving letters of complaint about the composition of the committee. "According to our interpretation," the Association for Patients' Interests wrote, only "three persons in the committee may act or speak on behalf of the patient [...] in contrast to eight persons who clearly represent the caregivers."[111] Another letter was sent by the organized paramedical associations with the request that they, too, be allowed to "contribute either directly or indirectly to the work of the committee."[112] More letters followed from organizations representing retirement homes, "parents around residential schools," and volunteer organizations for individuals with psychiatric problems. The chairman of the Association for Equal Rights for All Ways of Healing sent in a letter asking if their input was not desired. After all, the association represented a wide range of healing practices and had the goal of furthering the interests of patients in the alternative healing circuit.[113] The trade association Nefarma, meanwhile, wrote in to state that it hoped the pharmaceutical industry would also be permitted to offer its insights on the subject.[114] In February 1979, when the Committee for the Rights of the Patient was newly underway, its members decided to invite two more patient representatives, one from a national foundation for health education, the other from the Dutch Disability Council.[115] By June of that year, the Committee of Delegates concluded that people with learning disabilities also needed additional representation.[116]

It was a trend indicative of the difficulties the Central Council experienced in honoring the ideal of the *mondige* patient. The reality was that all sorts of patients existed, many with their own needs and interests, so how did one decide who got to talk? And excluding a specific patient group from a committee on patients' rights was like denying a suffragist her right to vote. The entire idea of the committee, many argued, was that patients would finally be treated as mature individuals whose voice would be heard in health care—so they most certainly should have their say on a committee that would set an important standard for the ways in which the doctor-patient relationship would be regulated in the Netherlands in the years to come. Any proposed policy measures, the ideal was, should be reached through a process of *participative decision-making*, in which the inclusion of patient representatives would make sure that patients' perspective was heard and— just as importantly—that the scales of influence would not tip unfavorably in the direction of caregivers. After all, vertical relations of dependence and subordination had to make way for horizontal relations of consultation and participation on all governance levels in health care: from the doctor-patient relationship to the conference tables of the Central Council.

Between 1980 and 1982, the Committee for the Rights of the Patient produced five policy reports on the realization of patients' rights in the Netherlands. Four of these reports offered policy proposals for the regulation of the doctor-patient relationship and were largely written from a juridical perspective.[117] In effect, the committee almost religiously avoided the word "ethics." As Van der Mijn explained in 1980 during a meeting of the Committee of Delegates, in response to a question about whether a paragraph on the duties of a general practitioner should not at least mention *some* ethical aspects:

> Indeed, it used to be that a good physician was identified as he who acts in accordance with the latest scientific and ethical insights. But since pluralistic views with regards to ethics have developed which can exist next to one another, such a moral assessment has become much more difficult. These days, a reference to ethics is omitted.[118]

For the secretary-jurist of the KNMG, the idea that a unitary professional ethos regulated the conduct of Dutch physicians had become an antiquarian notion in the year 1980. Both patient and physician had to look to the legislature for the codification of their principal rights and duties. And in the realm of law, it was better to avoid the pitfall of ethics.

In line with this approach, the word "ethics" was not mentioned a single time in the first four policy reports. Only in the fifth committee report did the E-word pop up again: in a document proposing measures for the public oversight of human experimentation in medicine. It was an odd report for the Committee for the Rights of the Patient: the only report out of five that dealt with a specific medical (research) practice and that outlined clear norms for its permissibility. It was a document that, as will become clear, the Central Council had initially not wanted to write, but that would go on to become the cornerstone document in the late twentieth century for the realization of Dutch research ethics committees.

CHAPTER 4

EXPERIMENTING *with* HUMANS

"Societal developments," biologist and philosopher Matthijs Visser concluded in an October 1979 issue of *Medisch Contact*, "have made a consumer, also one of health care, more *mondig* and critical. [. . .] The modern patient wants to know what is done with him or her."[1] What else is new, the weary reader might have thought at the close of the 1970s. By then, the notion of the mature patient made an appearance in journals like *Medisch Contact* almost every other week, with authors—doctors, legal scholars, philosophers, and others with a claim to a specific type of expertise—stating again and again that the modern patient no longer just accepted the authority of caregivers. In 1979, Dutch experts stood in line to profess they knew the expert's place in health care. But Visser did have something new to say. Despite all the talk of patients' rights, he wrote, one key element was still wholly neglected: the rights of human research subjects. Hardly any form of public oversight existed for human experimentation, for instance, even though "trust in experts has been shaken quite a bit" recently. True, expert review bodies had been proposed in recent years to strengthen the "internal surveillance" of human research studies. Yet Visser did not think such review bodies were appropriate for the governance of a scientific practice in an open, egalitarian society. "Expert thinking," he argued, "stands in the way of a satisfactory ethics review of biomedical experiments on humans, as scientific interest usually prevails above ethical interest." Hence, to keep the medical research establishment in check, committees consisting mostly of laypersons had to be installed to decide on the moral permissibility of human experiments. As "only democratic decision-making is acceptable," Visser argued, these committees had to operate as jury trials, allowing ordinary citizens to participate in the oversight of medical science. In the eyes of the biologist-philosopher (and later self-proclaimed bioethicist), the realization of patients' rights would not be complete in the Netherlands until the practice of human experimentation had been brought under external control.

This chapter examines the policy report written by the Committee for the Rights of the Patient in the early 1980s on the governance of "medical tests upon human beings." In comparison to the unrest in the United States and Great Britain, unrest over human experimentation in medicine had played only a minor role in "the backlash against professional society" in the Netherlands in the 1960s and early 1970s. In the late 1970s, however, this unrest suddenly did emerge, and resulted in an urgent request from the Dutch government to the Central Council for Public Health to include human experimentation in its deliberations on patients' rights.

In response to this request, the Committee for the Rights of the Patient recommended in 1982 that the Dutch government demand that experiments with humans only take place in the country if special review committees first gave their permission. What was more, these bodies had to include at least two "society representatives" to ensure that "seclusion and mystery make way for openness and transparency" in a democratic society.

In the 1980s and 1990s, this report came to function as the cornerstone document for the Dutch governance of human experimentation. In virtually all subsequent policy deliberations on the subject, the report was referred to as *the* blueprint for the appropriate oversight of human experimentation. From its publication onward, the Central Council report was preferred by almost all Dutch politicians over the Health Council reports previously written on the subject. Still, most parts of the report were written by Erik Noach, the pharmacologist who had lobbied since the early 1970s for the installation of more *expert* review bodies in the Netherlands. In effect, even though the 1982 Central Council report recommended that research ethics committees function from then on as tools of external control, it also continued to lobby for the protection and promotion of human experimentation itself. Only this time, the project of therapeutic reform went hand in hand with a narrative of egalitarian decision-making in a democratic society.

A Discernible Absence of Dutch Concern

Historians who have investigated the emergence of the patients' rights movement in the United States and Great Britain have often maintained that a series of exposés of unethical human experimentation inaugurated the quickly spreading public distrust in the autonomy of the medical profession in this period. Rothman, for instance, claims in his 1991 book *Strangers at the Bedside* that "the story opens in the laboratory, not the examining room": i.e., that the revelation of a number of human research scandals in the mid-1960s first "revealed a stark conflict between clinical investigators and human subjects, between researchers' ambitions and patients' well-being," a perception that almost singlehandedly "undercut an older confidence in the exercise of medical discretion."[2]

The defining moment that would have caused this pendulum to swing was a publication by Harvard anesthesiologist Henry Beecher in the June 1966 issue of the renowned *New England Journal of Medicine*. In this article, titled "Ethics and Clinical Research," Beecher discussed twenty-two clinical research studies—all published in recent years in prominent medical journals—that he believed to be ethically questionable.[3] His list included studies in which known effective treatments had been withheld in favor of placebos; invasive physiological studies with little to no benefit for the participating subjects; studies in which patients had been deliberately infected with disease; and studies in which no informed consent had been obtained. This "roll of dishonor" included the now-infamous Willowbrook State School study that had been running since the late 1950s, in which clinical researchers infected disabled children with hepatitis to study the disease's infectivity period.[4] It also included a study conducted at the Jewish Chronic Disease Hospital in 1962, in which elderly patients had been injected with cancer cells without their knowledge.[5] The study Beecher himself found most shocking was a clinical trial in which penicillin had been deliberately withheld from 109 soldiers with streptococcal infections, thereby causing two soldiers to develop acute rheumatic fever and one acute nephritis.[6]

Beecher was not the first to raise the alarm about unethical clinical research in the United States, but, according to Rothman, the significance of his publication was twofold for the emerging patients' rights discourse in the mid-1960s. First, it argued that unethical research studies were no exception to modern medical science. Beecher pressed the point that his twenty-two anonymized cases had all recently been published in "excellent journals" and were just a selection from a much larger pool of questionable studies.[7] Second, it made clear that mainstream medical researchers did not shy away in the postwar era from using human beings as research subjects "who were in one sense or another devalued and marginal [...] retarded, institutionalized, senile, alcoholic, or poor, or [...] military recruits, cannon fodder in a war against disease."[8] They used marginalized people in this way despite knowledge of the atrocities that had taken place in World War II in the name of medical science. "The thought that some would have agreed that deliberate infection was all right since the subjects were mental defectives," Beecher said at one point in reference to the Willowbrook State School study, "gives me the Nazi shudders."[9]

The admission that medical researchers regularly conducted experiments on disenfranchised social groups ensured in 1966 that Beecher's article "quickly became linked to the rights movements that were gaining strength in the 1960s."[10] Studies like the ones that took place in Willowbrook and the Jewish Chronic Disease Hospital were seen as evidence that weaker members of society were easily abused by medical elites who violated their rights and used them as guinea pigs for the elites' own advancement.

In 1972, this perception was further corroborated by the uncovering of the Tuskegee syphilis study: a study by the US Public Health Service in which the progression of untreated syphilis in impoverished African American men from Tuskegee, Alabama, had been monitored since 1932, even though penicillin had been available as an effective cure since the 1940s and other cures had commonly been used before then. For a period of forty years, these men had been offered free "medical care," hot meals and—so as to allow researchers to conduct autopsies—free burials in return for their participation. Yet, they were never told they suffered from syphilis and that actual cures existed for their illness. As a result, many of the men died, forty of their wives contracted the disease, and nineteen of their children were born with congenital syphilis.[11]

According to Rothman, such exposés of unethical human experimentation fostered a great distrust of the discretionary authority of the American medical profession and brought a rights discourse to medicine; i.e., the notion of informed consent first gained prominence in the context of the subject-researcher relationship in the United States. In addition, these exposés contributed to new "mechanisms for collective decision-making" in medicine.[12] In 1966, the US Surgeon General drew support from Beecher's article for a memo he had sent out to American hospitals and universities a few months earlier, announcing that applications to the Public Health Service for financial support for clinical research studies from then on had to "provide prior review of the judgement of the principal investigator or program director by a committee of his institutional associates."[13] In 1974, after the Tuskegee study, this prerequisite was codified into law by the National Research Act.[14] This new mechanism of communal ethics review, Rothman argues, later spread to the governance of medical practice as well in the United States. Hence, human research scandals played a key role in the rise of the American patients' rights movement, including the call for more public procedures of medical decision-making.

A similar case has been made for the emergence of the patients' rights movement in Great Britain. In the late 1950s, British medical tutor Maurice Pappworth had started writing concerned letters to medical journals he found to publish reports of questionable human experiments without much hint of any ethical reservations. When editors refused to publish Pappworth's letters, the medical tutor decided in 1962 to write a piece for a popular British magazine, listing dubious experiments on patients with a call for a "battle to defend the rights of all patients against the whims and ambitions of some doctors."[15] In early 1963, Duncan Wilson writes, this call led to the establishment of the British Patients Association, a high-profile social movement that in the 1960s "regularly challenged medical paternalism in letters to newspapers and professional journals."[16] Pappworth, meanwhile, kept on collecting medical research articles mentioning dubious experiments on humans, and published over two hundred of them in 1967 in the book *Human Guinea Pigs*.[17] Again, the physician berated the medical profession for its unwillingness or inability to prevent such studies from taking place, and he called for the active involvement of "medical outsiders" to bring them to a halt. British parliament had to demand that every regional hospital board install a "consultation committee" seating at least one lay member to review clinical research protocols. "The medical profession," Pappworth wrote, "must no longer be allowed to ignore the problems or assert, as they often do, that this is a matter to be solved by doctors themselves."[18]

Pappworth's call to arms, Wilson emphasizes, did *not* actually lead to more outsider involvement in or formal regulation of medicine in Great Britain in the late 1960s. When the British Parliament debated Pappworth's claims in May 1967, the responsible statespersons rejected any form of government involvement with human experimentation. Similarly, a year later, when the Patients Association demanded a public inquiry into the matter, the Ministry of Health rejected this proposal by stating that ethical questions were "for the profession to consider."[19] As a result, the governance of clinical research in Great Britain mostly remained a form of "club regulation" for quite some years to come. Still, Pappworth's work marked one of the "earliest and strongest critiques of medicine" in Great Britain and, as such, contributed significantly via its concerns over human research practices to a larger "backlash against professional society" and the concomitant rise of the British patients' rights movement in the 1960s.[20]

In the Netherlands, the situation was different. Contrary to the United States and Great Britain, the Netherlands evinced little public unrest over human experimentation in the 1960s and early 1970s. In the 1950s, still, antivivisectionists had at times made headlines with claims that unethical experiments were being conducted in Dutch hospitals and clinics. In the 1960s, however, such claims of experimental misconduct grew smaller rather than larger. Sporadically, the Dutch media did report incidents, but at no time did these reports result in prolonged public unrest.

In 1966, for instance, newspapers reported that pharmaceutical company Philips-Duphar had tested anti-flu tablets on residents of an "insane clinic" in Eindhoven: 250 out of 750 patients (as well as a few staff members) had been given these tablets instead of their yearly anti-flu vaccination to compare the immunity levels conferred by each treatment.[21] This report caused a stir. In the liberal newspaper *Algemeen Dagblad*, Senator Arie Querido strongly condemned the tests: whether or not the pills turned out to be harmless, he argued, a principal line had been crossed by conducting experiments on "the mentally disturbed." "Even if it is just sugar water," Querido was quoted to say, "the other end is the gas chamber."[22] In parliament, the Senator requested the government to forbid all human experimentation in state-supervised facilities in the Netherlands. Yet, despite this uproar, the matter was easily settled by an admission from the government that such practices indeed should not take place, a reminder it promised to convey to the Superintendent for Mental Health and the KNMG.[23] Afterwards, Dutch newspapers did not keep the scandal alive for much longer.

Foreign research scandals also occasionally made Dutch news in this period. Pappworth's *Human Guinea Pigs*, for instance, received widespread news coverage in 1967.[24] Similarly, when the British physician claimed during a radio interview in 1971 that uninformed and terminally ill patients were commonly used as test animals "not only in America but also in England," he could once again count on a significant amount of Dutch media attention.[25] In 1972, the Tuskegee syphilis study made headlines as well, although the resultant outrage was nothing compared to the storm of indignation which the study provoked in the United States.[26] However, when news of these scandals broke in the Netherlands, they were discussed as *foreign* problems by Dutch media and did not translate — at least in writing — into any heightened awareness that unethical human experimentation in medicine might present a significant problem for the position of patients "at home" as well. Similarly, none of these foreign scandals resulted in parliamentary questions or debate.

Likewise, in the Dutch crisis of medical ethics of the 1960s, concerns over unethical human experimentation in medicine only played a minor role. In the late 1950s and early 1960s, still, prominent physicians had warned that the number of questionable clinical research studies recorded in international medical journals was increasing rapidly, a development that gave rise to grave concern.[27] Yet, in voicing their concerns, these commentators had pointed largely to the United States: American physicians no longer knew right from wrong, American patients were in danger, American medical ethics was failing. When in the late 1960s a similar sense of crisis emerged about Dutch medical ethics, different concerns took center stage: new technologies raised questions about life and death, and changing social bonds demanded a new approach to the doctor-patient relationship. In medical journals and mainstream media alike, interventions such as abortion, artificial insemination, and euthanasia dominated—not human experimentation.[28]

In the 1970s, the proponents of a patients' rights approach to medical ethics did occasionally start to focus their attention on human experimentation. In 1970, for instance, Jaap Rang wrote a lengthy treatise on human experimentation for the booklet *Recent medisch ethisch denken II* (Recent medical ethical thinking II) in which he mentioned Beecher and the Jewish Chronic Disease Hospital study and emphasized that a research subject's informed consent was also in the Netherlands a sine qua non for the legal permissibility of human research studies.[29] A few years later, in 1975, Henk Leenen wrote two articles for *Medisch Contact* in which he, too, brought up Beecher and the Jewish Chronic Disease Hospital study and emphasized the absolute precondition of a subject's informed consent.[30] In addition, Leenen recommended the installation of local review committees that reported to a national council in which "at least the professional organizations, hospitals, medical faculties, independent scientific practitioners, and legal scholars" would take up seats.[31] In the United States, Leenen wrote in defense of this suggestion, a similar system had already been put in place.

In the Dutch parliament, Leenen's articles inspired members of parliament to ask why there was still no oversight system for human experimentation in the Netherlands.[32] The responsible state secretary of public health replied soothingly. Existing disciplinary laws offered medical examination boards the option to take repressive action if needed, the state inspectorate could keep an eye on things, and pharmaceutical products that were used experimentally first had to be registered with the Medicines Evaluation Board. What was more, "the possibility of being held liable in civil courts for any possible damages in the treatment of patients (resulting from experimentation) will surely prevent irresponsible experiments."[33] Nonetheless, since the House of Representatives had recently adopted a motion asking the government to study patients' rights in the Netherlands, the state secretary promised to ask the Council that would execute this study to take the position of patients in experimental treatments into account, too.[34]

Indeed, when the government finally contacted the Central Council for Public Health in 1977 to study the rights of patients, the request for advice contained a sentence stating that "the position of the patient in medical research and in teaching situations (demonstrations) *may deserve* consideration," a statement which in itself makes clear that human experimentation was still not considered a matter of immediate concern in the late 1970s.[35] In any case, human experimentation did not make the list of urgent topics that the Committee for the Rights of the Patient absolutely had to discuss—a list drafted by Leenen and Van der Mijn in early 1978. Hence, not even the author of the two articles that had provoked the Dutch parliament to ask questions about the governance of human experimentation in 1975 considered the matter sufficiently urgent in early 1978 as to make it part of the deliberations of a committee on patients' rights. In the Netherlands, no one really seemed to worry about human experimentation.

The Effect of Two Atypical Research Scandals

This dynamic changed in the spring of 1978. On the morning of Thursday, April 20, 1978, Dutch newspapers had big news to report: Leiden University would appoint criminologist Wouter Buikhuisen—an employee of the Ministry of Justice—as professor of criminology and penology and had offered him ƒ250,000 "from public funds" to conduct scientific research into the "biological characteristics of the delinquent."[36] With this money, the papers reported, Buikhuisen was planning to hire a neurobiologist, a psychophysiologist, and an endocrinologist to study the role of the nervous system in criminal behavior. It was news that caused a great public outcry. "Views from the nineteenth century threaten to return," one newspaper headlined: "Buikhuisen wants to conduct brain research on prisoners."[37] Even though the criminologist made a public statement two days later that he had no wish to deny the social determinants of criminal behavior and that he had no plans whatsoever to start putting electrodes in people's brains, it was the comparison with nineteenth-century Italian criminologist Cesare Lombroso and his infamous theory of criminal atavism that stuck in the media.[38]

In the influential left-wing magazine *Vrij Nederland*, the well-known literary critic Hugo Brandt Corstius soon started up a weekly column dedicated to tackling Buikhuisen's ideas.[39] According to Corstius, Buikhuisen was not only a perverted scientist—a Nazi ideologist, in fact—but also an incredibly stupid one who neither understood basic philosophy of science nor seemed aware of the latest publications in his own field of study. In the Dutch law journal *Nederlands Juristenblad*, meanwhile, legal sociologist Kees Schuyt strongly questioned "the scientific merit of the proposed study," which he considered to pose a distinct *moral* problem, similar to the way in which the therapeutic reform movement maintained that only "good science" could ever be "ethical science."[40] In addition, Schuyt maintained that the manner in which Buikhuisen planned to obtain his data was also morally problematic: would he conduct tests on prisoners, for instance, and, if so, how would he make sure they were in a position to give their free consent? And what about their privacy?[41]

In the Dutch parliament, Buikhuisen's appointment became the subject of an emergency debate requested by the Dutch Communist Party.[42] On April 26, 1978, 131 members of the House of Representatives came together for an exceptional event in Dutch parliamentary history: that afternoon, both the minister of education and sciences and the minister of justice were summoned to parliament to defend the appointment of a single professor at a Dutch university.[43] Political concern varied by party, but most politicians voiced deep concern about Buikhuisen's plans to conduct biosocial research on criminal behavior. A member of the Christian-Democratic Party emphasized it was essential that humankind not become subordinate to science and technology.[44] Representatives of the smaller progressive parties wanted the government to promise that weak members of society would not be abused by scientific elites and underscored the similarities between Buikhuisen's plans and the prevailing scientific ideologies in Hitler's Third Reich.[45] A member of the Labor Party, meanwhile, claimed that since Buikhuisen was supported with public funds, the Dutch parliament could hold the government responsible for his actions. So, how did the ministers plan to supervise Buikhuisen's research and what policy measures were they taking to safeguard the voluntary consent of imprisoned research subjects?

Dick Dees, member of parliament for the conservative-liberal party VVD, was also allotted time to speak. Moving away from Buikhuisen, Dees wished to direct attention toward "questions of a more general nature": the autonomy of Dutch universities, the freedom of scientific research and, crucially, the regulation of human experimentation. With regard to the first two domains, the liberal politician argued, a government had to practice caution. With regard to the third domain, however, things were different. After all, it was very well conceivable that a researcher, "driven by a desire to solve his problems," might cross the limits of what was tolerable. Yet what was the government now actively doing to protect the rights of research subjects? There was the Health Council advice from 1955, Dees noted, and questions had been asked in parliament in 1975. But as far as Dees could see, neither initiative had led to any direct action from the Dutch government. Could the two ministers clarify, perhaps, what had come of the government's plan to make human experimentation part of a study into the rights of patients in the Netherlands?[46]

In his address, the minister of education and sciences emphasized that this type of broad parliamentary discussion on the relation between science and society was a laudable initiative. After all, the subject under investigation did not so much concern the appointment of a single professorship but pertained to "the tree of knowledge of good and evil" and the fruits society might reasonably pick from it.[47] It was important to recall from time to time that "a societal frame exists for academia" and that scientists could not just hide away in their ivory towers without accounting for their actions. Still, the minister agreed with Dees that a government should practice restraint in interfering with academic freedom. The not-so-distant past had shown, after all, what could happen if "a state believes it can misuse the practice of science for its own purposes."[48] He had no intention, therefore, of interfering with the appointment of Buikhuisen. His colleague for the Ministry of Justice could affirm, however, that the Dutch government was willing to promote a study into the realization of legal safeguards for human research subjects. He would therefore once more request the Central Council of Public Health to make human experimentation a priority of the Committee for the Rights of the Patient.[49] Meanwhile, the Ministry of Justice would issue an interim arrangement to protect prisoners from undue experimentation, an emergency regulation that went into effect in June 1980 and prevented Buikhuisen from doing his study.[50] Hence, due to a single criminologist, the Dutch government in 1978 suddenly got serious about the governance of human experimentation—not because the criminologist in question had actually conducted any questionable experiments, but because too many people felt he had questionable ideas.

In December 1978, political pressure mounted even more when a second research scandal came to light. On Wednesday, December 13, newspapers reported that the Inspectorate of Mental Welfare was investigating "circulating rumors that 640 mentally retarded patients have been exposed for years to irresponsible and medically unnecessary diagnostic procedures in the context of scientific research."[51] In the Huize Assisië nursing home in Noord-Brabant—a facility run by friars—the general practitioner on duty was accused of having carried out all sorts of dubious tests on patients, including craniometry (measurements of the skull) and pneumoencephalography (an invasive procedure in which the cerebrospinal fluid around the brain is drained by a lumbar puncture to provide a more-defined brain structure on an X-ray).[52] Soon, newspapers also reported that one abdominal surgery and two castrations had likewise taken place, all without clear medical indication and all by the same general practitioner, who lacked the professional qualifications for doing so and who did not have the appropriate equipment needed for these operations in Huize Assisië.[53]

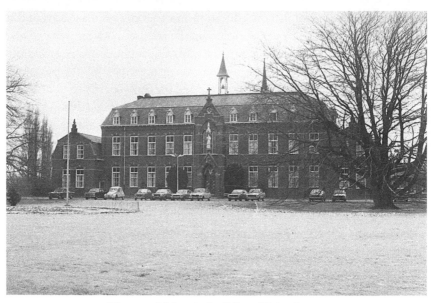

Figure 4. A historical still from Huize Assisië.
Photograph from the National Archive, The Hague.

In January 1979, the friar who had assisted the general practitioner in these "experiments" announced his resignation and went to live at a neighboring congregation.[54] Both the general practitioner and the medical director of Huize Assisië had to appear before a disciplinary court. In September 1980, they were fined ƒ10,000 each—at the time the highest financial punishment possible in the Netherlands.[55] The court could have taken away their licenses to practice medicine, but had decided against this course of action with the argument that no permanent damage had been done to the residents of Huize Assisië and because the defendants had already suffered great immaterial disadvantages from the widespread media attention that the case had generated. In addition, the court had taken into account that the general practitioner had worked as a missionary physician in Nigeria before he started his appointment at Huize Assisië and was therefore used to "operating independently."[56]

These events were not right away linked to the governance of human experimentation. In the media, the general practitioner was portrayed as an out-of-control cowboy who had operated in Assisië as he had grown accustomed to doing during his time "in the jungle."[57] Although his behavior was strongly condemned, he was framed as an exception who was in no way representative of Dutch medical practitioners more generally.

In early 1979, however, Huize Assisië became part of a two-piece article in *Medisch Contact* by the biologist-philosopher Matthijs Visser. What had occurred at Assisië, Visser affirmed, was not representative of Dutch medical science. Still, that did not mean there was no reason for concern. To prove his point, Visser had collected forty-five articles from the *Dutch Journal of Medicine* to show that, in the Netherlands as elsewhere, medical researchers were not careful enough in experimenting with patients. Articles did not always specify whether informed consent had been obtained or whether enough information had been provided to patients. Worse, some articles mentioned nontherapeutic studies that carried substantial risk, which raised the question of whether they should have been conducted at all.

To ameliorate this situation, Visser contended, the government had to take charge of the oversight of human experimentation in the Netherlands. Visser noted that some forms of "internal control" had been proposed in recent years, but these, he argued, were inadequate for the governance of such a sensitive scientific practice. After all, by virtue of their professional disposition, medical researchers were unable to reach unbiased ethical decisions: their interest in the progress of scientific research prevented them from "fully appreciating the rights of the research subject."[58] Hence, laypeople had to take on this role. People with no affiliation to medical research were "best able to impartially represent the public opinion on the admissibility of experiments."[59] "If we truly want to democratize health care, including biomedical research, and to protect the right to mental and bodily integrity of all patients and test subjects involved," Visser wrote in conclusion, "some things will have to be regulated by law."[60] Human experimentation had to be brought under *external control*.

In one of the next issues of *Medisch Contact*, the editor of the *Dutch Journal of Medicine* responded indignantly to Visser's piece. "It is interesting to note how more and more non-physicians concern themselves with the actions of physicians to check if they are ethical," the editor started off delicately. Really, he very much appreciated the enthusiasm, and all this under the banner of protecting the integrity of the patient. However, he continued angrily, as "Dr. Visser violates the integrity of at least 45 Dutch physicians, he is morally obligated to not just leave it at such gratuitous allegations, but to justify himself properly and understandably."[61] So perhaps the biologist could be so kind as to help the *Dutch Journal of Medicine* out and to identify these "sins against ethics" he had detected in its pages. For the "unsuspecting medical reader" simply could not find them, although—the editor concluded cynically—this was probably because "physicians are blind to their own mistakes."[62]

Other physicians and researchers also wrote in.[63] Most notable among respondents was Dirk van Bekkum, who was considered an authority on the subject of medical research involving human subjects. Trained as a physician and biochemist, Van Bekkum had been director of the Radiobiological Institute of the Netherlands Organization for Applied Scientific Research (TNO) since 1960. Under his leadership, the institute had made key international contributions to radiobiology, experimental leukemia research, bone marrow transplantation, and stem cell research. By the end of the 1970s, the radiobiologist had gained international renown as a leading medical scientist.[64]

In his reply, Van Bekkum remarked that as a result of "the emancipation from patient to client," people had increasingly started to argue that medical research had to be brought under public control. They were typically people, Van Bekkum noted, with "no personal experience in the field of medical research" who "carry on a theoretical discussion and try to realize regulation with the aid of foreign inspiration and information."[65] These people, however, tended to forget one crucial thing: contrary to the United States and Great Britain, the Netherlands conducted hardly any medical experiments with humans, as the field very much remained underdeveloped. The radiobiologist therefore called on all medical researchers to start speaking out and to help realize a workable system of oversight. If not, the danger existed that a field that was only just beginning to blossom would be unduly nipped in the bud due to overbearing concerns of medical outsiders. This curtailment, Van Bekkum warned, would ultimately be to the detriment of Dutch health care itself.

In parliament, Visser's article was received more enthusiastically. In May 1980, during a debate on the amendment of the Dutch constitution, the biologist's arguments were used to advocate "the inviolability" of the human body. "Visser shows," a parliament member stated, "that the introduction of new diagnostic and treatment methods has been neglected in the Netherlands, also compared to other countries."[66] It was a perspective that could count on overwhelming political support at the close of the 1970s. On June 25, the amendment was adopted unanimously by the House of Representatives.[67] And whatever the Committee for the Rights of the Patient was working on, it had to make human experimentation a priority now.

The New Function of Research Ethics Committees

The Central Council was not very enthusiastic about making human experimentation part of the Committee for the Rights of the Patient: a serious investigation, it argued, would have to include more than just the rights of patients in research, such as the need for such research or the means for its appropriate oversight.[68] After ongoing political pressure, however, the Central Council gave in, after which Leenen decided to establish a separate working group for this task. The topic was too specific and would take the committee itself too much time and work.[69]

Legal scholar and committee member N. de Jong was willing to chair this working group.[70] He was joined by four other committee members: an internist representing the KNMG, a medical inspector, a member of the National Hospital Council, and a representative of a patient organization who had recently published a book that dealt among other things with human experimentation.[71] In addition, a number of outsiders participated. In addition to two nurses, a pediatrician, and pharmacologist Erik Noach, two TNO employees took up seats: a biochemist who had chaired an American IRB in the 1970s, and Dick van Bekkum, head of its Radiobiological Institute and an authority on clinical research.

Hence, Leenen's decision to install a separate working group on the topic of human experimentation meant that, contrary to the Committee for the Rights of the Patient itself, only one patient representative took part in the working group's deliberations, which lasted from May 1979 to May 1981. In fact, with the exception of chairman De Jong, all working-group members were health care providers. Yet, if this disproportionate composition might have worried advocates of the patients' rights movement, the conclusions of the working group would likely have surprised them. In 1982, the Central Council recommended a regulatory regime for human experimentation that was stricter than any of the Health Council reports had ever been. From the first page onward, the Central Council put the rights and protection of human research subjects center stage.

First of all, the Central Council report made much more elaborate demands on the informed consent of research subjects than any of the older Health Council reports had ever done. No researcher was ever allowed to conduct medical experiments with human beings, including clinical trials, without having first acquired their informed consent. In addition, research subjects were always entitled to revoke their permission and to submit complaints if they felt that they had not been treated properly.[72] Also, experiments with humans could only take place if a research protocol lived up to "reasonable standards" regarding the objectives and execution of the proposed study; such standards included the duty of researchers to ensure an experiment had a positive risk/benefit ratio with only limited discomfort (both physical and mental) for its subjects, that the experiment honored subjects' privacy and personal integrity, and that in case a research subject was also a patient, the refusal to participate would not negatively affect his or her treatment plans.[73] Finally, individuals who found themselves in "a dependent position" could never participate in experiments, unless these experiments were geared directly toward the "special situation in which these persons find themselves," and then only if these could absolutely not be held without those individuals' participation.[74]

Secondly, the Central Council underscored emphatically that human experimentation had to be regulated by law. It referred multiple times to the articles of Rang, Leenen, and Visser and admitted that "although patient law is now establishing a place for itself in health care, the rights of sick and healthy research subjects in the biomedical and behavioral sciences are still hardly ever discussed."[75] What was more, due to the conflict of interest inherent in human experimentation, legal warrants were needed to protect the interests of research subjects. Finally, the Central Council made clear that medical researchers had to be held publicly accountable out of principle. Its report cited Visser's article in *Medisch Contact* multiple times, including statements like "biomedical research cannot escape the ever-increasing call for more societal influence on scientific research" and "the times have passed that a researcher could autonomously define his own field of research."[76] The report also wrote that "the progress of medical science cannot shield itself from social scrutiny, and seclusion and mystery have to make way for openness and transparency."[77] In a democratic society, the suggestion was, human experimentation out of principle required public control.

Thirdly, following these conclusions, the Central Council proposed to restrain the individual autonomy of researchers much more than any of the Health Council reports had ever done. The difference with the Health Council reports, according to the working group, was that the former had based their blueprints on a "yes, if" premise, while that of the Central Council was built on a "no, unless" principle. In less Delphic terms, the working group meant that the decision to start a human research study could not be left to individual researchers: such experiments could only ever take place after specially-appointed authorities had first given their permission. In addition, this authority had to be empowered to do follow-up checks to inspect whether researchers had actually stuck to the protocols they had submitted for review. If not, the authority should be authorized to halt studies midway.

This type of oversight, the working group maintained in its 1982 report, could best be realized by establishing "independent local or regional review committees" that would be tasked with assessing the permissibility of research protocols "with due regard for prevailing views and norms and this both scientifically and ethically."[78] These bodies had to be overseen by one national council that would register all approved research protocols, document developments in thinking about human experimentation, and direct the local and regional committees to review studies in a more or less uniform manner. In addition, it could check whether the local and regional committees operated as they were supposed to and, if needed, function as an appeal body for research studies that were declined by a local or regional committee.[79] Finally, this authority would publish a report about its activities each year that would explain developments on the terrain of medical-biological research "in a manner that is understandable for a larger audience, so that also in this way more openness and transparency are provided."[80]

Finally, in contrast to the 1955 and 1971 Health Council reports, the 1982 Central Council report recommended that such review committees consist not only of "experts on the terrain of medicine and medical-biological research," but should also include "a number of other experts, including an ethicist or pastor and a jurist, as well as a nurse and at least two laypeople who can function as society representatives."[81] The report did not elaborate why "an ethicist or pastor and a jurist" had to be included. During a working-group meeting, however, Noach had argued that including "someone with expertise in ethics" made sense because review committees had to evaluate the ethical permissibility of protocols. It did not matter whether this member was an ethicist, a theologian, a pastor, or "[person] who [busies] [themself] with norms of human behavior"; they just needed some sort of affinity with issues of morality.[82] The report did explain why the participation of a nurse was a good idea: she could be expected to offer a different viewpoint and, importantly, "her function ensures that she is often better informed of certain situations and has more direct contact with research subjects."[83] The inclusion of a nurse, in other words, was another important safeguard for the protection of research subjects.

Notably, the role of two "laypeople who can function as society representatives" was not defended in the policy report, nor had it been questioned in meetings.[84] However, the working group did discuss for some time how many laypeople should participate in the review of research protocols. In discussing Visser's and Van Bekkum's articles, Van Bekkum himself stated that he was quite optimistic about the installation of review committees consisting almost solely of laypeople. If expert committees had first evaluated the scientific quality of research proposals, it was fine if laypeople thereafter evaluated whether the protocols also respected the rights of research subjects. This committee makeup would ensure that laypeople would not be overpowered by experts and could really make their voices heard. Noach, however, argued that it was better not to segregate experts and laypeople. They would have to reach verdicts on the permissibility of research proposals *together*, not separately from one another. The majority of the working group agreed. As it was explained in the 1982 report: "The integration between the world of science and the non-scientific world is best achieved by mixed committees" in which "scientists and laypeople can both influence one another."[85] In theory, such integration offered another way to realize the ideal of mature citizens. Review committees would help establish "horizontal relations of consultation and participation" and function as tools of external control over medical experiments with human subjects. Or, as Visser later summarized this move (and critically questioned its merits) in *Medisch Contact*: with these additions, the working group hoped to move from a regime in which experiments were conducted "upon humans" to one where experiments would be conducted "with humans."[86]

The Old Function of Research Ethics Committees

To be sure, this new function of review committees did not displace one of their key older functions, as imagined by Noach et al. in 1971; i.e., the protection and promotion of human experimentation in medicine. In 1979, in fact, the deliberations of the working group had started off on a bit of a rough note. During the first few meetings, members had debated what types of interventions should be included in the category of medical experimentation. Like the Health Council committees before it, the working group soon concluded that it was not always so easy to distinguish between research and practice. When did an intervention constitute an experiment and when was it just a form of advanced care? Did observational studies count as experiments? Should interventions already routine in the United States but still experimental in the Netherlands be included? And what about the first time that a surgeon-in-training carried out an operation? After a little while, the working group decided to settle on a generic description: "Investigations consisting of the application of new or insufficiently tested resources and procedures in humans with the goal of determining whether new insights can be acquired or whether prevailing insights require revision."[87] Most members agreed this definition had to be understood as a guideline rather than a strict juridical category: it would be up to the committees to decide which activities warranted further investigation.

Van Bekkum, however, strongly disagreed with this description. Absent from the first three meetings, the radiobiologist sent in pressing notes to express his discontent. The fact that the definition included clinical trials especially frustrated him:

If one wants to classify this work as "experiments with human beings" one has to realize that therewith all introductions of new treatments and diagnostic methods, that is all innovation in health care, will come to fall under the term "experiments with human beings." [...] I do *not* think it is wise for a working group called "Medical Tests upon Human Beings" to address these activities, given the special interpretation that all outsiders and many physicians give to this label.[88]

By "special interpretation," Van Bekkum meant the recent public unrest over human experimentation. The label "tests upon human beings," the radiobiologist argued, had come to acquire a negative connotation in recent years. It now invoked images of the research scandals that had taken place in the United States or, worse, the Nazi concentration-camp experiments.[89] Clinical trials had to be kept away from any association with these atrocious events; otherwise, the already-fragile field would be shut down. In fact, Van Bekkum wrote, if the working group decided to proceed this way, he would be forced to break his ties with it.[90]

This remark provoked considerable dismay among the other working-group members. Noach insisted, however, that it was important to keep Van Bekkum on board, as he belonged to a relatively small group of Dutch experts who had any practical experience with the subject under investigation. During a subsequent meeting, the radiobiologist was present to explain his frustration: as things stood, he claimed, about 50 percent of all therapeutic and diagnostic interventions had never been tested on their efficacy. They only persisted out of tradition.[91] Hence, he concluded, the systematic conduct of clinical trials was direly needed to allow researchers to evaluate the merits of all these interventions (Van Bekkum very much was a therapeutic reformer). Plus, patients in clinical trials did not even need additional legal protection—they typically received "a top treatment by a top team, often with resources that are available nowhere else."[92] If anything, Van Bekkum scoffed, patients treated by physicians who just meddled about with therapies needed extra protection.

Some members objected that Van Bekkum seemed to forget that he was a "frontier scientist," a leading researcher who was at the center of new developments in medical science and who worked in state-of-the-art facilities with well-trained team members. His experiences were likely to be more positive than those of researchers in "hospitals and clinics, where all kinds of things happen under the guise of science." The participating medical inspector, in particular, argued that he at times encountered situations that made him think that "those [working] in clinics, especially, often have absolutely no realization of what it is they are doing exactly."[93] The elite scientist Van Bekkum, in other words, might be trusted to conduct clinical trials, but the same could not be said of the average physician. The regulation of clinical trials was needed to keep those "in the periphery" in check.

Noach agreed with Van Bekkum that the phrase "tests upon human beings" had become a bit of a taboo in recent years. In Leiden, he stated, they therefore preferred to speak of "patient-related research" rather than of clinical experiments.[94] He also agreed that patients who participated in clinical trials were usually surrounded with better safeguards than those who did not. Yet, he continued, turning to Van Bekkum, this difference arose partly because most clinical researchers acknowledged that such patients needed additional protection. Hence, the working group's goal should not be to keep clinical trials away from public regulation, but to ensure that *all* medical experiments with humans took place under similar conditions—and thereby to eradicate their negative public image.

According to the participating patient representative, the negative public image of medical experimentation was in large part due to "the high degree of seclusion and mystery in which these sorts of activities currently take place." Most laypeople did not know what to make of stories they heard, because the practice was often wrapped in a "dense fog." Hence, if the general public were to be made "more research-minded"—which the patient representative apparently also considered desirable—"more openness and insight has to be provided."[95] Noach agreed. Their group had to make clear that human research was "no unseemly activity" and "be as open as possible, to make the Dutch public more familiar with the phenomenon." If the saying "unknown, unloved" held true, people had to be introduced as soon as possible to *good* human experimentation.[96] This was an important duty *and* opportunity the working group had in writing a policy report on the public governance of this type of scientific research.

The entire working group, including Van Bekkum, agreed with this proposal. Its policy report would state the rights of research subjects in human experimentation, but would also emphasize that the practice itself, when conducted within bounds, was needed to realize the much-desired progress of Dutch health care and, importantly, was nothing to worry about. Thus, while the 1982 Central Council report frankly acknowledged that human experimentation had acquired a bad reputation due to American research scandals and the concentration-camp experiments, it stated simultaneously that *good* human experimentation should be understood as categorically different from such past wrongdoings. In fact, the report read, since "the words 'medical tests upon human beings' still invoke associations with abuses from the past" and "the working group has wanted to stay away from such negative images, it has preferred to speak in its reflections of experiments with human beings." This new label fitted the contents of the report better anyway, as the preposition *upon* unjustly suggested an "underlying position" of the research subject.[97] A healthy researcher-subject relation was not a vertical relation of dependence of subordination, but a horizontal relation of consultation and participation. Experiments took place *with* human beings.

The participation of "society representatives" served a similar function. In its 1982 report, the working group frankly stated that it hoped the inclusion of laypeople would help to erode the negative public image of human experimentation. More openness would show the general public that "experiments are useful and necessary and take place in compliance with rules and procedures."[98] To ensure this result, however, it was important for the participating laypeople to agree that human experimentation was in fact "necessary and permitted." They could not, like the old antivivisectionists had done, reject the practice altogether. Furthermore, they needed to be able to conduct themselves "in a reasonable manner." Not *every* layperson was qualified; a layperson had to have "a bit of quality and a certain interest" to be eligible for a committee seat. To ensure that the right society representatives were elected, therefore, Noach proposed that in practice laypeople would be chosen via a "co-optation procedure," whereby each of the sitting members, i.e., the *experts*, would be permitted to decide which laypeople were suitable to take part.[99]

Other elements of the 1982 Central Council report mimicked the older Health Council reports, too. The working group emphasized, for instance, that review committees had to seat enough experts to judge the scientific quality of proposals. For studies to be permitted, they had to adhere to "generally accepted scientific principles [...] including both the theoretical and methodological aspects as well as the organization of the study."[100] Hence, like the Health Council reports before it, the Central Council report also envisioned review committees to function like *epistemic filters*: they had to sift out methodologically good research studies from bad research studies. In meetings, Van Bekkum literally referred to review committees as "filters" with the appropriate "know-how" to judge research designs.[101] Now, however, the Central Council no longer invoked the maxim "only good science is ethical science," pivoting instead to the notion that "only good science is reasonable science." Sound science, as defined by a specific class of medical researchers, had become a patient right.

Likewise, the working group recommended an oversight system built around multiple local review committees; such a system, they contended, would benefit the intensification of clinical research more than a system built around a single national council, as the Health Council had suggested in 1981. Both Noach and Van Bekkum emphasized that the swift realization of medical progress demanded that ethics review never take more than a few weeks, meaning that enough committees had to be installed to guarantee that all review requests could be handled quickly. In addition, both men were convinced that local committees would hold a more workable middle ground between the public and professional regulation of human experimentation. According to Van Bekkum, the review criteria proposed by the Central Council could never be taken as *conditiones sine quibus non*, but as benchmarks to decide if a study was reasonable. Were the qualifications of researchers in order? Check. Did the host organization have the proper research facilities? Check. Did the review committee feel enough laboratory experiments had already been conducted? Check. These questions could only be answered by committees familiar with the actual research setting; no national authority could stipulate absolute criteria for them.[102] In research, Noach explained, "there are always imponderable elements at play" that could not be written down on paper. Hence, as only local authorities could truly know their "pappenheimers" (darlings), only they could emphatically decide whether the research(ers) being reviewed meant to do well—and thus reach informed and, crucially, *flexible* decisions.[103]

Hence, all in all, despite the fact that the 1982 Central Council report drew explicitly on articles such as those by Visser, its blueprint for the oversight of human experimentation differed crucially. Where Visser favored the participation of laypeople to institutionalize a healthy form of public distrust in medical researchers, the working group hoped their participation would restore public trust in the research establishment. Similarly, where Visser felt reviewers should operate as distant judges to reach impartial decisions, the working group stated that a close proximity to, and intimate familiarity with, research studies was needed to enable reviewers to reach objective decisions. And where advocates of the patients' rights movement typically emphasized the importance of univocal legal rules for human experimentation, the working group preferred to speak of flexible guidelines and the need to decide on a case-by-case basis if studies were permissible. Although the working group agreed, in short, that human experimentation in medicine demanded external control, it hoped much more than critical thinkers such as Visser that this control would safeguard the practice itself as well. According to the therapeutic reformers Noach and Van Bekkum, a moral need still very much existed in the Netherlands for *proper* human experimentation.

The Continued Relevance of the E-Word

After the working group finished its deliberations in May 1981, its report first had to be discussed by, consecutively, the Committee for the Rights of the Patient, the Committee of Delegates, and the Central Council itself (a matryoshka effect of the famous Dutch polder model) before it could be released for publication. Although the report was accepted fairly easily by the Committee for the Rights of the Patient, it ran into difficulties in the Committee of Delegates and the Central Council. In the Committee of Delegates, the Central Council president—presiding as well over the delegates— noted that even though the report presented an important and solid piece of work, hesitation had befallen him with regard to "the aspects of the subject which have to do with ethics." While the word had not been mentioned a single time in one of the other four reports put out by the Committee for the Rights of the Patient, it was used several times in that of the working group, which spoke of the "ethical and juridical aspects" of human experimentation and the need to ensure that such experimentation violated "neither ethical standards nor human rights."[104] The report nowhere specified what it meant precisely by "ethical standards," but in an appendix prepared by Noach, the pharmacologist justified this heuristic use of the E-word:

> Views of medical-ethical issues have gone through a rapid revolution in recent decades, which does not yet appear to be complete. For this reason, the stipulation of all too strict and detailed norms is premature and undesirable.[105]

Instead, the appendix continued, "a certain standard of norms needs to be developed through experience within each review committee over the course of its existence." Reviewers, Van Bekkum had argued in a working-group meeting, continuously had to "align themselves with prevailing views in a particular country [. . .] which are not static and will change from time to time." Tacit and fluid, such views could not be laid down in sterile legislation—they depended on the context of individual research studies and fell in the category of ethics.[106]

However, this casual use of the word "ethics" made the Council president nervous. As the report dealt with an "extremely sensitive matter," the president felt it out of order to freely invoke ethics when "the ethical discipline as such" had not been represented in the working group. Before the report was ready to be published, therefore, he first wanted to contact a number of ethicists and ask them what they thought of the document's "ethical merits."

Delegate Wim van der Mijn, the legal scholar representing the KNMG who was also vice-chairman of the Committee for the Rights of the Patient, objected. The report was in line with "prevailing views on medical ethics" and *his* constituency, the medical profession, had no problem with the language in the report. Besides, the working group had been asked to explore the juridical difficulties of experimenting with human subjects—not its ethical aspects—and it had done so. Every Council report had ethical aspects, so why make a problem out of this one? In Van der Mijn's opinion, the Council president was really attributing "a weight to ethicists above their significance." Another delegate wondered if the Council president did not, rather, want advice on how the report might be *read*. Hence, should he not be reaching out to public relations officers instead of ethicists? The Council president was adamant, however, that *ethicists* had to take another look at the report. The Committee of Delegates decided, therefore, to send the document to five authors who had published on medical ethics in recent years to check whether they could condone its contents.[107]

The responses of these authors varied, but they concurred that the report did not contain any statements that flagrantly violated ethical norms or values. This consensus satisfied the Council president, and thus the report could now be discussed in the Central Council. There, however, additional objections mounted. One member, a representative of a patient organization, claimed to have shivered when reading the report, as it emphasized so strongly the necessity of experimenting on humans while speaking only in veiled ethical terms about the researcher-subject relationship. In his opinion as a "medical outsider," the report came across as suspiciously "medical": its recommendations had been written from a technical perspective, whereas it should have been written from the perspective of patients' rights.[108] What was more, he was unimpressed with the composition of the review committees that the report proposed. Physicians dominated, while only a few seats had been reserved for those who would see it as their primary aim to secure the interests of patients. (This criticism was later echoed by Visser in *Medisch Contact*: the two society representatives only gave the biomedical research establishment "an alibi.")[109]

Both Leenen and Noach, who were present for comments at the Central Council meeting, assured the council that the experience they already had in reviewing research protocols taught them that there was no need to worry about these things. In practice, reviewers always worked things out in an open and congenial manner, whereby ample attention was paid to the rights of research subjects.[110] Leenen admitted that also he found the use of the term ethics in the report somewhat vague, but this vagueness, the jurist argued, was unavoidable. Ethical norms changed from time to time, so it did not make sense to try and nail them down in a policy report. He could guarantee, however, that the norms used in the report rested on a "widespread and international consensus."[111] Still, if the council insisted, Leenen was willing to tone down those parts of the report that sounded overly enthusiastic about human experimentation.[112]

With that admission and a few changes, the Central Council report was authorized for publication in March 1982. In the 1980s and 1990s, it became the single most authoritative blueprint for the governance of human experimentation in Dutch politics. Nonetheless, it would take another fifteen years for the Dutch government to present a legislative proposal based on the 1982 Central Council report. In effect, when the Dutch parliament in 1997 debated this legislative proposal for the first time, it was discussing a system of ethics review that had already congealed around the ideas of the people who had started to push in the 1980s for more *expert control* over human experimentation. In fact, when members of parliament once again brought up the need for more *democratic control*, the Dutch government increasingly found solace in turning to a new type of expert to resolve the tension between these two modes of governance: i.e., the ethicist. For although Van der Mijn had argued in the early 1980s that it was foolish to attribute a weight to ethicists above their significance, this new expert on the block came to fulfill a key function in the public governance of human research studies in the Netherlands in the late twentieth century.

PART III

PUBLIC ACCOUNTABILITY

CHAPTER 5

The CONTESTED RISE of the ETHICAL EXPERT

In 1988, ethicists Heleen Dupuis and Inez de Beaufort published the first Dutch textbook on "health ethics," the Dutch version of bioethics. Forty authors had contributed to the textbook, of whom seventeen identified as ethicists (most had originally studied theology), six were legal scholars, nine were physicians, and eight had other disciplinary identities.[1] This interdisciplinary approach was chosen because it corresponded to the "daily reality of health care." Nonetheless, the editors wished to make it clear that professional ethicists took the lead in moral thinking. As Dupuis and De Beaufort wrote in the introduction:

> Well, people could now say, is everyone thus actually an ethicist? Of course almost all human beings are morally thinking and acting beings. And ethics should not be an esoteric chunk of knowledge that is only available to a handful of "experts" who have mastered a secret language. Yet, to call everyone with a moral "private practice" an "ethicist" would be the same as to call everyone who manages a household wallet an "economist" and everyone who regularly flicks through a medical family encyclopedia a "medical practitioner."[2]

Ethics was a profession. Its practitioners possessed a specific skillset with which they were able to tackle the growth of moral problems in modern medicine. "The starting point of this book," the preface stated, is that "ethics *can* help, and can certainly indicate in concrete terms what direction has to be taken to address and solve a problem."[3] By 1988, in short, two of the most prominent Dutch health ethicists had grown confident enough of their field to assert that it was indispensable for a morally healthy health care system. Not consulting ethicists increasingly had to be considered unprofessional.

In the final two chapters of this book, I chart the demise of the participatory democratic ideal that had dominated Dutch discussions over research ethics governance in the 1970s. Against the backdrop of a rising neoliberal climate and the ongoing internationalization of medical science, new forms of reasoning about ethics review became popular in the 1980s and 1990s, reasoning that no longer emphasized the direct participation of laypeople, but rather the need for a proper legal framework and for uniform and transparent decision-making. Once again, a new relationship had to be forged between medicine, society, and the state—and the role therein of scientific experimentation.

In chapter 6, I show how professional ethicists in the 1990s came to fulfill a specific function for Dutch politicians responsible for hammering out this relationship. To set the scene, this chapter first traces the rise of health ethics in the Netherlands. Like its Anglo-American brother bioethics, health ethics is often argued to have emerged after the 1960s to hold the once-autonomous class of physicians, the *artsenstand*, publicly accountable. In a democratic society, after all, all reasonable people should have access to the norms governing medicine, not just a select group of anointed professionals. Within this framework, research ethics committees are often understood as one of the earliest successes of the health ethics movement. The two would have arisen as two peas in a pod: as twin responses to the growing societal critiques of medicine in the 1960s and 1970s.

Earlier chapters have shown, however, that ethicists in practice had little to do with the first ideas for ethics review in the Netherlands; nor did they, as scholars such as Stark and Hedgecoe have shown, in countries such as the United States and Great Britain. In this chapter, I show that the relationship is better understood the other way around: originally designed as a tool of internal control, research ethics committees became a battleground for health ethicists in the 1980s and 1990s to flesh out *their* fledgling professional identity and appropriate a public role. Underlying this debate was a question that had been fundamental in earlier decades as well, but now once more found itself a new answer: what forms of ethical reasoning about medicine and science are appropriate for public deliberation in a democratic society?

A Brand-New Authority on Medical Ethics

In 1982, the British philosopher Stephen Toulmin published the now-famous article "How Medicine Saved the Life of Ethics." In it, Toulmin asserts that in the first half of the twentieth century, ethical discussions in the United States and other English-speaking countries could be characterized by two elements. One, a neglect of substantive ethical questions among moral philosophers, who instead busied themselves with abstract metaethical questions. Two, a stalemate "in less academic circles" between dogmatists, who held on to codes of universal rules or the authority of religious teachers, and relativists, who emphasized endless anthropological and psychological differences in moral viewpoints. In effect, "ethics" had become a field that had lost all touch with concrete, practical issues.[4]

This state of affairs changed in the 1960s, when philosophers turned their attention to medicine. The fact that certain medical afflictions affect humans regardless of culture turned the attention away from moral relativism to a more "universal approach" to ethics, while the casuistic approach to medicine provided a template for moral reasoning: rather than focusing on the formulation of general rules or principles, it reintroduced into ethics the importance of practical reasoning about particular cases. Even more, their attention to medicine reminded philosophers of the fact that professional roles and relations bring along problems that cannot be generalized, but require specific moral attention and analysis.

In his article, Toulmin nowhere describes why philosophers started to pay attention to medicine in the 1960s. Often, the answer to this question has been the rise of new moral challenges due to new medical technologies, coupled with the uncovering of research ethics scandals in a time when an anti-authoritarian generation was coming to question the longstanding moral authority of physicians. "I suddenly saw that explicitly in the text of the [Hippocratic] Oath would-be physicians pledged they would not reveal the precepts of the profession to anyone outside the group," ethicist Robert Veatch writes in his recollection of the birth of American bioethics. "Nothing could be in greater conflict with the ways of knowing morality in the secular world where reason, empirical observation, or metaphorical social contract involving all reasonable people provided a basis for knowing the moral norms."[5]

In the last few decades, scholars from various fields have challenged this narrative. As historians Robert Baker, Dorothy Porter, and Roy Porter pointed out back in 1993: "It is nothing new for physicians to be confronted with novel and agonizing problems of unexplored biotechnical possibilities and uncertain public response."[6] Hence, the rise of new medical technologies in and of itself cannot explain the emergence of bioethics. Others have similarly challenged the link with the counterculture of the 1960s. Rather than questioning the authority of physicians, bioethics would have consolidated existing power mechanisms in medicine by helping to diffuse "the changes demanded by more radical, and more popular, social critics of the sixties."[7]

In reaction to these critics, Duncan Wilson proposes that we should look not only at changes in medicine itself in the 1960s, but also at changes in professions that later came to constitute the bioethics movement: i.e., law, philosophy, and theology. Following sociologist Andrew Abbott, Wilson proposes a "systemic view of professions," in which professional authority is understood in relational terms: i.e., if physicians could claim full jurisdiction over medical ethics until the 1960s, they did so in part because others did not, thereby effectively consolidating the moral authority of doctors and medical scientists.[8] So why was it that these other professions let go of their "hands-off" approach to medical ethics in the 1960s and 1970s? And how did they start making jurisdictional claims *as* ethicists?

Also in the Netherlands, the emergence of health ethics has often been explained as a "breaking of the bulwark" of the *artsenstand* by a group of outsiders who had become convinced in the 1960s and 1970s that the old monopoly of the medical profession on medical ethics had to be broken.[9] Medical ethics, Heleen Dupuis wrote in the 1988 *Handboek gezondheidsethiek* (Textbook of health ethics), used to be "ethics *of* and *for* the profession." But thanks to the rise of the *mondige* patient and a "storming of the gates of 'the Bulwark of the know-it-alls'" by ethicists and legal scholars, "medical ethics has [now] become everyone's business."[10]

This origin story, I argue in the following pages, is partly true. Health ethics did emerge in the Netherlands as an alternative to a medical ethics tradition that had almost solely addressed the role and responsibilities of physicians. Likewise, theologians, legal scholars, and philosophers did play a considerable part in the formation of this new paradigm, although the contribution of caregivers and policy officials should not be underestimated. However, to understand the rise of health ethics as solely an emancipatory movement of the 1960s and 1970s ignores that this development was closely related to the rise of ethics *itself* as a standalone academic discipline in this period, one that did not necessarily aim to democratize older ethics traditions (medical or otherwise), but to find a new way to speak with expert authority on ethical issues during a time in which traditional moral authority was waning.

The Fledgling Dutch Ethics Movement

In the 1980s, health ethics became the collective term in the Netherlands for a new academic field with its own professorial chairs, journals, and research institutes. Not everyone agreed the term did justice to this development— some preferred to call it biomedical ethics or bioethics; others persisted in arguing that the field should continue to use the older term medical ethics.[11]

Yet by the end of the century most agreed that health ethics had gained general currency in the Netherlands to refer to a field of study that closely resembled the international bioethics movement.[12]

According to many of its practitioners, health ethics had to be understood as a subfield of philosophy. As Inez de Beaufort wrote in 1985: "What is biomedical or health ethics? Put shortly: it is the application of 'normal' ethics, the philosophical reflection on norms and values, on moral problems in and around health ethics." From this definition it followed that physicians could not lay jurisdictional claims on health ethics on the basis of their profession. Their practical experience in seeing patients was valuable, but did not make them "mini-philosophers."[13] Professional ethicists were needed for proper reflection on the moral boundaries of health care.

However, this confident assertion belies an important historical element: until roughly the 1960s, ethics—as an academic field of study—had hardly been practiced by philosophers in the Netherlands. Instead, it had been the terrain of theologians, who, if they taught classes in ethics at all, usually had done so in terms of moral theology.[14] What sort of ethics were taught depended on the theologian. Orthodox theology professors were only permitted to teach the *zeden* (mores) according to scripture, while a modern theologist like Izaäk Jan de Bussy, professor of ethics and philosophy of religion at the Municipal University of Amsterdam from 1892 to 1916, taught students that moral beliefs had to be studied as the product of their historical and social context (de Bussy was a follower of sociologists like Durkheim, Lévy-Bruhl, and Simmel).[15] At Catholic seminaries, in turn, priests-to-be were trained to argue concrete cases with "reasonable moral arguments" and to study the proper relationship between church codes and national law—knowledge and skills they needed to take confessions from future parishioners.[16]

Occasionally, ethics was taught by professors of other disciplines as well. From 1815 to 1876, for instance, students who hoped to enter any theology department had to obtain a signed testimonial from the faculty of letters and philosophy certifying that they had formally studied "wijsgerige zedekunde" (moral philosophy). (Moral philosophy classes were usually taught by professors in speculative philosophy.) However, after the government revoked this requirement in 1876, the number of students studying moral philosophy underwent a sharp decline. From 1890 to 1928, the experimental psychologist Gerardus Heymans did teach ethics classes to explain why "moral people" were more likely to get married than "immoral people" (an "observation" that would explain the moral growth of the human species as a whole).[17] But

Heymans was an exception. By and large, until the 1960s, ethics professors were only appointed to Dutch theology faculties, while the term ethicist was mostly reserved for church authorities—not academics.

This state of affairs changed radically in the second half of the twentieth century. First, between 1967 and 1973, three philosophy faculties created chairs in "philosophical ethics," while in Utrecht, the theology faculty's professorial chair in "ethics and the encyclopedia of theology" was changed to one in "ethics, including philosophical ethics and the encyclopedia of theology"—and was now part of both the theology *and* philosophy faculties.[18] In the decades thereafter, all other Dutch universities created ethics chairs on their own philosophy faculties as well, with most schools establishing additional chairs in applied ethics on other faculties. Plus, those ethics professors who continued to be appointed to theology faculties increasingly started to argue that ethics had to be studied autonomously from theology and debated "with ethical not theological arguments."[19]

In the 1970s and 1980s, this amalgam of scholars began to communicate with each other in newly founded ethics societies and journals, and they increasingly identified as ethicists. While the field was now considered more closely related to philosophy than theology, most practitioners argued that the field had to be understood as an interdisciplinary one that was defined by its object of study (ethics) and that possessed a specific body of literature and skill set. Thus, in the 1990s, when academics were pressured by the Dutch government to organize themselves in national research schools, ethicists started a Research School of Ethics that stood separately from the Research School of Philosophy and the School for Theology and Religion.[20] Ethics, the message was, had become an academic field in its own right.

To explain the quick rise of their discipline in the 1970s and 1980s, Dutch ethicists often invoke Toulmin. According to Henri Krop and Koo van der Wal, older theoretical approaches in philosophy increasingly looked irrelevant and disdainful in the face of new moral problems: if philosophers wanted to make a real difference, they had to be willing to take on "practical problems."[21] Likewise, ethicist Bert Musschenga argues that developments in medical technology made Dutch theologians willing to take a more secular approach to their analysis of ethical problems: instead of locating moral truths in the Bible, they started to evaluate ethical cases by taking their specific context and participants into account.[22]

In the publications of Dutch philosophers and theologians of the late 1960s and early 1970s, their preoccupation with the dark sides of science and technology indeed stands out.[23] Yet, in most of these texts, especially those written by theologians, an important second reason for the need for new forms of ethical reflection can be detected as well. In Herman Heering's 1969 book *Ethiek der voorlopigheid* (Provisional ethics), for instance, which would become a standard text in the fledgling Dutch ethics movement, the Remonstrant theologian wrote, right after emphasizing the need to investigate whether "everything that is technologically possible should also occur," "the government by God's grace has been replaced with a democratic order in which everyone is supposed to bear co-responsibility. The entire sacred confirmation of morality is broken, orders and judgements are disputed and reviewed."[24] Likewise, in his 1969 book *Voorlopige diagnose* (Provisional diagnosis) on the need for new medical ethics, Catholic theologian Paul Sporken asserted: "Ever increasing is the group of believers who wish to have a say in ethical statements and who no longer accept these are imposed from above, isolated from communal opinions."[25] In other words, new forms of ethical reflection had also become urgent around 1970 because traditional moral truths were increasingly questioned in a secularizing society.

Sporken, in particular, was convinced that this growing plurality of voices in Dutch society demanded a more secular approach to (medical) ethics. The church had to learn to accept, the Catholic scholar wrote, that:

> Understanding the ethical demands of humanity is not a monopoly of the Christian community of faith. [...] A Christian ethics only deserves the name insofar as it is willing and open to listen to the revelation and salvation of God wherever it can be heard, where true humanity can be found.[26]

In fact, even though Sporken considered Christian ethics open to all people, he thought it best not to use the adjective "Christian" anymore, as it might put off a more secular readership. "It is explicitly not my intention," Sporken hastened to write in his *Voorlopige diagnose*, "to sell this introduction to medical ethics as theological ethics or moral theology."[27] An ethicist was at work here, not a theologian. Heering, who did use the term theological ethics, also increasingly favored a more secular approach to ethical reflection: moral truths were not to be located in Biblical commandments, he felt, but in human beings themselves.[28]

Importantly, however, this secular turn did not mean the two theologians—or ethicists—felt that everyone stood on an equal footing in ethical deliberations. Ethicists did have a certain type of *expertise*. They could function, for instance, Sporken explained in a 1970 talk for the KNMG, "as a luminary [voordenker] when it comes to thinking together." Ethicists' intention was not to claim jurisdiction over medical ethics, he added reassuringly, but they could light the way in getting a grip on the difficult ethical problems caused by techno-scientific advancement: "From his profession, the ethicist may offer a helping hand to physicians."[29]

To solidify the position of the ethicist, Heering in 1970 sent an invitation to all ethics teachers at Dutch universities. In 1964, the theologian had been closely involved in the establishment of the Societas Ethica, an international and interdenominational ethics society, and now wished to install a Dutch ethics society as well. "Because more and more is asked of ethics," Heering wrote in his invitation, "this contact and deliberation are increasingly wanted and needed."[30] All ethics teachers were therefore invited to talk about "the place of ethics" in academia, about the appropriate "division of labor" between ethicists, and about the "joint study and discussion of foundational as well as practical ethics." In addition, Heering hoped to discuss how ethicists could ensure that they were consulted by the government when "legal articles with clear moral aspects" were drafted.[31] At the meeting itself, Heering emphasized the need for ethicists — *not* theologians — to meet up regularly: "Developments in academia and society force us to. Ethics can no longer be practiced in isolation. Scholarly ethics is now confronted more than ever with concrete issues."[32] Those present agreed. On March 7, 1970, the Dutch Society of Ethicists was founded, with theologian, and now also — or even primarily — ethicist Heering as its first chairman.

A Guiding Light and Helping Hand

Theologians like Heering busied themselves with a strong rhetoric of public demand: swift societal changes *necessitated* the organization of ethicists, *called for* their involvement with public policy, and *demanded* that they secure a better academic position. Heering and his colleagues did not invoke many actual public cries to substantiate this apparent need for ethicists, but they seemed sure nonetheless that they had a key role to fulfill in binding society in a time when traditional authority was waning and moral problems were growing.

This conception of ethicists' professional identity found support among other professions in the early 1970s. In Dutch medical circles in particular, theologians like Heering and Sporken became welcome guests to help tackle the crisis of medical ethics that had developed in the 1960s. They were invited to publish in journals such as *Medisch Contact*, asked to speak at the General Assembly of the KNMG, and nominated to participate in expert advisory bodies such as the Health Council. In 1970, the KNMG even announced that it would start inviting experts from the fields of theology, law, sociology, and psychology to write regular essays on medical ethics. In short, the upper echelons of the Dutch medical profession, at least, seemed quite willing in the early 1970s to have a new type of expert function as a "luminary" in medical ethics. Hence, even though Dutch ethicists might have started storming the medical bulwark in this period, they found its doors wide open.

In 1974, Sporken was appointed to the medical faculty of the State University of Limburg (later Maastricht University) as the first Dutch professor in medical ethics.[33] In 1977, he introduced the term health ethics in his book *Ethiek en gezondheidszorg* (Ethics and health care). The old medical ethics, the theologian-cum-ethicist argued, had been formulated primarily for the doctor-patient relationship. Yet modern health care had become a complex network of caregivers and patients, all embedded in tightly knit social structures and all heavily influenced by their environment. Hence, an ethics had to be developed that no longer focused only on the responsibilities of doctors, but "that describe[d] and analyze[d] health care in all its various aspects, including the ethical norms that exist or are imagined therein, that clarifie[d] the images of man and society that lie at the root of these norms, and that critically assesse[d] this underlying vision on its humanitarian character."[34]

In 1977, the Health Council, too, introduced the term health ethics. In 1975, it had quietly disbanded its Committee for Medical Ethics after it had proven difficult to formulate a new ethics framework for "medical practice in a modern society." Yet in 1977, the Council president did decide to install a Standing Committee for Health Ethics that could "signal questions and developments in health ethics that should be studied by ad hoc committees," and "coordinate how various council committees approach facets of health ethics."[35] This new name, committee member Henk Leenen stated approvingly at the first meeting, allowed the standing committee to consider the social dimension of health care and to discuss the responsibilities of the government.[36]

Initially, the committee seated four physicians, two legal scholars, and two ethicists—a lecturer in theological ethics and the upcoming ethicist Heleen Dupuis, who had recently finished a dissertation with Heering on the notion of *mondigheid* as a basic ethical principle of modern society.[37] A little while later, Sporken joined the committee deliberations as well. This interdisciplinary composition was considered crucial to the workings of the committee.[38] Still, the ethicists were attributed a leading role. As its secretary—a physician—stated in 1981, without their input discussions were likely to "break down due to dilettantism, casuistry, and side-tracking."[39] Professional ethicists had to ensure that deliberations took place systematically and methodically.

In 1984, an Institute for Health Ethics was established in Maastricht, modelled after the American Kennedy Center for Bioethics at Georgetown University (in 1979, the Dutch-born obstetrician André Hellegers, director of the Kennedy Center, had held a passionate speech advocating the creation of a similar Dutch institute).[40] Steeped in Enlightenment rhetoric, its founders visualized the institute as a "palace of light," "a place where the light can shine on questions on life and health" that would help the Dutch people "to see what they are doing with their lives, world, and future," in the expectation that "people who are able to see will not be blind to the light."[41] Concomitantly, the institute's conception of ethical expertise was similar to the one formulated by Sporken in 1970: in a society in which traditional moral authorities were no longer accepted, ethicists could function as luminaries in thinking about ethics. Its staff, the institute's president stated in 1986, had been chosen to "form a selection of our 'secular pluralist society'"—a term he took from philosopher Tristram Engelhardt, author of *The Foundations of Bioethics*, who later famously stated that "in a secular pluralist society, health care policy requires a moral *lingua franca*, a general moral perspective that transcends particular moral and religious commitments."[42] The Institute for Health Ethics would labor to provide this lingua franca.[43]

Other institutes followed in the late 1980s and early 1990s. In 1988, a Center for Bioethics and Health Law was established at Utrecht University and, in 1993, a Dutch Society for Bioethics was inaugurated.[44] In the same period, multiple Dutch journals for health and bioethics were founded as well, of which the most prominent was the *Tijdschrift voor geneeskunde en ethiek* (Journal for medicine and ethics), which released its first issue in 1991.[45] In 1986, Heleen Dupuis was appointed as professor of medical ethics on the Leiden medical faculty. In 1991, Inez de Beaufort, who had in 1985 successfully defended a PhD dissertation on the ethics of human experimentation in medicine, was inaugurated as a professor of health ethics on the medical faculty in Rotterdam. In the years thereafter, most other Dutch medical faculties realized chairs in medical or health ethics as well.[46]

With this growing professional success, health ethics was increasingly recognized as a mature field of study in the Netherlands. Heleen Dupuis, in particular, gained national fame in this period as an expert commentator on ethical problems in health care and the biomedical sciences. Whether the topic of concern was the public discussion of euthanasia, AIDS, genetics, physical examinations, or the care of the elderly, Dupuis was interviewed and quoted by members of the media across the political spectrum.[47] Dupuis did not shy away from giving clear opinions on these issues. "It is criminal to endlessly prolong the life of hopeless coma patients," one paper would cite the ethicist.[48] "AIDS tests may also be carried out without the permission of the patient," another would quote her.[49] "Triple abortion [in a woman expecting quintuplets] was humane and prudent," a third would say, again citing Dupuis.[50] She was frequently invited to speak on television, served as the chairperson to the Dutch Society for Voluntary Euthanasia, and participated in many a government advisory body.[51] And in 1985, when the KNMG established two medical ethics committees—one solely dedicated to the topic of euthanasia—they welcomed a multitude of ethicists, including Dupuis.

Seen in this light, the suggestion can hardly be maintained that the Dutch medical profession, in contrast to the American and British ones, retained full jurisdiction over medical ethics in the second half of the twentieth century. Yes, the KNMG continued to play an important role in discussions over medical ethics, but that does not mean that "the Royal Dutch Medical Association [...] was able to negotiate physician-initiated euthanasia practices with Dutch legal authorities without involving 'bioethicists' in any major decision." Instead, the organization incorporated ethicists within its ranks—an interplay that was beneficial to both the Dutch medical profession, who thereby avoided the "adversarial" relationship that doctors had developed with ethicists in the United States, and to the newly established health ethics profession, for whom it served as a validation of the field's added professional value.

In 1988, Dupuis and de Beaufort explained in the *Handboek gezondheidsethiek*—the first Dutch textbook of health ethics—that ethicists were professionals with a specific skillset on offer: they brought terminological clarity, mapped moral problems, and applied normative theories to find solutions. In doing so, they could help physicians and others handle the growth of moral problems in medicine and society. Thus, the *Handboek* "not only provide[d] insight into the most important moral problems in health care by giving an overview of them, but also assist[ed] in how to tackle them."[52] Ethicists were no threat to physicians. They simply lit the way.

Storming the Bulwark of the Ethical Know-It-Alls

In the same period when health ethics was booming in the Netherlands, however, criticism of the discipline started to grow as well. Occasionally, these critiques came from medical professionals, who felt that ethicists made their practice needlessly difficult.[53] The most scathing criticism in this period, however, came not from caregivers or researchers but from philosophers, who vehemently disagreed with the intellectual claims and political function of the health ethics movement. The role that ethicists envisioned themselves to fulfill in a so-called secular pluralistic society, these philosophers started to argue in the late 1980s, was detrimental not only to the academic study of ethics, but to the democratic functioning of society as a whole. It was in this context that research ethics committees came to function as a battleground on which ethicists and philosophers could hash out their conflicting conceptions of the intellectual aspirations and political role of health ethics.

The core of these philosophical critiques was directed at a specific approach to health or bioethics that had grown popular in the 1980s and that facetiously came to be called "the Georgetown mantra" after the place where it was first proposed in the 1970s. This mantra, also called common morality principlism, is an approach to ethics that revolves around four principles: autonomy, beneficence, non-maleficence, and justice. According to its advocates, these principles are compatible with most outlooks on life—religious, cultural, or otherwise—and can therefore function as the moral lingua franca of a pluralistic society.[54]

In the Netherlands, this approach became known in the 1980s as "an ethics of minimum morality." Every person, theologian-cum-ethicist Harry Kuitert explained in the 1988 *Handboek gezondheidsethiek*, has their own "comprehensive moral system" that originates from, and is nurtured by, their social background and personal experiences.[55] Yet, in order to peacefully coexist with those who adhere to a different moral system, all people should be able to justify their actions via "a minimum morality that [...] posits those basic principles on which coexistence is based as inevitable obligations."[56] While such basic principles were general, in applying them to particular cases they became guiding ethical notions that should be acceptable to all members of a pluralistic society.

One of the first explicit critiques of this approach in the Netherlands was voiced in 1987 by philosopher and theologian Paul van Tongeren, at the time professor of "philosophy in relation to the Catholic tradition." According to Van Tongeren, moral philosophy was essentially a form of hermeneutics: an "art of interpreting or explaining what announces itself as meaningful to us, but that for whatever reason is distant, so that it has to be transposed and explained." Hence, the academic study of ethics consisted of "bridging this distance, so the meanings we suspect or just faintly discern [to exist] may occur in full form to us again."[57] This approach was everything the applied ethics tradition was not. In Van Tongeren's assessment, ethicists following the Georgetown mantra hardly investigated "that which can be heard" in moral instances: they simply assumed they already knew what was being said in order to apply their supposedly universal principles. In doing so, they failed to truly understand what was as stake in such instances.

A year later, philosopher Hans Achterhuis drew a similar conclusion in a scathing review of the *Handboek gezondheidsethiek*. According to Achterhuis—today one of the Netherlands's most well-known philosophers—the textbook had to be read as a "specific language game in which terms like *mondigheid*, self-determination, and choice take center stage."[58] But while this language game was presented as a moral lingua franca, it was in fact a highly liberal discourse that displaced other ways of knowing, such as more historically and sociologically informed critiques of modern health care by critical thinkers such as Ivan Illich and Michel Foucault. The authors simply accepted, for instance, that a core ethical problem of modern health care was the scarcity of medical goods and services, without analyzing what function a term like scarcity fulfills in capitalist societies.[59] Hence, the textbook ignored the fundamental question of how some issues and not others come to be socially recognized as ethical problems—and thereby reproduced the very problems it believed to be solving. Health ethics, Achterhuis concluded, could hardly be called a reflexive field of academic study.

These critiques marked the beginning of a storm of denunciations of health ethics in the late 1980s. In 1990, the physician-philosopher Henk ten Have dedicated his entire inaugural lecture as "professor of philosophy related to the Catholic outlook on life" at the State University of Limburg to the misconceptions on which he believed health ethics to be based.[60] Ethicists like Dupuis, Ten Have observed, were popular in the media and on government advisory bodies. "Apparently our society has a need for such spokespersons, who offer orientation, directions, a sense of security for confusing and difficult situations of which we do not know ourselves what to make of them." Yet "what really happens to ethics when it lets itself get seduced to fulfill this role?"[61] It became a form of "moral engineering," a term Ten Have borrowed from American ethicist Arthur Caplan.[62] Like engineers, ethicists would try to surgically dissect and fix moral problems by simplifying moral choices and designing standardized pathways for them. Like engineers, they would be preoccupied with spectacular technological problems and have a desire for homogeneity to streamline ethical decision-making in health care.[63] "However complex a case may be," Ten Have argued, "however difficult the decision is to deal with, the ethicist aims to offer certainty and solutions" by appealing to principles that could easily be translated into policies, rules, and regulations.[64]

But what problems did health ethics solve, really? Ten Have recounted something that had struck him when taking a bioethics course in the United States in the 1980s. "At the same moment an elaborate plea was being held in the course room for the primary importance of individual freedom and respect for autonomy, outside in the public park a few dozen beggars could be discerned who possessed nothing more than a plastic bag or grocery trolley."[65] Why, the philosopher asked, did bioethicists write article after article about the importance of informed consent, while they could hardly be heard in any discussion of the relation between economic inequality and life expectancy? The reason was that bioethics had created a profile for itself in the 1960s as a modern, "neutral" alternative to older religious perspectives on medicine. In this quest for a more secular ethics, principles like autonomy and non-maleficence had been presented as the only sensible "moral Esperanto" of a pluralistic society. Consequently, only specific types of issues came to be understood as moral problems—e.g., informed consent—while others were neglected or designated to be political: a matter of weighing interests or counting heads.[66]

In part, the grievances of these philosophers concerned the feeble intellectual position of health ethics. On what foundations did principles such as autonomy and non-maleficence rest? What tools did ethicists possess to apply such principles consistently and unambiguously to individual cases? Did these principles not just function as catchall terms, abstract enough to make any moral argument one wanted? The Georgetown mantra, in other words, would function as the emperor's new clothes, with doctors and policymakers as the emperor and ethicists as the shrewd weavers and philosophers, of course, as the only children sane or daring enough to point out the emperor was, in fact, naked.

To a large extent, however, these philosophers' grievances also lay with the political function they believed health ethics to fulfill, and the way they perceived it to push other perspectives to the margins of political debate. In 1993, this view was articulated by philosopher Hub Zwart—a student of Van Tongeren—in his dissertation, which detailed how health ethicists sought to reach "ethical consensus in a pluralistic society."[67] Health ethicists, Zwart argued, typically acknowledged that their claims rested on a feeble intellectual foundation. Their point was not that principlism produced truth claims, but that it could rest on a reasonable consensus among most participants in moral deliberations, which was all that could realistically be expected in a pluralistic society. Health ethics thus predominantly advocated a *procedural* approach to ethics: as long as people were guaranteed their right to speak and were willing to utilize this right in "a reasonable manner"—i.e., by participating in conversations, sustaining their opinions with arguments, and listening to others—the minimum morality needed for peaceful coexistence would eventually surface in moral deliberations. The deliberation process itself was primary, not its outcome.[68]

However, Zwart also argued, while this doctrine was presented as a neutral procedure, it was in reality an attempt to pass off a liberal ethics as the only ethics suitable for a pluralistic society. By constantly using the threat that all other ethical perspectives might result in conflict and warfare, adepts of principlism effectively labelled these perspectives as threats to peaceful coexistence.[69] "The liberal perspective [on moral discussion]," Zwart wrote, is "*de jure* broadminded, but *de facto* restricted."[70] Ethicists' supposed ability to broker consensus was in practice an instrument of social control.[71]

Notably, the foremost example used by most of these philosophers in illustration of their criticism was the participation of ethicists in research ethics committees. Ethicists, Van Tongeren argued, had to explore fundamental questions as to why a society would invest in a practice like human experimentation and how such a practice related to "what we really are after in life."[72] They should *not* help to decide in concrete cases, on the basis of a limited number of guidelines and abstract principles, whether these practices were permissible. Research ethics committees, Ten Have also stated, were a typical example of moral engineering that helped to legitimate medical science. A professor in obstetrics had recently stated that an experiment with a new abortion pill did not present any ethical problems, since it had been approved by an ethics committee.[73] This statement, Ten Have argued, offered a clear example of how a procedural approach to ethics was an obstacle to substantive reflection: "Once procedures are agreed upon, they obtain, in accordance with the model of law, an alibi function. Ethics as a process of continuous reflection on medical action is therewith halted."[74]

The philosopher who perhaps most strongly shared this view was Gerard de Vries, who published a series of highly critical pieces in the early 1990s on the political function of health ethics.[75] According to De Vries, research ethics committees were a typical example of how "routines have come into existence [in health care] that meet the classic requirements of modern, bureaucratic organizations, formulated by the sociologist Weber: competencies are strictly regulated, intercourse takes place in writing, judgement is in principle impersonal." This bureaucratic framework had great advantages for all involved: it gave legal protection to researchers, research subjects, those who financed research, hospital boards, etcetera. It even "provide[d] ethics with a well-functioning memory," making it possible for researchers to compare new cases with older ones and for research ethics committees to compare notes. Yet it also ensured, De Vries remarked sarcastically, that reviewers did not even have to *think* anymore. They only had to follow procedure. "If the forms are not filled in correctly," the dictum was, "the medical ethicist cannot do his job."[76]

In other words, health ethics had not become successful because it provided a necessary moral check on the activities of caregivers and researchers. It had become successful because it provided the status quo with a means of legitimizing activities such as human experimentation—without requiring that the debate be opened up to a greater number of critical voices. Health ethics, in short, had become an indispensable greaser for techno-scientific machineries. In doing so, de Vries concluded, it undermined democratic decision-making: under the flag of ethics, moral issues were increasingly *depoliticized*, maneuvered outside of the political arena to be "solved" by a group of anointed experts.[77] Van Tongeren felt the same. If moral problems had become difficult to solve in a pluralistic society, he wrote, the solution was *not* to defuse them by having a small group of ethicists draw up some sort of minimum morality: "I see no other possibility than that rules are drawn up in the political and legal arenas, realizing that they are ethically provisional or inevitably without ethical legitimization." Ethicists had to know better than to try and "give a political compromise the pretense of ethical legitimization."[78]

The Determined Rebuttal of the Ethical Engineers

Not surprisingly, representatives of the Dutch health ethics movement did not quite agree with their critics. In 1991, Dupuis wrote a scathing review of Ten Have's work for the *Dutch Journal of Medicine* in which she insisted that the newly appointed professor must have completely lost sight of reality. His portrayal of health ethics was so off the mark that it could not even be called a caricature. Ten Have had gotten it wrong in every possible way.[79]

In 1991, the ethicist Frans Jacobs, who had written his dissertation on why a liberal ethics is the only ethics that meets the demands of a pluralistic society, responded to Van Tongeren.[80] Jacobs admitted that many ethicists nowadays played a role resembling the one vicars used to fulfill, i.e., that of "passing normative judgements from an authoritative position."[81] This behavior was annoying (Jacobs specifically referred to "Ms. Dupuis" as one offender) and the role not one that ethicists could legitimately fulfill. Yet, the haughty dismissal by Dutch philosophers of the applied ethics tradition was equally annoying and, worse, possibly even dangerous. After all, Jacobs claimed, common morality principlism was not formulated out of some sort of intellectual laziness, but to accommodate for moral beliefs that differed from those of the dominant cultural group in a pluralistic society. This kind of accommodation was incredibly difficult, yet essential for developing an ethical framework for peaceful, tolerant coexistence.

Now more than ever, Jacobs continued, society needed such a framework. Pollution, nuclear energy, the arms race—they were all examples of the life-threatening consequences of techno-scientific advancement. These potentially volatile circumstances demanded moral guidance, guidance that could no longer in a secularizing society be offered by Christianity. Hence, applied ethics found its right to exist in this demand: that society simply *needed* scholars who could ask meaningful questions and guide moral thinking about these developments.

Dupuis and De Beaufort agreed with this analysis. In 1985, De Beaufort had already stated that she firmly believed that ethics, as an academic discipline, should serve to formulate answers to the urgent and complex moral questions faced by society: "In this she finds her ultimate justification, otherwise she is just an academic pastime."[82] In their 1988 textbook, Dupuis and De Beaufort repeated this point. While philosophers might keep their hands clean by sitting in their ivory towers and savoring their intellectual abilities, ethicists made an actual difference in the world by getting their hands dirty in taking on real-life moral problems.

In 1992, the upcoming ethicist Frans Brom offered another fiery defense of this point. At the time, Brom worked at the Utrecht Center for Bioethics and Health Law, but was contracted by the Ministry of Agriculture, Nature, and Food Quality to help develop policies for new techno-scientific developments in these fields. According to Brom, ethicists were no engineers: they did not replace moral deliberation with technocratic solutions. Instead, they acted as mediators, to ensure that all the participants in policymaking correctly understood one another.[83] Ethicists offered conceptual clarity, pointed out elements that were not yet considered problematic, and brought up ethical viewpoints which they believed were unjustly ignored in deliberations. In doing so, they enabled policymakers to "pursue better, because more rational, policies."[84] Plus, in order to speak truth to power, intellectuals actually had to *speak* to those in power, which could not be done from a tall ivory tower.

The core message of these rebuttals was that ethicists *did* have an important public role to fulfill and that, given the many ethical problems faced by modern society, the refusal to contribute to solving these problems was both unwarranted and irresponsible. As long as a societal need existed for their reasoned input, neither philosopher nor ethicist had the luxury to rummage around the halls of academia and twiddle their thumbs. "A world threatened with extinction clings to the life buoy of applied ethics," Jacobs wrote in 1991, "which is thereby saved from extinction caused by irrelevance and sterility."[85]

Of course, an important part of the philosophers' critique of health ethics had not just been the political function of ethicists, but the feeble foundations of their intellectual claims. Even if the ethical problems faced by contemporary societies were substantial, why would the judgements of ethicists be any more relevant than those of the average citizen? The most systematic answer to this question was offered in 1991 by ethicist Theo van Willigenburg in his book *Inside the Ethical Expert*.[86] In 1996, Van Willigenburg would become professor of medical ethics in Amsterdam and, in 1991, ethics professor on the philosophy faculty at Rotterdam, where he served as dean as well until 2005.[87] Even in 1991, however, Van Willigenburg was already one of the most visible faces in the Dutch applied ethics field.

Notably, like the critics of common morality principlism, Van Willigenburg also rejected the Georgetown approach to ethical analysis. The idea that moral judgements about real-life ethical problems could be reached by applying moral rules or principles, he argued in *Inside the Ethical Expert*, was logically problematic. After all, before an ethicist could know which principles to apply, (s)he first had to qualify the case as being of a certain moral kind, e.g., as a problem in which the autonomy of individuals was at stake or in which the principle of beneficence might apply. As only the principles themselves could provide this sort of indication, principlism was basically a form of circular reasoning.

Rather than dismissing applied ethics, however, Van Willigenburg proposed a case-oriented approach to moral reasoning. When people encountered situations that they experienced as morally problematic, he explained, this uneasiness was often invoked not by recognizing that the situation violated a general principle, but by a moral intuition: a direct and immediate reaction to a particular event. This "intuiting" was nothing else than interpreting an issue according to specific moral patterns that organized how people perceived the world around them: moral glasses that made them see certain things and not others. These patterns could differ by community and individual and, importantly, change or dissolve upon careful reflection. Yet, according to Van Willigenburg, "satisfying interpretative grids" could be found for specific moral problems by collecting enough real and hypothetical cases to enable their comparison, and by generating patterns from them to allow for the satisfactory intuiting of future cases.[88] Hence, rather than a deductive approach to applied ethics (i.e., principlism), Van Willigenburg proposed an inductive approach involving the production and application of "statistical regularities."

Similarly, as the Dutch philosophers had done, Van Willigenburg also invoked research ethics committees to develop his perspective on moral reasoning. In the past decades, the ethicist argued, these committees had gained extensive experience in the moral evaluation of practical cases. Contrary to what some believed, their moral reasoning process did not proceed deductively through an application of moral principles or declarations. Instead, committees typically deliberated by invoking cases they had previously dealt with, revisiting the arguments and concerns that had been put forward in those instances. Principles played a role, e.g., by setting the parameters within which discussions took place, but "fine-graded assessment in moral thinking [wa]s performed by a process of comparison of the problem case to other real and hypothetical cases."[89] This modus operandi, Van Willigenburg explained, was a perfect institutionalized example of how moral reasoning worked in practice.

Professional ethicists worked in a similar manner: due to the simple fact that they could busy themselves full-time with moral issues, the patterns at their disposal for interpreting moral cases tended to be larger and more finely graded than those of the average layperson. "The large repertoire of interpretative patterns stored as part of the expertise of the ethical practitioner" made them more "*sensitive* to the new (type of) problem, which means that (s)he is able to respond more promptly and accurately to the important cues in the case."[90] To be sure, this expert ability did not mean that the judgements of ethicists were objectively better than those of laypeople. An objective yardstick to measure the accuracy of ethical judgements did not exist. Still, ethicists' conclusions went beyond mere opinions or beliefs. First, because their "hard drive" was filled with a wide knowledge of past cases, in addition to a sufficient understanding of ethical theories and principles. And, second, because their skill in moral reasoning and analysis — their "software" — allowed them to extract the morally relevant dimensions of past cases and explain in a consistent manner how these past examples applied to new ones. "Depending upon the quality of the reasoning process underlying a moral conclusion," Van Willigenburg concluded, "one is justified in holding that one does not just 'believe', but that one 'knows.'"[91]

Ethical expertise, Van Willigenburg wrote in response to Ten Have, consisted not of "a kind of 'Greenpeace-like' activism [. . .] against the dominant 'technocratic' ideology in modern medicine."[92] Ethicists' contribution was intellectual, not political. Thus, if ethicists were asked to take part in a research ethics committee, their role was not "to put into the pillory the 'pernicious power' of the pharmaceutical industry," but to assist in thinking through the research proposal under examination with their knowledge of past cases and ability to argue them consistently.[93] "Ethical practitioners need to be critical," Van Willigenburg concluded, "not as activists or reformers, but as experts who take their discipline seriously as a discipline of reason."[94] Doing so was not selling out, in his assessment; it was filling the only role that ethicists could sensibly fulfill.

A Standstill in Academic Debate

In the early 1990s, diverging views as to the abilities of ethicists were increasingly experienced as a full-on factional struggle in the Netherlands. In 1993, at a meeting of the Center for Bioethics and Health Law, Van Willigenburg and Van Tongeren again crossed swords over the issue of ethicists' potential contribution to "the manner in which moral issues are addressed by policymakers, [...] physicians, and other caregivers."[95] Van Willigenburg opened the debate by stating that he had decided to appropriate the title of "ethical engineer." In recent years, the ethicist argued, the term engineer had frequently been thrown at applied ethicists to demean their activities. Like plumbers, they would be in the business of mindlessly repairing leakages without investigating their cause. Besides offering an unjustly negative portrayal of plumbers, Van Willigenburg countered, this jab also incorrectly described the work of ethical engineers. To be an ethical engineer meant precisely to take a careful, step-by-step approach to considering the many aspects of moral problems, and thereby to enable well-considered ethical decision-making. It meant coaching participants in moral deliberations to make valid arguments and to "ensure a necessary argumentative hygiene" in the decision-making process.[96] Critics of this approach argued that the ethical engineer was not critical enough; that he did not ask fundamental philosophical questions. Apparently, moral questions could only be answered by pondering human existence. "I find such an approach wicked," Van Willigenburg stated. "It tries to find answers with far-reaching reflection on a philosophical-theoretical level, while we live in a time in which it is very naïve to assume that philosophy [...] can still give answers to 'fundamental' issues such as 'how we should look at existence.'"[97] Philosophers wanted to tackle a dilemma such as whether traffic victims might be used as organ donors by exploring how this question in and of itself betrayed a mechanical vision of life. They wanted to make all sorts of historical connections and think up cultural criticisms. Yet in doing so they *never* got around to answering the actual question. Perhaps, the ethicist suggested delicately, it was time for these critics to get out of their comfy armchairs and, instead of reading another book, take up an internship in a hospital or government office to help investigate dilemmas with which real people actually struggled.

Van Tongeren's response was equally forbidding. Van Willigenburg's perspective, the philosopher felt, bespoke an "almost shocking anti-intellectualism."[98] The dismissal of asking overly difficult questions and reading books could only be a "commercial mask" meant to persuade "no-nonsense managers" to hire ethicists, for such an approach had little to do anymore with any actual academic study. The philosopher had no objection in principle to the type of engineering that applied ethicists were so enthusiastic about. Yet, he continued, "Whatever it is that Van Willigenburg is doing, it is not philosophy anymore. And, insofar as ethics is a philosophical discipline, it cannot be ethics anymore either."[99] In the long run, Van Tongeren contended, scholars such as Van Willigenburg would bring about the demise of moral philosophy as a whole.

This struggle over the professional identity and public function of ethicists was by no means resolved in the early 1990s.[100] For most of the decade, the hermeneutic perspective kept on being denoted as the Nijmegen school of ethics, while the applied ethics perspective was referred to as the Utrecht school. In 1994, when national research schools started to emerge in the Netherlands, the Nijmegen group joined the Research School of Philosophy, while the Utrecht group joined the Research School of Ethics. Other academic approaches circulated as well in this period. Scholars like De Vries, for instance, who identified neither with the hermeneutic nor with the applied ethics perspective, joined the Research School of Science, Technology, and Modern Culture, which brought together scholars in Science, Technology, and Society studies.[101] And from the mid-1990s onward, the ethics of care became quite popular in the Netherlands—as a normative approach that opposed the dominance of notions such as autonomy and non-maleficence and instead introduced terms such as dependence, vulnerability, and mutual responsibility.[102] Still, by 1997, the dispute between the Nijmegen and Utrecht ethicists continued to be understood as one of the most dominant fracture lines in the Dutch academic practice of ethics.[103]

Hence, when viewed solely from the angle of academic debate about the (non-)existent epistemic foundations of their discipline, the factional struggle in Dutch ethics reached a standstill in the late twentieth century: members of neither camp could convince their opponents of their point of view. When viewed from a broader political and institutional perspective, however, one of the two schools made much more headway than the other in the 1990s. For while the debate was academic, it was heavily influenced by the growing political involvement with medicine and science seen in this decade. And just as the architects of the first Dutch research ethics committees had favored a particular way of knowing in medical science in the 1950s and 1970s, the expanding regulatory role of the Dutch state in this period favored a specific conception of ethical expertise, especially in the governance of human experimentation. Consequently, when the Dutch parliament in the late 1990s finally came to debate the public role of research ethics committees, ethicists were increasingly brought on stage as key actors in the democratic oversight of medical science. They were ethicists of a specific breed and color.

CHAPTER 6

PUBLIC GOVERNANCE *in a*

PLURALISTIC SOCIETY

Around half past eight on the evening of September 3, 1997, the Dutch parliament began its deliberations on the "medical research involving human subjects" bill, a proposal that had been in the works since 1982. Ad Lansink, a member of the largest Christian party in parliament, was the first to take the floor. "Mr. Speaker!" Lansink began formally, "the fight against disease [. . .] remains both a task and a mission, also for science and technology." Yet not everything scientific could be labelled as progress; a growing number of questionable research studies served as ringing reminders of this fact. Hence, now more than ever, Lansink continued, "society and the government have a duty to ascertain whether all research is permitted when held up to the norms and values that should bind a pluralistic society."[1] The Christian politician was not too sure, however, whether the current government, an administration made up solely of secular parties, shared the same concern. The review committees described in the bill, for instance, would also have to decide on socially contentious studies such as embryo experiments or experimental gene therapy. But these committees were not expected to include a single layperson, and did not in any way have "to take the ethical and religious plurality of society into account."[2] Really, how could "a committee that does not have to account to anyone" decide on studies about which hardly any ethical consensus existed?[3] What sort of public function did research ethics committees fulfill in a democratic society?

This chapter examines the realization of the Medical Research Involving Human Subjects Act (WMO), which has regulated medical research with humans in the Netherlands since 1999. In 1982, after publication of the Central Council report "Medical Experiments with Human Beings," the expectation was that the government would make haste to legislate such research. As Heleen Dupuis aptly put it in the fall of that year: "The matter of ethics committees, as expressed in the report of the Central Council for Public Health, is pretty much one of the only things about which a reasonable consensus exists in our country."[4] Yet the realization of a legal framework would take another seventeen years.

In this chapter, I explain that this inertia has to be understood in light of changing political winds in the 1980s and 1990s, which once again threw into question which forms of collective reasoning are suitable for the public governance of ethically contentious issues in medicine and science. This inertia did not prevent many Dutch research institutes, pressured by the ongoing internationalization of medical science in this period, from establishing their own research ethics committees. In this process, however, they often paid more attention to the *strategic* and *bureaucratic* functions of research ethics committees than to their possible *democratic* function. Hence, when the Dutch parliament finally got to debate a first version of the WMO bill in 1997, members were, to their frustration, debating a practice that had already congealed around different governance ideals than necessarily democratic ones.

In this context, the Dutch government increasingly found solace in the aid of the professional ethicist, whom they believed capable of speaking with expert authority on behalf of a pluralistic society. Ethicists themselves had by no means resolved their disagreements over the identity and political function of their profession by the late 1990s. Yet their role was one warmly welcomed by politicians, who continued to struggle with the public governance of medicine and science in a democratic society.

The Prolonged Absence of a Legal Framework

In April 1982, one month after publication of the Central Council report, the Dutch parliament unanimously adopted a motion stating that with the publication of that report, a large enough consensus now existed in the Netherlands to allow the government to take legal measures.[5] It was time the government started preparing a bill for the regulation of human experimentation.

The state secretary responsible for this task moved swiftly. In 1984, he was already able to report that his "human experimentation" bill, modelled largely after the 1982 Central Council report, would be submitted before the end of the political year. In 1985, however, his expeditious plans were brought to a halt by a change in political winds that came blowing in from the very government he was a part of. As in other countries, neoliberal initiatives to reduce government spending and regulations came to dominate Dutch politics in this period. In 1982, the Christian-Democrat Ruud Lubbers—often called the Dutch Margaret Thatcher—had won the elections with the slogan "more market, less government." Lubbers stayed in office as prime minister until 1994, marking a twelve-year period dominated by attempts to reduce "the public 'mania for organization.'" The Dutch health care system, for instance, was characterized by Lubbers and his supporters as an overwhelming bureaucracy providing little leeway for professionals to act efficiently and in the interest of patients. Rather than imposing top-down state regulations, therefore, the Lubbers government nurtured the bottom-up powers of the market—a neoliberal politics that went hand in hand with initiatives of privatization and deregulation.

This frame proved to be an ill fit for a bill that proposed to greatly restrict the autonomy of researchers via the installation of numerous ethics committees from which researchers would have to ask formal permission before they could start a human research study. In 1985, therefore, the minister of justice and minister of interior affairs vetoed the first Dutch human experimentation bill on the grounds that it did not fit the government's attempts at deregulation.[6]

This rejection inaugurated a lengthy period in which various Dutch government bodies were unable to reach an agreement over what sort of oversight was best for the governance of human experimentation. Where some legislators advocated a reactive system, wherein the state would respect the autonomy of researchers and only intervene if wrongdoings were suspected, other legislators maintained that the precarious position of research subjects demanded a proactive system, one requiring the prior permission of thereto-installed public review boards.

An additional political difficulty was posed by the fact that *human* experimentation in this period increasingly came to include discussions over the permissibility of embryo and fetal research as well, research about which hardly any consensus could be said to exist in the Netherlands. Then, in 1990, the Dutch Council of State, the country's highest advisory body, published advice that was extremely critical of the fact that the government wished to allow for research with "incapacitated individuals," i.e., people legally incapable of giving their informed consent.[7] Various international conventions, including the International Covenant on Civil and Political Rights, prohibited any form of research with such individuals; those prohibitions had been adopted to prevent any future recurrence of the atrocities committed in the Nazi concentration camps.[8] Yet, many medical researchers in the Netherlands did want such studies to be possible, in the hope of curing diseases specific to these groups. The Dutch government in this period wanted to allow for such research as well.

With every new hurdle, the statespersons responsible for the human experimentation bill decided that they wanted to undergo another round of deliberation and policy advice rather than send a proposal to parliament. In effect, the first oral treatment of the bill did not take place until September 1997, fifteen years after the Central Council had published its report.

This slow trajectory gave rise to many concerns and frustrations in the 1980s and 1990s. Members of parliament filed motions pressuring the government to make haste with its legislative plans, as the Netherlands was turning into "a true paradise for experiments" that had long since been prohibited in countries such as the United States.[9] In *Medisch Contact*, legal scholars pondered what would come of the regulation of more-controversial biomedical research, such as recombinant DNA technology, if the government could not even pass a human research act. The Netherlands was quickly becoming "a 'free state' for experiments [...] which are refused elsewhere."[10] In addition, general practitioners warned that "the Netherlands is (becoming) an international testing ground for all sorts of experimental research."[11] Increasingly, doctors were receiving requests from big pharmaceutical companies to enroll their patients in clinical trials in return for financial rewards or lucrative gifts like computers.[12] The deputy superintendent of public health confirmed these claims: in the past few years, the state inspectorate had received multiple complaints about advances of "Big Pharma," which had been drawn to Dutch general practice because of its lack of systematic oversight.[13] Although the inspectorate tried to fill this lacuna the best it could, the deputy superintendent wrote—half apologetically, half angrily—"it can only effectively perform this task if a legal basis exists for it."[14] Yet the Dutch government remained unwilling or unable to realize a proper legal framework for human experimentation.

Developments on the Ground

The absence of a Dutch law for human subjects research does not mean that no research ethics committees were established in the Netherlands in the 1980s and 1990s. Quite the contrary: from the early 1980s onward, they shot up like mushrooms from the ground, for reasons intimately related to the ongoing internationalization of medical science in this period.

In 1976, the first official Dutch research ethics committee was inaugurated at Leiden University, titled the Committee for Medical Ethics. The Leiden CME gave advice on various issues of ethical concern, but its foremost task was the review of human research protocols, executed under the auspices of the Leiden medical faculty and university hospital. This review board, which would become the prototype for almost all other Dutch research ethics committees in the 1980s and 1990s, was the brainchild of a medical scientist who had held a professorial chair in pharmacology at Leiden since 1963 and who by 1976 had become quite the national authority on the governance of human experimentation: the founder and first chairman of the Leiden CME was none other than pharmacologist Erik Noach.

In Leiden, Noach had been involved in the communal ethics review of clinical research since 1965, when the Institute of Radio Pathology and Radiation Protection first asked the medical faculty to establish a committee that could offer advice on the permissibility of certain human experiments.[15] While no official ethics committee was established in this period, the faculty did occasionally ask Noach and two other physicians to evaluate human research protocols.[16] Although it is not entirely clear why this development took place, a letter posted in 1967 by the faculty's board of trustees to the US Department of Health, Education, and Welfare offers a likely reason. Written in the context of a grant application, this letter served to reassure the United States government of the following:

> [...] In 1965, the Faculty of Medicine at the University of Leiden instituted a committee to investigate all proposed experimental procedures involving humans which are to be undertaken by the members of the faculty.[17]

This claim was quite an exaggeration, as Noach and colleagues by no means evaluated all or even most human research protocols in Leiden. However, in 1966, in the midst of public outrage over the many questionable clinical experiments that were regularly taking place in American hospitals, the US Public Health Service (PHS) had made "prior review of the judgment of the principal investigator or program director by a committee of his institutional associates" an official eligibility requirement for those who wished to receive PHS grants. Soon thereafter, this policy was also adopted by the US Food and Drug Administration (FDA) and the US Department of Health, Education, and Welfare.[18] In theory, these policies mandated that Dutch researchers hoping to receive grant money from the PHS also needed to have their human research studies monitored by "a committee of [...] institutional associates"—a requirement that explains the reassuring letter of the Leiden medical faculty to the Department of Health, Education, and Welfare: i.e., as part of an attempt to gain access to American money.[19]

In November 1973, the Leiden medical faculty received another request from a physician to install a research ethics committee. The reason, this physician wrote, was that medical research increasingly seemed to be subject to ethical demands internationally: publications, for instance, "are [now] sometimes made dependent on the existence of a written verdict of an ethics committee." Hence, it would be helpful if the faculty could install a committee that "can operate as official conscience and warranting agency."[20] Again, the faculty council commissioned a response from Noach, who suggested that it might be a good idea to establish an official committee for this purpose.[21] In June 1976, this suggestion led to the instalment of the Leiden CME, often taken to be the oldest Dutch research ethics committee.

The Leiden CME was not the only research ethics committee active in the Netherlands at the end of the 1970s. In 1973, a committee had been established at the Free University of Amsterdam which gave advice about clinical pharmacological research as well as about euthanasia and abortion cases.[22] In 1977, a survey conducted by TNO showed that a "committee for research subjects" had recently been established at the University of Rotterdam and that small informal review groups were now active at the universities of Nijmegen and Utrecht. TNO, however, was skeptical about the actual functioning of these committees. "With the exception of Leiden," an internal memo stated in 1977, "the situation with regards to monitoring the use of human subjects is so miserable at the Dutch teaching hospitals and medical faculties that it does not appear sensible to trust the judgment of these self-styled local committees."[23] By the end of the 1970s, in short, research ethics committees were still hardly a familiar phenomenon in the Netherlands.

This state of affairs changed spectacularly in the 1980s. In June 1981, the University of Groningen proudly announced in *Medisch Contact* that "after Leiden now Groningen also has its CME."[24] In 1985, Noach could report that already twenty ethics boards were active in the Netherlands.[25] Merely one year later, the legal scholar Lucas Bergkamp counted sixty-three of them. In a few years' time, Bergkamp predicted, their total would likely amount to more than a hundred.[26] Sure enough, by 1989 their grand total was estimated to lie around 150.[27]

Commentators in the 1980s at times puzzled about the sudden exponential growth of Dutch research ethics committees in the absence of any legislation. Nonetheless, various likely reasons exist for their growth. First of all, in 1984, the Dutch government made the existence of an "independent medical review committee" a requirement for hospitals to participate in the Dutch health insurance funds. To be sure, this measure only required hospitals to install a review committee, not for medical researchers actually to pay it a visit—let alone ask for its permission. Yet the government hoped that hospital boards would stimulate the functioning of such committees via the magic of corporate liability: i.e., in case things went south, hospital insurance would only pay up if researchers had first required permission for their studies by an in-house review board.

Secondly, the history of the Leiden CME indicates that internationally changing grant and publishing policies had an important effect as well. Indeed, when Bergkamp in 1986 asked twenty-five Dutch research ethics committees why they had been established in the early 1980s, grant and publishing policies scored high on their lists.[28] By then, Anglo-American journals and funding bodies in particular had made the written approval of an ethics board a requirement for funding or article submissions involving human experimentation—a development that was soon copied by Dutch funding bodies.[29]

Other financial incentives likely had a similar effect. In 1981, the FDA reached an agreement with the US Department of Health, Education, and Welfare that mandated institutional review for all FDA-regulated activities involving human research subjects.[30] From then onward, clinical studies that involved medicines, vaccines, medical devices, or other products regulated by the FDA could not commence before an institutional review board had given its permission. Although these regulations were not directly applicable to studies conducted outside the United States—as "standards of protection for human subjects may vary from country to country, and the United States should not impose its standards on other countries"—it is likely that pharmaceutical companies active in the Netherlands also decided to comply with these conditions to sell their products on the lucrative American consumer market.[31] Similarly, in the 1980s, the European Economic Community (EEC) started to develop harmonization requirements for products traded within its member states. In 1990, this development resulted in the position paper "Good Clinical Practice for Trials of Medicinal Products in the European Community," which stipulated the need for prior ethics review of human research protocols.[32] While this document at the time had only the status of a "compelling recommendation," it contributed significantly to the explosive rise of Dutch research ethics committees in the late twentieth century.

As a result of these developments, a dense and at times impermeable forest of research ethics committees had sprung up in the Netherlands toward the end of the 1980s. These committees operated under various guises—interchangeably called institutional review boards, medical ethics committees, independent review councils, or ethics committees—with hardly any rules for their composition. Anyone, really, could claim the existence of a Dutch research ethics committee in the late 1980s. People did. In 1987, for instance, a few months after the deputy superintendent of public health had warned that insufficient oversight mechanisms existed in general practice clinics, *Medisch Contact* published a letter by two members of an unnamed research ethics committee, huffing angrily that "the state inspectorate apparently is not aware of the fact that an objective review option most certainly does exist." Did the deputy superintendent not know, they asked, that the Independent Review Board Foundation was active in the Netherlands outside of hospital walls? And that it had been brought into existence by the research community to "advocate the importance of assessing the ethical and legal acceptability of extramural experimental research in an impartial manner, irrespective of any institution and without any commercial intention"?[33] Well, clearly the deputy superintendent did not. From which one might either conclude that he was not that well informed about the concerns he chose to write about, or that the Dutch system of ethics review had become a bit inscrutable toward the end of the 1980s, to say the least. As a result, even though research ethics committees had been envisioned to restore much-needed public trust in the Dutch research establishment at the start of the decade, they themselves were increasingly becoming an object of distrust toward the end of it.

Calls for Uniformity and Attempts at Professionalization

Between 1986 and 1988, legal scholar Lucas Bergkamp researched the daily functioning of Dutch research ethics committees.[34] In two three-hundred-page reports, he analyzed all rulings made by twenty-two committees in a single year, and wrote up his findings of their assessments of three protocols they had reviewed on his request, in which he had included a number of "methodological, ethical, and informed-consent problems."[35] His analysis made clear that review standards differed in the Netherlands: not all committees under investigation had reviewed the methodological quality of protocols, most had different rules for the required competence of researchers, and all showed little consistency in their evaluation of informed-consent procedures. The cause for all this "variation and inconsistency," Bergkamp argued, was the large number of committees active in the Netherlands, which made it impossible to "avoid big differences in composition, procedures, and especially employed standards of evaluation."[36] This state of affairs, he concluded, was "one of the most important problems which the review system by medical ethics committees currently has to cope with."[37]

Back in 1985, health ethicist Inez de Beaufort had already called for "supervision, coordination, and a certain degree of uniformity" in the jumble of research ethics committees she saw springing up in the Netherlands. This uniformity was needed to avoid frustration and delays in multicenter trials, but also to maintain the trust of researchers in the professionalism of ethics review, and to make sure that researchers would not put committees under pressure "with the argument that her 'difficult attitude' blocks a collaboration with other institutions, while another committee, note well, has already given positive advice."[38] In 1986, Bergkamp added "the danger of shopping" to this list: researchers could very well go round the existing committees until they had found one willing to give any research protocol its blessing.[39]

To realize this uniformity, various attempts at self-regulation were undertaken in the 1980s and 1990s. In 1983, Noach and Dupuis had already started organizing a postgraduate course at Leiden about the "ethics review of medical experiments with human beings," with all those active or interested in reviewing human research protocols invited to attend.[40] In 1984, the Institute for Health Ethics in Maastricht started to offer training courses for members of ethics committees, teaching them the ins and outs of reviewing protocols. In 1987, the Dutch Hospital Council and KNMG even founded a "national station of support" with information and support for anyone involved in reviewing "experimental human and patient-related research."[41] And in 1991, the two organizations joined forces with an informal partnership of research ethics committees to found the Dutch Society for Medical Ethics Review Committees (NVMETC), which was to bring together experts in ethics review, influence national developments in this area, advance cooperation between local committees, and foster reliable and professional review procedures.[42]

What thus more or less took place in the Netherlands in the 1980s was a process of attempted professionalization of a trade that had barely existed a decade before. The competent ethics reviewer adhered to a communal set of standards and practices, sat in on training sessions to refresh his or her reviewing skills, and was a member of a national society that oversaw the conduct of its members. In these attempts, much emphasis was put on the importance of expertise. Ethics committees needed professionals who knew what they were talking about, and who were equipped to take on the growing number of protocols submitted for review every year. Unwanted variation could only be combatted by implementing nationwide standards that would be applied uniformly by qualified reviewers. Once reviewers were properly trained, it would no longer matter whether a protocol was submitted in Leiden or in Groningen: professional conduct would guarantee that the outcome of all reviews would be sufficiently similar if not the same.

This notion of the expert-reviewer did not sit well with the inclusion of laypeople in research ethics committees. As a participant at a Dutch conference on "the task and function of medical ethics committees in scientific research" pointed out in 1989: "We must prevent that all and sundry can take up a seat in these committees and join in on conversations they don't understand."[43] Laypeople, by definition, were not professional reviewers.

Still, for these advocates of proper expertise, reason for concern was on the horizon. In the 1990s, due to ongoing commotion over the permissibility of research studies with embryos, fetuses, or incapacitated individuals, multiple political parties started to argue that the diversity of moral beliefs in Dutch society *should* be fairly represented on research ethics committees. For what sort of ethics did these committees really prescribe and promote? And what sort of expertise did their reviewers possess to help them solve ethical dilemmas about which no reasonable consensus could be said to exist in the Netherlands? It was this tension between expert and democratic oversight that remained to be resolved when the Dutch parliament in 1997 was finally able to debate the long-awaited human experimentation bill.

The Definitive Departure of the Society Representative

Responsible for the human experimentation bill in 1997 was Minister of Health, Welfare, and Sport Els Borst-Eilers—often called Els Borst. Today, Borst is remembered as one of the most influential Dutch politicians of the late twentieth century, with her signature validating more than a hundred Dutch laws.[44] Most famously, she was responsible as minister of health in 2001 for the passing of the Termination of Life on Request and Assisted Suicide (Review Procedures) Act, more commonly known as the Dutch euthanasia law, an event that made headlines and waves the world over.[45] After her tragic death in 2014, the many eulogies commemorating her life without exception lauded her efforts, both as physician and politician, to help resolve many of the medical ethics dilemmas that had dominated public discourse since the 1970s.[46] "Few have made such a great contribution to the debate about medical ethics in the Netherlands," the website of *Medisch Contact* read in 2014.[47]

During her time as medical director, Borst had already begun to concern herself with the governance of human experimentation. In 1983, for instance, she was asked to speak about "the ethics review of medical experiments with human beings" at the first postgraduate course on the topic organized by Noach and Dupuis. In her lecture, Borst lauded the institutional functioning of review committees, which she believed to "fit [...] the current era of the *mondige* patient critical of governments and modern clinical medicine."[48] What was more, when she became vice president of the Health Council in 1986, Borst served as chairperson to both the Standing Committee for Health Ethics and the Core Committee for Ethics and Medical Research (KEMO), the latter of which was established in 1989 on government request to provide policy advice on "ethical, legal, and juridical questions of a general nature" relating to "socially relevant" developments in medical research.[49]

Hence, when Borst became minister of health in 1994, she already had quite some experience under her belt to put to use in one of the longest-running political dossiers bequeathed to her: the human experimentation bill. Borst remained minister until 2002, as part of the two governments led by Wim Kok, usually referred to as the Purple Coalitions due to their union of the Dutch labor party PvdA (red) and the conservative-liberal party VVD (blue). Borst was a member of the third party that completed these governments: the progressive social-liberal party D66.[50] None of these parties had a religious grounding, which made "Purple I" the first Dutch government since the introduction of proportional representation in 1917 in which no confessional party participated. This makeup had its effect, particularly when it came to regulations that were considered "morally contentious." Before Kok's two terms had come to an end, prostitution had been legalized in the Netherlands, as had same-sex marriage and euthanasia.

The latter issue in particular divided the secular and confessional parties in the Dutch parliament like few other dossiers ever had, with Borst not-infrequently cast in the role of irreverent statesperson. In 2001, she even faced a motion of no confidence signed by all the Christian parties in the Dutch parliament, because she had been recorded in an interview about the completion of her euthanasia bill to have clenched her fist, smiled, and said "It is finished"—the same last words Jesus spoke on the cross, as recorded in the Bible.[51] This rift ran so deep that, when Protestant politician Arie Slob spent a few days in the headquarters of D66 in 2012, he asked "half-jokingly, but also seriously" for the portrait of Borst to be turned to face the wall whilst he was there.[52]

In the parliamentary debates over the human experimentation bill, emotions did not run as high. Yet there, too, a divide existed at times between secular coalition parties and Christian opposition parties. Principal dissent manifested itself, in particular, over the permissibility of nontherapeutic experiments with incapacitated individuals. As the Christian-Democrats explained their rejection of this section of the human experimentation bill: "Every human being, created in the image of God, has an intrinsic value, which cannot be reduced to his health or intellectual capacities nor to the importance he has for a third party or society as a whole."[53] In addition, much more than secular parties, Christian parties pushed for democratic representation in advisory councils such as KEMO, because they feared that experiments with fetuses and embryos would be approved more easily if nobody from the pro-life movement could have a say.[54] Particularly during the 1990s, "the importance of ethical pluralism in a democratic state" became an oft-heard statement by Christian parties in debates over regulations pertaining to medical ethics.

Borst was in favor of nontherapeutic research with legally incapacitated individuals. However, she started off her involvement with the dossier by making what she later said was a political misstep, causing the topic to become a subject of heated debate once more. On the evening of October 3, 1995, Borst confirmed on national television that she was planning to allow for nontherapeutic research with incapacitated individuals. She defended this decision with the example of Alzheimer's disease. As the media reported the next day: "According to Borst, the testing of a pill against Alzheimer's disease is only possible on demented elderly people. In the interest of medical research, she finds it conceivable that drugs in the future will be tried out on these patients."[55]

One day later, the Alzheimer's Foundation reported that it had received "a flood of calls from worried relatives of Alzheimer's patients."[56] "Who decides that only drugs will be applied that are meant to do something about this dementia? As a layperson, you cannot keep a check on this," a concerned wife was recorded to have said. Geriatricians also blamed Borst: "Since the statement of Minister Borst on October 3, it seems that a majority of politicians and the public are turning against the possibility of experiments with the legally incapacitated."[57] Similarly, parliament members could not point out quickly enough that such practices were not what they had in mind when talking about nontherapeutic experiments with legally incapacitated people. In a leading newspaper, the Christian-Democrats were quoted to have "great difficulty with the plans of Borst," who was "now really starting to overstep the boundaries."[58]

The turmoil over Borst's remark ensured that the oral treatment of the human experimentation bill started off with substantial discontent among Dutch politicians.[59] How could Borst guarantee that researchers would always operate in the best interest of research subjects when the latter had few to no means, either legally or mentally, to make their objections heard? And, importantly, how could laypeople keep an eye on this process if they had no access to the review committees outlined in the bill?

The fact that the human experimentation bill did not require any laypeople to take part in the review of research studies became another point of contention in the indignation over Borst's misstep. In its 1996 form, the bill provided for a two-tier system with a limited number of local committees that were to be managed by one central committee. The central committee had to consist "in any case of one or more physicians and of persons who have expertise in the fields of pharmacology, nursing, the behavioral sciences, law, the methodology of scientific research, and ethics"—and could recognize only those local committees which "in any case consist of one or more physicians and of persons who have expertise in the field of law, the methodology of scientific research, and ethics."[60] Hence, the proposal made no room for "society representatives" or for laypeople in general.

Most political parties in the Dutch parliament objected to this exclusion. The Labor Party argued that it robbed the bill of its social basis, the Green Party argued that the position of the research subject needed strengthening, while the Conservative-Liberal Party felt that a patient representative had to take part to ensure the interests of this group.[61] The Orthodox Protestant Party, in turn, stated that lay representation was "needed to take the diversity of ethical views in society into account," a concern which was voiced by the reformed parties and Christian-Democrats as well (collectively, these four confessional parties took up about 25 percent of the Dutch House of Representatives).[62]

In her reply, Borst admitted that she did not see much use for the participation of laypeople. First of all, she argued, anyone taking part in the review of scientific research could only ever contribute in a meaningful way if they had a deep enough understanding of the protocol under review. Yet, in order to do so, reviewers needed so much expertise that it was questionable whether they were really laypeople anymore.[63] Secondly, if laypeople participated in order to represent interest groups such as patients or research subjects, they would undermine "the independent assessment of a research protocol" and increase the danger that "personal or commercial interests [would] influence the assessment of protocols."[64] Thirdly, Borst considered it redundant to let laypeople participate to ensure that "opinions from outside medical circles are expressed" or that "reviewers do not start to identify with researchers." The need to counteract the dominance of researchers, she argued, was already fulfilled by the contribution of "experts on the terrain of law, research methodology, and ethics."[65] Hence, she was inclined to dismiss the whole issue of lay representation.

Members of parliament, however, were not so easily persuaded, and they used their right of amendment to propose that the WMO should mandate that at least one member of the Dutch Patient-Consumer Federation participated on each committee.[66] These representatives did have a specific type of expertise, the members argued, as they were experts in being patients and research subjects, roles that comprised an essential piece of the jigsaw puzzle that made up the review of human experimentation in medicine. Borst was not convinced, as she felt a nurse also possessed this type of expertise, but she was willing to meet parliament halfway: she would not change the bill to include a lay representative, but she would add the stipulation that all committees had to appoint one person "to specifically review scientific research

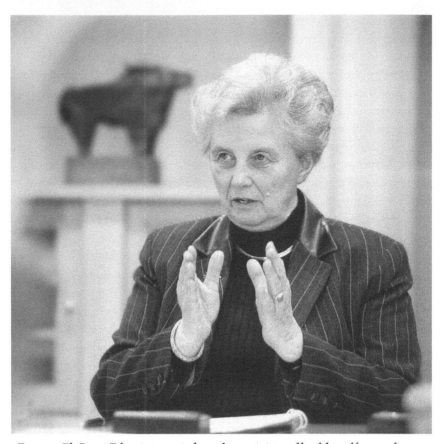

Figure 5. Els Borst-Eilers in 2000, in her role as minister of health, welfare, and sport. Photograph by Bart Versteeg.

from the perspective of research subjects."[67] This person could be a nurse, patient representative, or someone else—as long as they took part in order to watch over the position of research subjects, not to represent an interest group. With this concession, and its acceptance by parliament, the "society representative" of the 1970s saw its definitive departure.

The Fulcrum Function of the Ethical Expert

Of course, this inclusion did not address the objection that the committees should also fairly represent the diverse ethical and ideological viewpoints in Dutch society. Borst, however, had a different solution for this concern. In reply to the questions posed by the Christian parties, she pointed to the requirement in the bill that someone "with expertise in the field of ethics" would take up a committee seat. "From this person it should be expected," she explained, "that he in particular will make visible which visions and arguments exist with regard to a specific subject in our pluralistic society."[68] Not all members of parliament were immediately convinced. "It is a bit unclear why an ethicist should have a seat," the Protestant politician André Rouvoet remarked, "if he only serves to clarify what attitudes exist in society with regard to a particular subject." "Why should an ethicist do this and not a social scientist, for example?" Rouvoet continued. "It seems to me, that if you ask an ethicist, he brings along his own opinion."[69] "You have ethicists in all sorts of shapes and sizes," a politician from another reformed party remarked. "That does not detract from their scientific quality, but it says precious little about how representative they are."[70]

In part, the confessional parties pressed this hard on the position of ethicists because the Dutch parliament was simultaneously debating the composition of the ethics committees that would be installed if Borst's euthanasia law were to go into effect. The idea was that these committees would also include an ethicist, something about which the confessional parties were skeptical, as most felt that euthanasia could under no circumstances be considered ethical. So it mattered quite a bit what type of ethicist would be asked to take up a committee seat. In these related debates, Borst said of the role of the ethicist:

> A good ethicist is trained in careful reasoning and clear analysis [...]. That is his contribution. If you have a strong personal opinion which prevents you from ever considering pros and cons, you should not take up a seat in such a committee. And otherwise you must at times also be sure to take away from your own feelings and personal beliefs and just make an objective judgment.[71]

Hence, Borst envisioned ethical experts as analysts, able to weigh the opinions of others in a careful and objective manner and to offer clarification and consistent lines of reasoning. As such, they made committee deliberations more rational (logical) and therewith more reasonable (fair, sensible). In addition, Borst maintained that "a good ethicist" was able to bring together different types of experts with different types of temperaments:

> During my time at the Health Council, I have always benefited greatly from the presence of ethicists in committees. They were the people who, when it comes to thinking lucidly [...] were often the strongest committee members. A legal scholar argues very carefully and formally, while a doctor often argues with quite a lot of emotion. In those instances, an ethicist was clearly the neutralizing factor.[72]

Borst's ethicists, in other words, helped to make deliberations more humane without becoming overly emotional, and excelled in navigating difficult discussions through troubled waters. They did not offer strong moral opinions themselves, but mediated those of others, allowing people with conflicting viewpoints to reach harmonious decisions.

This conception of ethicists' potential contribution to euthanasia committees could easily have been transported to their role in research ethics committees as well. Borst never did so, however, for reasons that remain unclear. In the 1980s and early 1990s, the participation of ethicists in research ethics governance had mostly been accepted as self-evident. Both the 1981 Health Council advice and the 1982 Central Council report had recommended the inclusion of ethicists without much explanation, although the Central Council did speak interchangeably of the need for either an ethicist or a pastor. And while it was not the case that all the committees established in the 1980s seated ethicists, the suggestion that ethics review might also take place without ethicists was never actively questioned in these years.[73] Hence, the sobering truth may well be that Borst's department never really thought through the role of the ethicist until it was pressured to defend the notion in parliament, with the euthanasia debates taking place just after those on the human experimentation bill.

Dutch statespersons did at times, however, use the inclusion of ethicists strategically. In 1992, for instance, the state secretary then responsible for the human experimentation bill was already using the requirement of ethical expertise to counter questions in parliament about lay representation. The latter was not needed, he argued, as "it may be expected especially from the ethicist [that he will] take an approach from the perspective of protecting the research subject."[74] When this argument met with loud protest, however, as ethical expertise was argued to differ from lay representation, the state secretary just as easily dropped discussion of this function in subsequent memorandums and debates.[75] Borst, likewise, at times maintained that "a good ethicist" was defined by the ability to "just make an objective judgement," while she at other times stressed that ethicists had varying ideological and religious backgrounds that influenced the way in which they reviewed research protocols. She did so, for instance, in the solution she devised to pacify the unrest over research with incapacitated individuals. The WMO, she promised, would require that such studies take place only if permission had first been acquired by the central committee, which would include "ethicists from diverse ideological and religious backgrounds."[76]

Hence, when it came to the evaluation of socially contentious research studies, it suddenly *was* desirable to base one's judgement on the sociocultural background one represented—the sort of membership that Borst had explicitly rejected in debates over the participation of laypeople. And while she stated emphatically on other occasions that a good ethicist "takes away his own feelings and personal beliefs," these personal beliefs now served as an eligibility requirement for ethicists to participate in the central committee. Still, as they were experts, they were expected to do all this in an independent and objective manner. Ethicists did not represent interest groups; they presented the viewpoints of various social groups. In doing so, they acted as the fulcrum that balanced democratic governance with expert control—an apparently ideal solution for the public governance of a scientific practice in a pluralistic society, as it allowed the practice to be regulated without the participation of the unruly "all and sundry."

The Political Struggle to Deal with Ethical Issues

Ethicists who have known and worked with Els Borst maintain that it is quite plausible that her portrayal of the ethicist as a neutral mediator was nothing more than a strategy to guide the WMO and euthanasia act through parliament. Yet at the core of these debates did lie a fundamental question, i.e., that of "how a democratic polity should reason together about morally and technically complex questions."[77] This question, formulated by Benjamin Hurlbut in his 2017 book *Experiments in Democracy*, is one of the core questions that has dominated political thinking in technically advanced democracies in the late twentieth century. Depending on the country, different answers have been found. Even though research ethics committees today have become a worldwide phenomenon, for instance, those who may participate in them continue to differ by country.[78]

Bioethicists, of course, have increasingly claimed a seat at the table in the public deliberation of such "morally and technically complex questions"— a development that, as the previous chapter has argued, is closely connected to the demise of more-traditional moral authorities in the second half of the twentieth century. Yet this historical perspective, which focuses on the waxing and waning of professional authority from the perspective of academic disciplines, only tells half of the story. What we need in addition is a better appreciation of the wider cultural and political context that facilitates such jurisdictional claims of academic expertise. Why was it, as Hurlbut notes, that bioethics in the late twentieth century became an "important new element in the repertoire of democratic governance"?[79]

According to Wilson, the success of British bioethics in the 1980s neatly "dovetailed with the Conservative government's neo-liberal belief that professions should be exposed to outside scrutiny to make them publicly accountable" and, later, with New Labour's similar enthusiasm for public oversight and "empowered consumers."[80] John Evans similarly links the success of the American bioethics movement to a changing political climate in the 1980s and 1990s: its dominant intellectual framework, i.e., common morality principlism, should be understood in the context of growing state intervention in ethics. According to Evans, the political appeal of this framework was twofold: "First, government authority in Western liberal democracies such as the United States needs to be transparent to the citizens. Second, this government is bureaucratic."[81] Thus, on the one hand, the suggestion that a moral lingua franca could be formulated for a pluralistic society offered the allure of inclusivity and openness: "the public can feel it understands the decision being made on its behalf, giving the decision legitimacy."[82] Yet at the same time, the wealth of guidelines and procedures that have come to be associated with bioethics was desirable from a bureaucratic perspective—an argument similar to that made by Dutch philosopher Gerard de Vries in 1993.[83]

In the Netherlands as well, the rise of health ethics was closely related to growing government attention in the late twentieth century to the ethics of medicine and science. In 1988, the same year the first Dutch textbook for health ethics was published, a government report on "the limits of care" included a short, but intriguing statement: "Ethics," page 15 announced matter-of-factly, "is in."[84] The report was part of a series of policy reports on Dutch health care and listed five boundaries the state would have to deal with in the coming years.[85] The second was the "boundary between what may and what may not be considered ethically permissible."[86] Because individuals increasingly occupied a central place in society, page 15 read, and because new technologies made all sorts of health interventions possible, "the interest in medical ethics, or better put health ethics, is growing." "Ethical reflection [...] on what is good and evil, on what is permitted and what is unacceptable [...] can rejoice in growing public and political attention."[87] Ethics, in the Netherlands, was *en vogue*.

Page 15 also noted a second development. Despite the individualization of society, "it is becoming increasingly clear that it is a task for all of us, and then particularly for the government, to weigh the interests of groups of patients against each other." The state, it seemed, was increasingly called upon to take a hands-on approach in the governance of ethically contentious issues in medicine and science. In the past, the report explained, the government had often refrained from taking a stance on such issues, thereby endlessly postponing the development of public policy. But while "this sometimes seems morally defensible, it can also lead to ill-fated compromises or more seriously to indecisiveness, hidden selections, or veiled priorities."[88] The government was determined, therefore, to take a more active stance in the public governance of health ethics.

In January 1988, the Ministry of Welfare, Health, and Culture had already sent a memo to parliament with "an inventory of medical-ethical themes" and a discussion of the role of the government.[89] More and more often, the document explained, the question was asked whether the far-reaching technical possibilities in medicine did justice to the interests of patients, and those of society more generally. Protecting these interests was an important duty for a government—hence, the memo. Still, the ministry did not have any concrete policy measures to handle these concerns. Instead, it would confine itself to "closely following the advancing medical technology" and "to introduce legislation and regulation" only when needed, thereby ensuring that enough room would be left to the "self-regulating activities of the profession." The Dutch government in the 1980s was still a government operating under the motto "more market, less government."

At the time, this conclusion provoked a disappointed response in the Dutch parliament. One member of the Christian-Democratic Party, for instance, strongly disagreed that the time was not yet ripe for government policy and stated that he did not believe in "the self-regulating activities of the profession." A member of the Orthodox Protestant Party, meanwhile, declared that the memo proved the absolute impotence of the government in dealing with medical ethics. Unanimously, the Dutch parliament pressed the Ministry of Health to "provide guidelines and set borders," an issue they kept on addressing in the months thereafter.[90]

In 1989, the Christian-Democrats raised the issue again. Matters of ethical concern in health care, they argued, were now only discussed in local ethics committees and often only reactively, when problems had already been exacerbated and needed immediate resolution. "We call this laundering after the fact. It is practicing ethics on an incidental basis." Instead of "being a slave to such developments," the government had to actively anticipate them. "Medical technology should not determine ethics, it should be the other way around."[91] A few months later, the conservative-liberals voiced the same concern: "Scientific developments are now going so fast that politics is constantly behind the times." A permanent state council had to be established, therefore, to "keep a finger on the pulse" and to allow the government to react immediately when necessary.[92]

In all of these calls, the need for state interference was justified along two familiar lines. One, the speed and ferocity with which new techno-scientific developments announced themselves demanded government attention, as they presented large and unprecedented ethical problems to society. Two, in a pluralistic and increasingly secular democracy, older authorities and structures for handling such problems—such as the Church, professions, or the famous pillars that had organized Dutch society along ideological-religious lines until the 1960s—could no longer offer solutions that would be accepted by the majority of the population.[93] Instead, citizens now looked to the state to settle ethical conflicts via official regulations, a role which consecutive Dutch governments increasingly felt compelled to take up in the 1980s and 1990s, despite the growing popularity of liberal and market-based approaches to the governance of health care, the sciences, and other sectors.[94]

The million-dollar question was, however, *how* the government could take on this role. In 1988, the Ministry of Health proposed to have the Health Council regularly inform parliament about new developments in medicine and ethics. The Standing Committee for Health Ethics, the memo argued, "concerns itself with continuous reflection on the ethical and juridical aspects of medical developments" and could thus conduct crucial "pre-work" in ethical thinking about medicine and health.[95] The government would then only take an official position *after* the reports of this committee had been debated in parliament.[96]

Not everyone in the Dutch parliament, however, responded well to this proposal. If the Health Council were to take on this role, the Christian-Democrats maintained, the Standing Committee for Health Ethics really had to include laypeople.[97] After all, a committee consisting only of experts could not draw up reports on ethical dilemmas that included the opinions of all social groups. Similarly, two Protestant parties expressed concern that the expert composition of the Health Council did not do justice to the various religious and ideological viewpoints in Dutch society.[98] The conservative-liberal party VVD, in turn, objected that the power to make ethical decisions should ultimately be left to politicians, not experts.[99]

The concern that an expert body like the Health Council might hamper democratic decision-making was voiced repeatedly in the late 1980s and early 1990s. In 1990, for instance, the sociologist Pim Fortuyn, who would later become an ardent critic of the Purple Coalitions and one of the most (in)famous politicians the Netherlands has ever known, pointed out in a policy report on the functioning of public advisory bodies that the Health Council had increasingly started to publish ethical opinions in recent years—something that it did not have a mandate to do.[100] Similar concerns were voiced in parliament. In 1991, during a debate on "the ethical aspects of scientific and technological research," the Christian-Democrats complained that the Health Council's role meant, in effect, that the initial framing of issues of medical-ethical concern often took place behind closed doors, by a small circuit of insiders who frequently participated on the same committees and who proposed similar solutions each time, to the detriment of broader societal and political debate.[101] The left-wing Labor Party agreed. Citing Achterhuis and Van Tongeren, its representative pondered, "How do we prevent that discussions are only held by 'experts'? By experts, I think first of all of so-called ethicists."[102] These experts typically had a "narrow understanding of ethics" that was too easily used to justify new developments and explain away societal concerns. "I think we should prevent ethics committees from functioning in such a way that they legitimize research just because some people have looked at it," the representative continued. "As Achterhuis says, these committees too often function as a problematic buffer between the controversial practices of scientists and societal critiques."[103]

Philosophers like Achterhuis, Van Tongeren, and De Vries were popular among Dutch politicians in the early 1990s.[104] The government had to prevent ethics from being used as "a greaser to get society to accept [scientific] insights," the minister of education, culture, and sciences comforted parliament in 1991. Scientific studies always had to be "socially and humanly relevant" and possible ethical concerns had to be considered in a broad societal setting before a study could be executed, not when its outcomes were forced upon society as a fait accompli.[105] To achieve these ends, the influence of citizens had to be increased and expert opinions minimized. Hence, if philosophers such as Achterhuis had one influence on Dutch politics in the early 1990s, it was that any form of expert interference with "policy and ethics" came to be eyed with suspicion (not just a *specific* academic approach to ethics). As conservative-liberal senator Dian van Leeuwen-Schut said sharply in 1993, citing De Vries: "Ethicists are intellectuals, not policymakers. Political decisions have to be made in the political arena. [...] It cannot be the case that ethicists tell policymakers already at the start of the ride what decisions have to be reached."[106]

Still, these critical views on the political role of ethicists were not shared by all politicians and policymakers, especially not as the decade progressed. In 1991, for instance, the soon-to-be minister of health Els Borst voiced a rather different point of view. Borst, who was at the time vice president of the Health Council, strongly disagreed that the advisory body should refrain from including ethical opinions in its reports. Of course, she wrote, a scientific advisory body could never have the last word on ethically contentious issues. This had to be left to elected officials. The problem was, however, that "many debates in the Netherlands about the ethical aspects of gene therapy, embryo research, and prenatal diagnostics are neither here nor there because participants do not have the right facts." The input of experts was needed, therefore, she argued, as "ignorance and intense emotions just are not good ingredients to reach a meaningful moral consensus." This argument did not just hold for the technical side of new biomedical developments: "For good debates in- and outside of parliament [. . .] some preliminary work in the field of health ethics (and law) is indispensable as well." Ethical experts, Borst maintained, were capable of raising the level of debate by offering termino-logical clarity and mapping moral problems. In doing so, they created "the possibility for well-informed societal discussions and a proper consideration by government and parliament."[107]

In 1993, a similar viewpoint was articulated by a senior policy official at the Ministry of Welfare, Public Health, and Culture, in an article on ethical issues and public policy. "Ethics," this official wrote, "is not just practiced by ethicists, but by everyone who concerns himself with these sorts of issues. Ethics is thus also practiced by policy officials and politicians." Nonetheless, she added quickly, "The ethics practiced by these individuals, who are usu-ally laypeople, would soon get bogged down if they were not to be assisted by professional ethicists, who have the tools needed to investigate moral issues in a way that systematic reflection truly takes place and that substanti-ated policy choices become possible."[108] At the Ministry of Welfare, Public Health, and Culture, this insight increasingly prevailed. The state secretary, for instance, had started to organize meetings in which policy officials dis-cussed ethical issues; these meetings were led by professional ethicists. In addition, officials were encouraged to stay in close contact with ethicists at seminars, in the hallways at conferences, and in government advisory bod-ies. A new idea, the policy official continued, was to also start hiring ethicists as government officials. "The ethicist," she concluded enthusiastically, citing Van Willigenburg, "facilitates the policymaker, as it were."[109]

That same year, the state secretary himself also suggested that, despite the unpopularity of ethicists among politicians, good reasons existed to include them in policymaking. In reply to the demand of Van Leeuwen-Schut that the role of ethicists in policy circles be immediately rolled back, the state sec-retary stated in parliament:

In itself, this [demand] is correct, but a surprising development has occurred. In the domain of government control we aspire to a smaller role for the government and for good reasons. [. . .] Yet in the domain of medical ethics we are witnessing an opposite trend. As medical tech-nologies and their implications grow, a sharper need crops up for legis-lation in the medical ethics domain.[110]

While this response does not directly address the criticism levied by van Leeuwen-Schut, it provides a clue as to why statespersons would be interested in including ethicists in policy. In a time when the government was increasingly being called upon to resolve ethical issues, to seek input from those who concerned themselves professionally with such issues became an alluring route, even if doing so went against the grain of popular opinion. This, at least, was the suspicion of Labor politician Joop van den Berg, who remarked in a 1993 article on the "place and task of parliament in ethical discussions" that the Dutch political system just was not historically equipped to deal with difficult ethical issues. For most of the twentieth century, the country had been separated politically and socially into its infamous pillars: Catholicism, Protestantism, socialism, and liberalism. Each pillar had had its own social institutions, and politics had been dominated by the idea of "sphere sovereignty": each pillar was ruled by its own authorities as much as possible. Hence, Van den Berg continued, "in the age of pillarization [...] a culture of decision-making [was] developed with an interest in restricting the political agenda. [...] To ensure its stability and acceptance, the political arena [had done] best to abstain from highly charged normative issues."[111] Ethical issues that ran across pillars preferably had not been discussed in parliament at all, and in instances where such discussion really could not be avoided, experts had been called in to prepare a position that the government could adopt. This approach had allowed politicians to defend decisions by deferring to expert opinions rather than ideological arguments and to thereby depoliticize the treatment of ethical issues. Despite the recent de-pillarization of Dutch society, Van den Berg concluded, this pacifying approach to policymaking had remained popular. Dutch politicians just did not know how to handle ethical issues any other way.[112]

The Use of Ethical Expertise in Liberal Democracies

Van den Berg's analysis—which assumes some sort of immaterial collective psychology to underlie Dutch politics—is difficult to ascertain from concrete historical sources. What is true, however, is that the Netherlands is famous for its *polder model*, a consensus-based approach to policymaking. Stemming from the suggestion that people in the Low Lands have always had to "cooperate despite differences" to ward off the ever-present threat of the sea, the term polder model points to the idea that, as long as all parties are heard, pragmatic policy solutions can be found that may be supported by everyone involved, even if participants would not have come up with the same solutions individually. The polder model flourished in particular in the 1990s under the Purple Coalitions of Wim Kok, which favored a managerial approach to government: i.e., rather than developing policy with a specific ideology in mind, the government had to take a businesslike approach to steering societal processes. Policy decisions had to follow from pragmatic consideration of the situation at hand, not from pushing political interests.[113] Internationally, this approach became popular in the late 1990s as the "Third Way": an approach to politics, advocated by leaders such as Bill Clinton and Tony Blair, that tried to reconcile right-wing and left-wing ideologies and move beyond traditional political fault lines in liberal democracies.[114] As Clinton famously said of Kok at a 1999 Washington conference on the Third Way phenomenon: "He was doing it all before we were."[115]

Experts fulfilled a key role in this political philosophy: rather than representing the interests of specific groups, they would be trained to analyze problems objectively and to present public policies neutrally to those responsible for them. This, certainly, was the philosophy of Els Borst's party D66, which had been founded in the 1960s as a pragmatic alternative to religious-ideological approaches to politics. Public policy, this party maintained, should be problem-based (i.e., they should follow from a consideration of specific problems) and had to be justified with reasonable rather than religious-ideological arguments. While D66 defended a direct approach to democratic decision-making, this conviction went hand in hand with a belief in the enlightening impact of education and expertise: as long as citizens were well-informed, they could be expected to make reasonable choices when called upon to do so.[116]

Hence, despite the critical attitude of Dutch politicians toward ethical experts in parliament, four Dutch ministries were found willing in the 1990s to cofinance a "stimulation program for policy-relevant ethical research" that had academics helping to develop policies for "the many large and unprecedented ethical problems" faced by society in an era of swift technological advancement.[117] With a budget of over ƒ9 million, this program subsidized sixty-seven "ethics and policy projects," giving a swath of young scholars the opportunity to obtain PhDs in ethics.[118] Although it offered funding for both fundamental and applied ethics studies, the latter proved much more popular, as it was more likely to engage with concrete policy questions. According to one of the program directors, this measure had the effect that the applied ethics field in particular grew in the Netherlands in the 1990s, in contrast to the hermeneutic approach advocated by philosophers.[119]

The same went for the various ethics committees that were established by the Purple Coalitions for the public oversight of ethically contentious issues in medicine and science. All required the inclusion of people with appropriate ethical expertise. Today, seventeen research ethics committees, five euthanasia committees, and about twenty-five animal research committees are active in the Netherlands.[120] Since 2014, the central committee overseeing the local research ethics committees has also stipulated that ethicists may participate in ethics review only if they hold degrees in theology, philosophy, humanism, or ethics; have "demonstrable knowledge of health ethics, proven by a dissertation and relevant recent publications in peer reviewed journals"; and have at least three years of work experience in health ethics in the five years leading up to their participation on a committee.[121] Hence, Dutch public policy now guarantees professional ethicists a spot in the public regulation of a number of highly ethically contentious medical (research) practices—an honor quite exceptional for a humanities discipline. This guarantee not only ensures that the expertise of ethicists is brought to bear in discussing difficult ethical cases, it also provides a strong incentive for medical (research) centers to hire ethicists to support their medical and scientific staff.

These public policies favor a specific type of ethical expertise. While none of them mentions what specific type of ethical expertise is suitable for people participating in ethics committees, the institutional function of these bodies is a better fit for the applied ethicist than for the hermeneutic philosopher. The ethical evaluation of human research protocols, for instance, focuses on the protection of research subjects within the confines of the Dutch law. Thus, committees are in principle not permitted to reject studies because they would unjustly profit Big Pharma or harm the environment.[122] As Van Willigenburg put it in 1991: "The task that the ethical consultant takes up sometimes excludes certain forms of criticism."[123] Yet this was precisely why scholars like Van Tongeren and Ten Have had been convinced that ethicists should not take up a seat on (research) ethics committees. For ethicists unwilling to accept the role of consultant, in other words, not much of a role is left in these public review bodies. In that sense, De Vries was right in 1993, that rather than health ethics having disciplined the *medical* field, the bureaucratization of medicine contributed to disciplining the *ethics* field.

In the last decades, this type of criticism has frequently been launched at the health ethics and bioethics professions, by both scientific researchers and humanities scholars. When scientists make themselves heard, it is often to complain that ethicists needlessly halt scientific progress with their obsession over rigid principles and red tape. Humanities scholars, on the other hand, have continued to state that health ethics and bioethics predominantly function as greasers for techno-scientific machineries. In recent years, as I laid out in the introduction to this book, this criticism has also become popular among historians, who claim that research ethics committees are an example of how bioethics shields the biomedical research establishment from harsh societal critiques.

However, for the history of Dutch ethics review at least, it is doubtful how much truth there is to this finger pointing. For one thing, as previous chapters have shown, it royally overplays the involvement of ethicists in the realization of research ethics committees. For another, it attributes much more power to ethicists than they have ever had in the oversight of human experimentation in the Netherlands. To this day, ethicists remain just one voice among a larger group of experts, of which the vast majority still come from the biomedical sciences. Moreover, quite a few health ethicists themselves have been very critical of the institutional functioning of ethics committees. In 2001, for instance, Heleen Dupuis, famous doyenne of the Dutch health ethics movement, cried out that Dutch ethics committees had turned into "bureaucratic straightjackets" in which moral pathos was replaced by "managerial arrogance and a mania for organization."[124] While she meant something different by this criticism than De Vries had when he argued that the bureaucratization of medicine produced ethicists who did not have to think anymore, both critics shared an uneasiness over the standardization of ethical discourse in ethics review.

Most importantly, the narrow focus on professional ethics ignores the role of the government in bringing about this "ethics bureaucracy." In 1982, in the Netherlands, the Central Council for Public Health had preferred to speak of the *ethical* evaluation of medical research, as the stipulation of too-detailed *legal* norms might stifle a practice that was continuously developing. It was perfectly fine to include laypeople in this process, as long as they acted "reasonable" and were accompanied by experts with a thorough understanding of the studies under examination. Yet over the course of the 1980s, voices began to argue that only legal rules and expert judgement could ensure uniform decision-making. If the government wanted to exercise proper control, it had to be crystal clear as to what was and was not permissible. Without exception, all Dutch governments in the late twentieth century favored this approach: whereas professionals could be expected to consistently assess protocols according to agreed-upon rules, laypeople—the unruly "all and sundry"—would infuse unpredictable and thus uncontrollable elements into the review process.

In adopting this policy perspective, the Dutch government never gave a substantial defense of why ethicists should be included in the evaluation of human research studies. Only when it became clear that parliament would not pass the WMO without an assurance that the plurality of societal viewpoints would be brought to bear in ethics review, were ethicists brought onto the stage as "obvious mediators" between expert and democratic governance. In making this claim, the Dutch government made eager use of a specific approach to ethical reflection that had become popular in the 1980s, and actively chose one way of knowing in the ethics discipline above others. But in reality, it more than anything else paid lip service to the applied ethics tradition. Ethicists who now take up seats on Dutch research ethics committees remain, even if they want to, hardly able to fulfill the once-imagined role of "luminaries" who speak the moral lingua franca of a pluralistic society. For only their physical presence was ensured in 1999 by the WMO—by a government that had a specific use for ethicists in a time when citizens were increasingly looking to the state to resolve ethical issues, and that wanted to claim democratic control over a scientific practice without actually needing to let these citizens actively participate in its governance.

CONCLUSION

On the evening of July 22, 1964, the American comedy writer Allan Sher-man performed his new song parody of Prokofiev's "Peter and the Wolf" for a buoyant audience at Boston's Tanglewood Music Center. The parody relates the story of the young composer Peter, who has just finished creating a beautiful new melody, but who, as a resident of communist Russia, needs to have it approved by the commissars of music prior to its release. The com-missars, who of course all lack Peter's talent, demand his song be changed to sound more like existing tunes: Tchaikovsky's Swan Lake, Beethoven's Fifth Symphony, Brahms's "Lullaby." After a while, Peter slinks off, battered and disillusioned, with a song stamped "not approved" and time in the clink to rethink his sins. Luckily, all turns out well in the end, as a savvy recording-company owner hears Peter whistling his song, recognizes its potential, and thence, "in spite of the number one Chief Commissar, Peter [became] big-ger than Ringo Starr."

Since 1964, "Peter and the Commissar" has gained fame as a celebration of American individualism and free-market capitalism that reigned supreme during the Cold War. Yet as Sherman also rhymes, "Now the Commissar in this story is Russia, but that is just for purposes of discussion. One finds this type no matter where one lives, we call them junior executives." For the thing is, the comedy writer maintains:

> [...] These people on committees, they sit there all day
> And they each put in a color, and it comes out grey
> Grey is a nice color, but not if you have ever seen
> Orange or red or yellow or blue or green
> And we have all heard the saying, which is true as well as witty
> That a camel is a horse that was designed by a committee.[1]

Today, the saying "[design] by committee" has gained general usage in the English language to refer to a defective trait of bureaucratic decision-making: a lack of vision and originality that would stifle innovation. In the sciences, certainly, this practice of "new Marxism" has often been argued to inhibit any form of "true progress."[2]

Objectivity in Ethics Review: A Fickle History

In 1998, to convince the Dutch parliament of her vision for ethics review, Els Borst stated confidently that an orderly review system could be realized as long as reviewers "just [made] an objective judgement." This statement harbors the belief that ethical decision-making in medicine and science can proceed almost scientifically itself: i.e., as long as certain experts are brought in and certain methods are followed, objective judgements can surely be reached. Yet historians of science know objectivity to be a fickle concept, one that has not always dominated conversations of how knowledge is acquired or judgement is passed, and that, even since it has achieved dominance has nevertheless still been subject to change through time and space.[3] In the history described in this book, the pattern is no different. In every instance in which ethics review was proposed as a suitable tool for the oversight of human experimentation, objectivity played a crucial role—in that only those people considered capable of passing an objective judgement on the permissibility of protocols could participate in their review. But what it meant to pass an objective judgement, and who could reasonably be expected to pass it, shifted substantially in the latter half of the twentieth century, with strong implications for the forms of oversight that were felt appropriate for human experimentation.

Originally, in the 1950s, when ethics review was first proposed in the Netherlands, the communal review of tests upon human beings was meant to alleviate two concerns about the ability of physicians to objectively assess the permissibility of these studies. The first was a moral concern: due to a growing pressure for physicians to advance their careers with scientific research, the temptations to engage in tests that did not primarily benefit the wellbeing of patients were becoming too strong. The individual physician came to be thought of as too involved to be able to *impartially*—and thus objectively—determine whether risky interventions could be justified. The second was an epistemic concern: due to the growing specialization of medical knowledge, it had to be doubted whether the average physician was still capable of conducting studies that would truly bring about medical progress. This concern, under the banner "only good science is ethical science," was understood to be a moral one as well. Peripheral members of the medical profession increasingly had to be considered incapable of *accurately*—and thus objectively—assessing the scientific value of medical research studies. Together, this layered mistrust in the capacities of individual researchers led to the formulation of a need to install committees that would seat experts who were not directly involved in the study under review, but who were still competent enough to determine its scientific worth.

That these expert reviewers had to be impartial with regard to the study under consideration did not mean at the time that they also had to be socially or physically distant from the research setting. Erik Noach, in fact, in all his thinking about research ethics committees in the 1960s and 1970s, repeatedly emphasized that it was essential for reviewers to be intimately familiar with the local context in which an experiment was conducted: only this closeness allowed them to truly assess whether a researcher had the right motives for a study and whether the right facilities were in place for the study to proceed responsibly. Only immersion, in short, enabled an *informed*—and thus objective—assessment of the permissibility of an experiment.

In the 1980s, however, with the mushrooming of research ethics committees in the Netherlands, this notion came under pressure. Increasingly, individual committees came to be eyed with suspicion. After all, how could those who *were* physically distant from the research setting ascertain whether local committees were actually impartial and accurate in reviewing protocols? "Variation and inconsistency," as legal scholar Lucas Bergkamp worded this suspicion in 1989, were the biggest problems that Dutch ethics review had to deal with. Only standardized procedures could squash these individual idiosyncrasies, and only standardization would ensure a *consistent*—and thus objective—assessment of research protocols.

Initially, these new objectivities were primarily intended to overcome drawbacks of the growth of the medical science system in the twentieth century: the increase of scale had undermined older rules of trust in determining whether an individual researcher or local group of reviewers were impartial and accurate. Distance and unfamiliarity between parties resulted in new ways to assess researchers'—and later reviewers'—ability to be objective and thus new modes to govern their conduct. Communal structures and procedures were hoped to enable this strengthening of internal control.[4] Yet in this same period, key changes took place in the broader societal appraisal of the medical science as well, and soon ethics review became imbued with another register of objectivities that served to assert external control over medical research.

In the 1950s, still, only members of an *artsenstand* free from state interference had been argued capable of reaching *uncorrupted*—and thus objective—judgements about the permissibility of medical tests upon humans. By the 1970s, however, the trained judgement of the medical in-group had come to be suspected to muddy rather than to clarify the vision of physicians. In effect, ethics review was reimagined as a public control mechanism that had to be wielded by ordinary citizens—as only they were truly uncorrupted and thus able to render objective judgements—to realize participatory decision-making structures in health care.

Yet this notion of objectivity did not last either. In the 1980s, laypeople themselves became an object of distrust, not only because they were believed not to understand enough of science to pass informed judgements upon it, but also because each of them were perceived to represent just one of many opinions in a pluralistic society, making participation by only a few of them haphazard and circumspect. Hence, ethics review had to become devoid of all perspectives—*aperspectival*, as it were—and thereby more objective.[5]

In Dutch policy circles in the late twentieth century, this political desire to realize aperspectival review procedures for the conduct of human experimentation was wed to the earlier notion that *consistent* review procedures were needed to ensure objective decision-making. As long as reviewers were capable of parting with their own personal beliefs to place themselves in the point of view required by the review process—i.e., "to just make an objective judgement"—they would succeed in consistently applying the carefully designed procedures for the adequate assessment of protocols, which would in turn enable a full escape from perspective. In other words, regardless of the colors put in by the people on committees, the end result would turn out grey—which was exactly what was needed to ascertain that decision-making about ethical issues proceeded impartially and democratically. If reviewers just followed procedure, no social group or moral perspective would unduly profit from the public governance of human experimentation in a pluralistic society.

This conception of ethical decision-making permitted the Dutch government in the late twentieth century to kill two birds with one stone. On the one hand, it enabled the state to assert that it did not leave medical researchers to their own devices—an autonomy that they had proven incapable of handling, was irresponsible with regard to the amount of power they held, and did not befit a democratic order anyway. Physicians and scientists would have to learn to accept that they did not only have to justify their actions to colleagues and perhaps patients, but to the general public, by means of the government, as well. Yet at the same time, the suggestion that this public scrutiny would proceed *objectively* enabled the government to assert that it infringed neither upon personal beliefs in a pluralistic society nor upon the freedom of inquiry that befitted an open society. After all, any state had to avoid acting as a "master of morality," as the boundaries between democratic and dictatorial governance were notoriously fluid. Hence, ethics review was not about bringing researchers under societal control, just about holding them publicly accountable. Researchers would have to submit protocols to publicly authorized review bodies, but the decision of whether these protocols could be executed would not result from unruly deliberations but from a fair application of uniform procedures by appointed administrators. The government itself, in fact, was to refrain from any further interference in the practice. Decisions were to be made only by *neutral*—and thus objective—reviewers.

Ethics in the Governance of Medical Science

As part of these transformations, two related changes took place in the way in which ethics was understood to function in the governance of medical science. First, the *locus* of ethical authority changed. In the 1950s, still, the vocational identity of the *artsenstand* reigned supreme in Dutch discussions of medical ethics. Medical-ethical expertise, the argument went, was *tacit* and only acquired via full immersion in the discipline: only members of the in-group possessed the honed moral compass needed to sense what was ethically just in medicine.[6] From this self-professed epistemic ideal, it followed that the governance of medicine was also first and foremost a professional affair. As only the lived experience of a physician conferred an understanding of the ethically right thing to do in medicine, the input of outsiders was potentially dangerous. In the 1960s and 1970s, the ideal of exclusive professional objectivity came under attack. By virtue of being a thinking subject, the mantra now became, every conscious individual had access to (medical) ethics. The professional identity of physicians, in fact, would be an obstacle to them in grasping the ethically right thing to do in medicine.

In the 1980s and 1990s, new epistemic ideals were formulated that aimed to do away with *all* perspectival views on morality. The idea became popular that more-objective moral decisions could be reached via "an escape from perspective." This moral lingua franca—or "view from nowhere," as Thomas Nagel once put it—would ensure more impersonal and therefore more objective decision-making in a pluralistic society.[7] Ironically, on the back of this new ideal, the locus of attributed ethical authority again changed in the Netherlands in the 1980s and 1990s—at least in policy circles concerned with the governance of medical research involving humans. Even if a moral lingua franca could be formulated for a pluralist society, the argument now became, some people could be expected to master this language better than others. A new notion of disciplinary objectivity arose, one in which the ethical viewpoints of professional ethicists were taken to be more trustworthy than those of laypeople. Even though elected officials were said to remain responsible for ethical decisions at the level of government, they could be expected to make more rational decisions with the help of ethical luminaries.

Often, this first change in the way that ethics was understood to function in the governance of medicine is explained by, and justified with reference to, the changing societal role of medicine and science in the second half of the twentieth century. In an age of growing medical powers and egalitarian social structures, the once-uncontrolled freedom of medical researchers to do as they please had to be reeled in. Yet around roughly the same time, a second change in the governing function of medical ethics was realized that seemingly had the opposite effect: after World War II, the existing Dutch medical ethics discourse was actively adapted to accommodate for and stimulate human experimentation. Traditional medical ethics, with its emphasis on *primum non nocere* and the primacy of a personal bond between patient and physician, was argued to no longer suit modern medicine. Therapeutic reformers started a lobby to convince clinicians that their concerns regarding patient participation in controlled trials were often unfounded and at times even unethical. In this lobby, research ethics committees were imagined to function as *epistemic filters* that would heighten both the quality and quantity of human experimentation in medicine. To enable a rational therapeutics to emerge, everybody—doctor and patient alike—had to participate in experimental investigations. Hence, even if the professional powers of individual researchers had to be reeled in, the freedom of the profession as a whole to conduct more research studies had to expand. A moral need existed for human experimentation, which meant that a new ethics discourse had to be formulated that enabled researchers to take some risks with individuals to benefit society as a whole.

Perhaps surprisingly, the popularity of this utilitarian logic was hardly hampered by the emergence of a patients' rights frame in the 1960s and 1970s. While this new framework brought about a more critical assessment of the individual researcher-subject relationship, it did little for a more critical assessment of the societal position of biomedical research as a whole. Thus, even when undesirable research studies were proposed, as in the case of criminologist Wouter Buikhuisen in 1978, the Dutch government maintained that an open society should guarantee "freedom of inquiry." In these instances, science was formulated to constitute a societal good that should proceed as free from political interference as possible. A government could only set the basic parameters in which a scientific practice like human experimentation could take place, not meddle with its actual content.

Still, it is of course far from the truth to state that the Dutch government acted in an epistemically neutral manner toward human experimentation in medicine. In the 1950s, by supporting the view that the experimental tradition itself was sound and that only excesses had to be prevented, it helped to protect experimental medicine from antivivisectionists who felt that all of modern medicine constituted an unethical experiment. In the 1970s, it refused to support ethics review on the grounds that it might hamper clinical research. In the 1980s, it adopted the idea that research ethics committees should function as epistemic filters to halt proposals that did not live up to agreed-upon standards of methodological quality. And in the 1990s, it stated outright in parliamentary debates that members of research ethics committees were prohibited from using their position to criticize Big Pharma or from taking the negative environmental effects of research studies into account — effectively excluding those voices of a pluralistic society whose moral criticisms of human experimentation went beyond that of the standard patients' rights frame. In effect, a specific type of medical research became much more ingrained in Dutch society by the end of the century than it had ever been before, with a government actively promoting certain ways of peering into the world and not others.

It is important to point out that this function of ethics review is not the result of some hushed-up power play on behalf of a medical in-group who hoped to protect a scientific practice they secretly knew could not stand the light of day. That ethics committees should function as epistemic filters was publicly and repeatedly defended by multiple generations of self-appointed therapeutic reformers convinced that only this way would the Dutch state be able to protect citizens from dubious research activities. Sure, reformers such as Nelemans strategically used their multiple professional identities to realize these ideals: in their roles as policy advisers, they pushed the government to further one way of knowing, while in their academic work they presented this growing state interference as an abstract, external force. When called upon, however, reformers usually were quite willing to defend why they believed it was good for the state to provide leading experts in the field with hard power to steer the conduct of the average practitioner.

In this same vein, it also has to be made explicit that, despite the frequent rhetorical positioning of science as a republic of equals in which "freedom of inquiry" remains one of the highest goods, this political ideal hardly does justice to some of the most dominant control mechanisms through which late-modern science has been *designed* to function.[8] While it has become somewhat popular today among scientists to complain that ethics review has brought a form of neo-Marxism to the once-free republic of science, research ethics committees were invented not so long ago by these same critics' predecessors to *enable* scientific progress.[9] This earlier generation of therapeutic reformers believed modern medicine was facing a crisis—but not one of individual researchers who failed to follow clear ethical guidelines. Rather, the crisis they perceived was one of scientific knowledge and how it could be generated and used in medicine.[10] Thus, to prevent medical science from descending into chaos or being corrupted by undue influences, gatekeepers were necessary to police the borders of the field.[11] In other words, that committees had to strictly inspect research designs was not an unintended consequence of design by committee in a bureaucracy full of red tape; it was a *built-in* mechanism to enforce a specific epistemic perspective in clinical research and practice.

The Continued Lure of Expert Governance

In the past as well in the present, the at-times inflexible and inefficient elements of this bureaucracy have been blamed on the (bio)ethics profession that arose alongside ethics review in the 1970s and 1980s.[12] Motivated by a false sense of moral righteousness, the criticism goes, these new commissars have brought about a tangle of red tape in the governance of the medical sciences, frustrating scientific innovation. Yet simultaneously, and just as loudly, (bio)ethicists have been (and are) accused of functioning as a lubricant for the medical research establishment, allowing those in charge to push through any scientific innovation without too much societal resistance.

Of course, it is crucial for any discipline to exercise reflexivity with regard to its professional functioning, and thus also to critically consider its political role in enabling certain forms of governance and not others. Yet as I have argued in chapter 6, for those who want to criticize ethics review as a frustrating example of design by committee, it seems more prudent for them to raise their voices at a mode of public decision-making that has gone hand in hand with the rise of a new political order in the late twentieth century. At this time, both in the Netherlands and internationally, politicians in liberal democracies struggled with the question of how to handle ethically contentious issues in the rapidly developing fields of medicine and science, while societies were secularizing, older moral authorities no longer held sway, and political discourse was dominated by neoliberal ideals of deregulation and public management. Here, research ethics committees, which had previously been imagined to function as councils of wise men, as epistemic filters, and as juries of critical laypeople, came to be imagined as rational instruments of semi-public oversight: the government would set the terms under which research ethics committees could operate, but the execution of their tasks would be left to *experts*, predominantly from within the scientific field itself.

This state of affairs allowed politicians to claim public control over human subjects research, without actually having to admit to undue interference with the freedom of inquiry necessary to scientists in an open society, and without actually having to include a plurality of societal voices in the rendering of ethical judgements.

According to historian of science Theodore Porter, this use of experts is a typical feature of large-scale liberal democracies: i.e., in political cultures where politicians are themselves constantly pressured to account for their actions, those in charge tend to justify policies with an appeal to "the rule of rule" rather than to explicit moral arguments. Referring to rules and procedures allows one to deflect claims of arbitrariness and bias and is a perfect way of "making decisions without seeming to decide." This perception is reinforced by the fact that only those *skilled* in the application of rules may exercise this judgement. Trained bureaucrats know better than to voice personal beliefs when evaluating protocols. Such officials are in the business of following procedure, meaning that any other bureaucrat, as long as they are properly trained, can be expected to reach the same conclusion. This combination of the procedural with expert decision-making, Porter argues, has become "especially compelling to bureaucratic officials who lack the mandate of a popular election, or divine right" in modern democracies. It is the sort of objectivity that "lends authority to officials who have very little of their own."[13]

Of course, the legal rules by which human research is regulated today in the Netherlands have been subject to extensive consideration in the Dutch parliament, which has ultimately used its legislative powers to pass the WMO. Hence, the contemporary Dutch governance of human experimentation *is* the result of a careful democratic process, one in which Dutch citizens, by means of their government, have set the terms under which the practice may take place. Experts only administrate these rules and may do so only in publicly approved ways.

Still, looking back on the Dutch history of governing human experimentation, the extent to which politicians have relied on expert advice to decide what policies are best is striking. From the Health Council committees of the 1950s and 1970s to the Central Council effort in the early 1980s and the ad-hoc committees on research with legally incapacitated individuals in the mid-1990s, all of these bodies permitted experts to set the frame within which human experimentation would be debated in parliament and to determine what types of policies could be considered suitable for its regulation. What is more, in all these years, the statespersons responsible for the regulation of human experimentation not only seemed perfectly happy with this expert-driven approach to the definition of public problems, they also actively appeared to invoke expert authority when challenged to take up a normative stance on the permissibility of human subjects research, in an attempt to depoliticize the issues at hand: i.e., this or that policy decision did not just follow from the opinion of *politicians*; it had been officially advised by *experts*.

In the Netherlands, this history has eventually resulted in a carefully constructed public ethics administration, one that is dominated by the rule of expert consensus and built around two—and *only* two—premises: for protocols to be permitted they (1) have to be methodologically sound, and (2) contain sufficient safeguards to protect the rights and safety of participating research subjects. If the correct procedures have been consistently followed and the correct rules justly applied, judgements are considered fair—and thus objective. In those instances, no undue perspectives are taken to have corrupted the review process—thereby implying that such decisions have democratic approval, *even* if no actual democratic process was involved in evaluating the protocol. Nonetheless, just in case these procedures and rules should prove insufficient, ethicists have been elevated to function as fulcrums between the expert and democratic governance of human experimentation. That is, they are so elevated in theory—when the public governance of medicine and science is debated in parliament.

In practice, it is better to describe Dutch ethics review as a late-modern liberal-bureaucratic tool for reasoning together about medicine, science, society, and the state; one that permits both science to progress and citizens to sleep soundly. That is, the sort of progress that fits the mold of *good* science, and the sort of citizens *reasonable* enough to understand that this mold is *necessary* and *inevitable*—and thus not subject as such to democratic debate. After all, only good science is ethical science. And ethical science, when confined to the realm of patients' rights, can only be good.

ACKNOWLEDGMENTS

Throughout the years, this book has taken on many identities, in the form of unreadable first drafts for chapters of my dissertation, articles that were never published, and scraps of paper that I was fully ready to throw into some bonfire, dance around maniacally, and never look at again. I could never have imagined that it would one day be published by the University of Chicago Press, and it most certainly would not have been, were it not for the support of a great many people. First of all, of course, my daily supervisor Frank Huisman, who helped me come up with this project and who read every draft of this book (of which there were too many!). And also Bert Theunissen, who gave me an academic home when I was feeling quite lonely, and whose support over the years continues to be of invaluable importance.

Most parts of this book were written in the joyful company of Ivan Flis, Steven van der Laan, Jesper Oldenburg, and Fedde Benedictus at the Utrecht Freudenthal Institute. Ivan, without you, this book would not be what it is today. I also learned much from the many lunch and hallway conversations with Hieke Huistra, David Baneke, Daan Wegener, Rienk Vermij, Chaokang Tai, Maaneli Derakhshani, Guido Bacciagaluppi, and Toine Pieters. Hieke, thank you for your many thoughtful questions and comments about my work—you were and remain a great source of authority (even if I do not always listen). Thanks also to the Utrecht *Isis*-team, especially to Floris Cohen, Ad Maas, Desiree Capel, and the marvel that is Joan Vandegrift, all of whose guidance and enthusiasm have made me a better historian of science.

At Maastricht University, where I started this project, I was lucky to teach classes for a number of years with Geert Somsen, Raf de Bont, Hans Schouwenburg, Thomas Mougey, Bart Zwegers, and Simone Schleper. Our weekly meetings on how to teach the history of science to humanities students taught me a great deal and made the visits to Maastricht something to look forward to. The great questions of Ernst Homburg, who was kind enough to attend multiple presentations of mine about this project, made me rethink some key elements of this book. Tsjalling Swierstra, even though you were not my daily supervisor, your sharp questions sat in the back of my head every time I started writing another chapter. Thank you for your help.

Since finishing a first version of *Ethics by Committee*, I have been warmly welcomed by the Department of Medical Ethics, Philosophy, and History at the Erasmus Medical Center in Rotterdam. Timo Bolt, Floor Haalboom,

Ruben Verwaal, and Martijn van der Meer, you are not only great historians of medicine, you are great partners in crime as well. Timo, thank you for everything you do to ensure that we budding historians can prosper as academics. Thanks also to all other departmental colleagues for the stimulating work environment. Hannie Aartsen, Suzanne van de Vathorst, Krista Tromp, and Ineke Bolt, our conversations have given me important new insights about the practice of ethics. You are all a joy to work and teach with! Thanks also to Inez de Beaufort and Maartje Schermer, two very different heads of department, who are both equally impressive in their own right.

My work has very much benefited from the lively history of science and medicine community in the Netherlands. Mart van Lieburg was kind enough to invite me to the Trefpunt Medische Geschiedenis and to introduce me to a number of enthusiasts of the Dutch history of medicine. The Woudschoten conferences were a great place to meet with historians of science from Belgium and the Netherlands, as were the international conferences organized by the European Association for the History of Medicine and Health, the History of Science Society, and the Society for the Social History of Medicine. I am very fond of the conversations I have had there with Frans van Lunteren, Heiner Fangerau, Kaat Wils, and Joris Vandendriessche. The same goes for the biennial PhD conferences at Rolduc and the Glind, and the cozy dinners and drinks with our Shells and Pebbles editorial team.

As a member of the WTMC Graduate School I had the pleasure of attending a number of workshops and summer schools with scholars working in the Dutch STS field, and of discussing my ideas with them. I feel lucky that I got to be a part of this community, in addition to the informal Dutch community of PhD candidates and postdocs working on the history of science and medicine. Many of them have already been mentioned, but I would fall short if I did not also mention Jeroen Bouterse, Ingrid Kloosterman, Abel Streefland, Friso Hoeneveld, Jorrit Smit, Sebastiaan Broere, Didi van Trijp, Roland Bertens, Nele Beyens, and Pieter Huistra. Listening to them talk about their work has taught me much about my own.

At the start of this project, I was lucky enough to visit the Centre for the History of Science, Technology, and Medicine at Manchester University, where Duncan Wilson took the time to talk with me for hours and hours about the history of bioethics, and John Pickstone took me to pubs and dinners and gave me a great collection of books. I still think fondly of those conversations and am very proud that Duncan came to the Netherlands for a workshop that was organized in honor of my PhD defense in June 2018. The same goes for Laura Stark and Nancy Tomes, both of whom I greatly admire. Laura, I think we both know that this book will be published in part because of your support. Nancy, not only are you a great historian of medicine, you are also a wonderful person. Thank you for all the advice (and blankets!) that you have given me. Karen Darling, editor at the University of Chicago Press, thank you for your kind and thoughtful comments and enthusiastic e-mails. Thanks also to the anonymous reviewers for their feedback, to Jessica Wilson for her attentive and smart copy editing, and to the team at UCP for their support—they have all made the manuscript much better. And Helena Tinnerholm Ljungberg, thank you a great deal for inviting me to Uppsala, for organizing a wonderful international workshop on the history of research ethics committees, and for the great many Zoom sessions we have had since then discussing our shared interests in political history and 1970s beards.

Finally, I would like to thank my friends and family for their love and support. Not all of you always understood what all this poring over books, going to archives, and obsessing about the past would amount to. But all of you always accepted and encouraged my quirky interests and digressions (or you managed to hide it remarkably well). I dedicate this book to my parents. Mama and papa, thank you for your endless trust and enthusiasm, for believing that I would finish this book even when I did not, and for always reminding me that other things are much more important. Syl and Luuk, thank you for giving me a second family. Hanne and Cas, your existence makes everything better.

Pim, when I first wrote these lines, you were preparing me dinner, as you did almost every day that I was working on this book and getting home late. Today, you are sitting across the table in our little COVID-born home office, staring at your screen, as you have done for the better part of this year. Seeing you smile encouragingly every time I was ready to give up on finishing this book has gotten me over the finish line. You are the best person to never read my work.

NOTES

INTRODUCTION

1. M. A. van Dongen, "Experimenten op Mensen," *Medisch Contact* 35 (1980): 170.

2. Willem Otterspeer, *The Bastion of Liberty: Leiden University Today and Yesterday* (Leiden: Leiden University Press, 2008).

3. For "obligatory passage points," see Michel Callon, "Some Elements of a Sociology of Translation: Domestication of the Scallops and the Fishermen of St. Brieuc Bay," *Sociological Review* 32 (1984): 196–233.

4. See Anita Guerrini, *Experimenting with Humans and Animals: From Galen to Animal Rights* (Baltimore, MD: Johns Hopkins University Press, 2003).

5. Charles E. Rosenberg, *The Care of Strangers: The Rise of America's Hospital System* (New York: Basic Books, 1987); John Harley Warner, *The Therapeutic Perspective: Medical Practice, Knowledge, and Identity in America, 1820–1885* (Princeton, NJ: Princeton University Press, 1997); Andrew R. Cunningham and Perry Williams, eds., *The Laboratory Revolution in Medicine* (Cambridge: Cambridge University Press, 1992).

6. Erika Dyck and Larry Stewart, eds., *The Uses of Humans in Experiment: Perspectives from the 17th to the 20th Century* (Leiden: Brill Rodopi, 2016); Susan E. Lederer, *Subjected to Science: Human Experimentation in America before the Second World War* (Baltimore, MD: Johns Hopkins University Press, 1995); Martin S. Pernick, *A Calculus of Suffering: Pain, Professionalism, and Anesthesia in Nineteenth-Century America* (New York: Columbia University Press, 1985); Sydney Halpern, *Lesser Harms: The Morality of Risk in Medical Research* (Chicago: University of Chicago Press, 2004); Ronald L. Numbers, "William Beaumont and the Ethics of Human Experimentation," *Journal of the History of Biology* 12, no. 1 (Spring 1979): 113–35.

7. One country which did have regulations for human experimentation before World War II was Germany. See Barbara Elkeles, "The German Debate on Human Experimentation between 1880 and 1914," in *Twentieth Century Ethics of Human Subjects Research: Historical Perspectives on Values, Practices, and Regulations*, eds. Volker Roelcke and Giovanni Maio (Stuttgart: Franz Steiner Verlag, 2004): 19–33; Daniel S. Nadav, "The 'Death Dance of Lübeck': Julius Moses and the German Guidelines for Human Experimentation, 1930," in *Twentieth Century Ethics of Human Subjects Research*, eds. Roelcke and Maio, 129–35.

8. Wet van 26 februari 1998, houdende regelen inzake medisch-wetenschappelijk onderzoek met mensen (Wet medisch-wetenschappelijk onderzoek met mensen).

9. See Joseph S. Nye, Jr., "Soft Power," *Foreign Policy* 80, twentieth anniversary issue (Autumn 1990): 159–71; Joseph S. Nye, Jr., *Soft Power: The Means to Success in World Politics* (New York: PublicAffairs, 2004).

10. Laura Stark, *Behind Closed Doors: IRBs and the Making of Ethical Research* (Chicago: University of Chicago Press, 2012): 5.

11. See Anne Hardy and E. M. Tansey, "Medical Enterprise and Global Response, 1945–2000," in William F. Bynum et al., *The Western Medical Tradition, 1800–2000* (Cambridge: Cambridge University Press, 2006): 405–534; James Le Fanu, *The Rise and Fall of Modern Medicine* (New York: Basic Books, 2012); John V. Pickstone, "Production, Community and Consumption: The Political Economy of Twentieth-Century Medicine," in *Medicine in the Twentieth Century*, eds. John V. Pickstone and Roger Cooter (Amsterdam: Harwood Academic Press, 2000): 1–19.

12. Marilyn Strathern, ed., *Audit Cultures: Anthropological Studies in Accountability, Ethics and the Academy* (London: Routledge, 2000); Michael Powers, *The Audit Society: Rituals of Verification* (Oxford: Oxford University Press, 1997); Cris Shore and Susan Wright, "Governing by Numbers: Audit Culture, Rankings and the New World Order," *Social Anthropology* 23 (2015): 22–28.

13. Adam Hedgecoe, "'A Form of Practical Machinery': The Origins of Research Ethics Committees in the UK, 1967–1972," *Medical History* 53 (2009): 331–50, at 331.

14. See also Adam Hedgecoe, *Trust in the System: Research Ethics Committees and the Regulation of Biomedical Research* (Manchester: Manchester University Press, 2020).

15. Hedgecoe, "A Form of Practical Machinery," 332.

16. Stark, *Behind Closed Doors*.

17. Zachary M. Schrag, *Ethical Imperialism: Institutional Review Boards and the Social Sciences, 1965–2009* (Baltimore, MD: Johns Hopkins University Press, 2010).

18. In 2021, a special issue of the *European Journal for the History of Medicine and Health* will be published that traces the rise of ethics review in a number of European and North American countries. For the Netherlands, one research article has previously been published, in addition to a few witness accounts. See Patricia Jaspers, "Controversial Issues in the History of Dutch Research Ethics Governance," *Journal of Policy History* 23 (2011): 74–93; F. A. Wolff, ed., *Geneeskunde en ethiek in harmonie: Liber amicorum voor Prof.Dr E.L. Noach bij diens 80ste verjaardag op 21 November 2001* (The Hague: Pasmans Offset Drukkerij BV, 2001); D. P. Engberts, Y. M. Reidsma, and A. R. Wintzen, eds., *Dilemma's getoetst: Liber amicorum voor prof. dr. H. M. Dupuis en prof. dr. P. Vermeij* (Leiden: UFB Universiteit Leiden, 2003).

19. Ezekiel J. Emanuel et al., eds., *The Oxford Textbook of Clinical Research Ethics* (Oxford: Oxford University Press, 2008).

20. See James Jones, *Bad Blood: The Tuskegee Syphilis Experiment* (New York: Free Press, 1981); Susan M. Reverby, *Examining Tuskegee: The Infamous Syphilis Study and its Legacy* (Chapel Hill: University of North Carolina Press, 2009).

21. I borrow the term "object lessons" from Stark, *Behind Closed Doors*, 7.

22. The notion of signposts is derived from Thomas F. Gieryn, *Cultural Boundaries of Science: Credibility on the Line* (London: University of Chicago Press, 1999).

23. Kamerstuk Tweede Kamer (parliamentary document of the House of Representatives) 1991–1992, no. 22588, sec. 3, 2.

24. Thomas S. Kuhn, *The Structure of Scientific Revolutions*, 4th ed. (Chicago: University of Chicago Press, 2012): 137. See also Marga Vicedo, "Introduction: The Secret Lives of Textbooks," *Isis* 103 (2012): 83–87; Kathryn M. Olesko, "Science Pedagogy as a Category of Historical Analysis: Past, Present, and Future," *Science & Education* 15 (2006), 863–80.

25. Frits Gonggrijp, "Commissies gepasseerd: Bloemenhove liet experimenten toe na late abortus," *De Telegraaf*, December 21, 1979: 7.

26. Brief van de Hoofddirecteur Gezondheidszorg aan de Hoofdafdeling Staats- en Strafrecht, Ministerie van Justitie, February 25, 1980, National Archive, The Hague, DG Volksgezondheid, access no. 2.15.65, inv. no. 2456.

27. See, for example: "Bloemenhove experimenteerde al op levend-geaborteerde kinderen," *Nederlands Dagblad*, December 22, 1979: 2.

28. E. O. Gunning, Tijdsein, N1, 20.50 uur. Dr. Gunning (Voorzitter Nederlands Artsenverbond) over medische proeven op levend geaborteerde kinderen, National Archive, The Hague, 2.15.65, inv. no. 2456.

29. These letters can be found in the National Archive, The Hague, access no. 2.15.65, inv. no. 2456.

30. H. Hoffman, "Géén experimenten Bloemenhove-kliniek: Bloedmonsters genomen van foetaal weefsel," *Het Vrije Volk*, December 28, 1979: 7.

31. Gonggrijp, "Commissies gepasseerd," 7.

32. David J. Rothman, *Strangers at the Bedside: A History of How Law and Bioethics Transformed Medical Decision Making*, 3rd ed. (New Brunswick, NJ: AldineTransaction, 1991/2003): 11.

33. Rothman, 10.

34. Robert Baker, *Before Bioethics: A History of American Medical Ethics from the Colonial Period to the Bioethics Revolution* (Oxford: Oxford University Press, 2013): 316–17.

35. Baker, *Before Bioethics*, 317.

36. Albert R. Jonsen, *The Birth of Bioethics* (Oxford: Oxford University Press, 1998). See also Peter Singer, "Introduction," in *Applied Ethics*, ed. Peter Singer (Oxford: Oxford University Press, 1986): 1–9; Robert Baker, "From Metaethicist to Bioethicist," *Cambridge Quarterly of Health Ethics* 11 (2002): 369–79.

37. Jonsen, *The Birth of Bioethics*, 157.

38. Robert M. Veatch, "The Birth of Bioethics; Autobiographical Reflections of a Patient Person," *Cambridge Quarterly of Health Ethics* 11 (2002): 344–52, at 344.

39. Charles L. Bosk, review of *Strangers at the Bedside: A History of How Law and Ethics Transformed Medical Decision Making*, by David J. Rothman, *Contemporary Sociology* 20 (1991): 831–33, at 832.

40. M. L. Tina Stevens, *Bioethics in America: Origins and Cultural Politics* (Baltimore, MD: Johns Hopkins University Press, 2000): x.

41. John H. Evans, *The History and Future of Bioethics: A Sociological Review* (Oxford: Oxford University Press, 2012): 75. See also John H. Evans, "A Sociological Account of the Growth of Principlism," *Hastings Center Report* 30 (2000): 31–38.

42. Roger Cooter, "Inside the Whale: Bioethics in History and Discourse," *Social History of Medicine* 23 (2010): 662–73, at 665 and 662. See also Roger Cooter, "The Resistible Rise of Medical Ethics," *Social History of Medicine* 8 (1995): 275–88; Roger Cooter, "The Ethical Body," in *Medicine in the Twentieth Century*, eds. Pickstone and Cooter, 451–67.

43. Stark, *Behind Closed Doors*, 8.

44. Stark, *Behind Closed Doors*, 162.

45. Duncan Wilson, *The Making of British Bioethics* (Manchester: Manchester University Press, 2014); Harold Perkin, *The Rise of Professional Society: England since 1800* (London: Routledge, 1990).

46. In his analysis, Wilson draws on Michael Moran, *The British Regulatory State: High Modernism and Hyper-Innovation* (Oxford: Oxford University Press, 2003).

47. See also Jenny Hazelgrove, "British Research Ethics after the Second World War: The Controversy at the British Postgraduate Medical School, Hammersmith Hospital," in *Twentieth Century Ethics of Human Subjects Research*, eds. Roelcke and Maio, 181–97.

48. Stark, *Behind Closed Doors*, 8.

49. Zachary M. Schrag, "Review: *Behind Closed Doors: IRBs and the Making of Ethical Research* by Laura Stark," *American Journal of Sociology* 118 (2012): 494–496, at 496.

50. Joseph R. Gusfield, *The Culture of Public Problems: Drinking-Driving and the Symbolic Order* (London: University of Chicago Press, 1981): 3.

51. Cooter, "Inside the Whale," 669.

52. "It could be otherwise," or ICBO, has become a popular phrase in Science, Technology and Society Studies (STS) to denote the value of historical, anthropological, and sociological scholarship.

53. George J. Annas and Michael A. Grodin, eds., *The Nazi Doctors and the Nuremberg Code: Human Rights in Human Experimentation* (Oxford: Oxford University Press, 1992); Paul J. Weindling, "The Origins of Informed Consent: The International Scientific Commission on Medical War Crimes, and the Nuremberg Code," *Bulletin of the History of Medicine* 75 (2001): 37–71.

54. Andreas Frewer and Ulf Schmidt, eds., *History and Theory of Human Experimentation: The Declaration of Helsinki and Modern Medical Ethics* (Stuttgart: Franz Steiner, 2007).

55. Henry K. Beecher, "Ethics and Clinical Research," *New England Journal of Medicine* 74 (1966): 1354–60.

56. Maurice H. Pappworth, *Human Guinea Pigs: Experiments on Man* (London:

Routledge and Kegan Paul, 1967). Also: Maurice H. Pappworth, "Human Guinea Pigs: A Warning," *Twentieth Century* 171 (1962–1963): 66–75.

57. See, for example: H. A. M. J. ten Have, R. H. J. ter Meulen, and E. van Leeuwen, *Medische Ethiek* (Houten: Bohn Stafleu van Loghum, 2003). Stark calls this the "critical event narrative." See: Laura J. M. Stark, "Morality in Science: How Research is Evaluated in the Age of Human Subjects Regulation," (PhD diss., Princeton University, 2006): 32.

58. Wilson, *The Making of British Bioethics*, 50. See also David Reubi, "The Will to Modernize: A Genealogy of Biomedical Research Ethics in Singapore," *International Political Sociology* 4 (2010): 142–58; Duncan Wilson, "What Can History Do for Bioethics," *Bioethics* 27 (2013): 215–23.

59. See Wilson, *The Making of British Bioethics*; Nikolas Rose, *The Politics of Life Itself* (Princeton, NJ: Princeton University Press, 2007); Reubi, "The Will to Modernize," 142–58.

60. Susan E. Lederer, "Research Without Borders: The Origins of the Declaration of Helsinki," in *History and Theory of Human Experimentation*, eds. Frewer and Schmidt, 145–64; Robert Baker, "Transcultural Medical Ethics and Human Rights," in *Ethics Codes in Medicine: Foundations and Achievements of Codification since 1947*, eds. Ulrich Tröhler and Stella Reiter-Theil (Aldershot: Ashgate, 1998): 312–31; Ulrich Tröhler, "The Long Road of Moral Concern: Doctors' Ethos and Statute Law Relating to Human Research in Europe," in *History and Theory of Human Experimentation*, eds. Frewer and Schmidt, 27–54.

61. For the term "reference culture" see Joris van Eijnatten, "Beyond Diversity: The Steady State of Reference Cultures," *International Journal for History, Culture and Modernity* 3 (2015): 1–8.

62. Baker, *Before Bioethics*, 278.

63. H. D. C. Roscam Abbing, "Genetische experimenten met mensen: Wetgever quo vadis?," *Medisch Contact* 41 (1986): 533–35, at 533. The attraction for clinical researchers (and companies conducting clinical research) of lower- and middle-income countries' lack of regulation over human subjects research has been discussed in detail in Adriana Petryna's groundbreaking *Global Pharmaceuticals* (2006) and *When Experiments Travel* (2009). There is little indication that similar exploits occurred in the higher-income Netherlands, even though some commentators did worry it might. See Adriana Petryna, Andrew Lakoff, and Arthur Kleinman, eds., *Global Pharmaceuticals: Ethics, Markets, Practices* (Durham, NC: Duke University Press, 2006) and Adriana Petryna, *When Experiments Travel: Clinical Trials and the Global Search for Human Subjects* (Princeton, NJ: Princeton University Press, 2009). See also Melinda Cooper and Catherine Waldby, *Clinical Labor: Tissue Donors and Research Subjects in the Global Bioeconomy* (Durham, NC: Duke University Press, 2014).

64. Stark, *Behind Closed Doors*, 133.

65. Other scholars have conducted such research. In 1975, Bradford H. Gray published a book about the daily practice of United States institutional review boards, an

ethnographic approach which has since been repeated by other scholars, for the United States and for other countries as well. See Bradford H. Gray, *Human Subjects in Medical Experimentation: A Sociological Study of the Conduct and Regulation of Clinical Research* (New York: Wiley-Interscience, 1975). See also Maureen H. Fitzgerald, "Punctuated Equilibrium: Moral Panics and the Ethics Review Process," *Journal of Academic Ethics* 2 (2005), 315–38; Jan Jaeger, "An Ethnographic Analysis of Institutional Review Board Decision-Making" (PhD diss., University of Pennsylvania, 2006); Adam Hedgecoe, "Research Ethics Review and the Sociological Research Relationship," *Sociology* 42 (2008): 873–86; Lura Abbott and Christine Grady, "A Systematic Review of the Empirical Literature Evaluating IRBs: What We Know and What We Still Need to Learn," *Journal of Empirical Research on Human Research Ethics* 6 (2011): 3–19; Stark, *Behind Closed Doors*; Robert L. Klitzman, *The Ethics Police?: The Struggle to Make Human Research Safe* (Oxford: Oxford University Press, 2015). For those interested in the present-day functioning of Dutch research ethics committees, see Patricia Jaspers, Rob Houtepen, and Klasien Horstman, "Ethical Review: Standardizing Procedures and Local Shaping of Ethical Review Practices," *Social Science & Medicine* 98 (2013): 311–18.

66. Sheila Jasanoff, *The Fifth Branch: Science Advisers as Policymakers* (Cambridge, MA: Harvard University Press, 1990). Also: Sheila Jasanoff, *Designs on Nature: Science and Democracy in Europe and the United States* (Princeton, NJ: Princeton University Press, 2005).

67. Schrag, *Ethical Imperialism*. See also Charles L. Bosk and Raymond De Vries, "Bureaucracies of Mass Deception: Institutional Review Boards and the Ethics of Ethnographic Research," *Annals of the American Academy of Political and Social Sciences* 595 (2004): 249–63; Kevin D. Haggerty, "Ethics Creep: Governing Social Science Research in the Name of Ethics," *Qualitative Sociology* 27 (2004): 391–414; Will C. van den Hoonaard, *The Seduction of Ethics: Transforming the Social Sciences* (Toronto: University of Toronto Press, 2011).

68. Ethics review of humanities studies remains uncommon in the Netherlands. Only in the last five years have ethics committees for these research studies started to pop up in response to changing funding policies at the EU level and changing publishing policies of international academic journals.

69. See the special issue of the *European Journal for the History of Medicine and Health* (referenced in note 18). See also Adam Hedgecoe, "Scandals, Ethics, and Regulatory Change in Biomedical Research," *Science, Technology, and Human Values* 42 (2017): 577–99; Paul J. DiMaggio and Walter W. Powell, "The Iron Cage Revisited: Institutional Isomorphism and Collective Rationality in Organizational Fields," *American Sociological Review* 48 (1983): 147–60.

70. See Mark Bevir, *Governance: A Very Short Introduction* (Oxford: Oxford University Press, 2012).

71. Bruno Latour, *Reassembling the Social: An Introduction to Actor-Network-Theory* (Oxford: Oxford University Press, 2005): 174.

1. Notulen van de vergaderingen, March 11, 1954, 2, National Archive, The Hague, Gezondheidsraad 1920–1956, access no. 2.15.33, inv. no. 547.

2. Jan Wester, "Advies van de voorzitter van de Gezondheidsraad," October 10, 1955, National Archive, The Hague, Gezondheidsraad 1920–1956, access no. 2.15.33, inv. no. 548.

3. Robert Baker, "Transcultural Medical Ethics and Human Rights," in *Ethics Codes in Medicine: Foundations and Achievements of Codification since 1947*, eds. Ulrich Tröhler and Stella Reiter-Theil (Aldershot: Ashgate, 1998): 312–31; Ulrich Tröhler, "The Long Road of Moral Concern: Doctors' Ethos and Statute Law Relating to Human Research in Europe," in *History and Theory of Human Experimentation*, eds. Andreas Frewer and Ulf Schmidt (Stuttgart: Franz Steiner, 2007): 27–54.

4. Gert H. Brieger, "Human Experimentation: I. History," in vol. 2 of *Encyclopedia of Bioethics*, ed. Warren T. Reich (New York: Free Press, 1978): 684–92; Susan E. Lederer, "The Ethics of Experimenting on Human Beings," in *The Cambridge World History of Medical Ethics*, eds. Robert B. Baker and Laurence B. McCullough (Cambridge: Cambridge University Press, 2009): 558–65.

5. Anita Guerrini, *Experimenting with Humans and Animals: From Galen to Animal Rights* (Baltimore, MD: Johns Hopkins University Press, 2003); Andreas-Holger Maehle and Ulrich Tröhler, "Animal Experimentation from Antiquity to the End of the Eighteenth Century: Attitudes and Arguments," in *Vivisection in Historical Perspective*, ed. Nicolaas A. Rupke (London: Croom Helm, 1987): 14–47; Erika Dyck and Larry Stewart, eds., *The Uses of Humans in Experiment: Perspectives from the 17th to the 20th Century* (Leiden: Brill Rodopi, 2016).

6. Simon Schaffer, "Self Evidence," *Critical Inquiry* 18 (1992): 327–62; Lawrence Altman, *Who Goes First: The Story of Self-Experimentation in Medicine* (New York: Random House, 1986); Londa Schiebinger, "Human Experimentation in the Eighteenth Century: Natural Boundaries and Valid Testing," in *The Moral Authority of Nature*, eds. Lorraine Daston and Fernando Vidal (Chicago: University of Chicago Press, 2003): 384–408; Andrew Wear, "The Discourses of Practitioners in Sixteenth- and Seventeenth Century Europe," in *The Cambridge World History of Medical Ethics*, eds. Baker and McCullough, 379–90.

7. Paola Bertucci, "Shocking Subjects: Human Experiments and the Material Culture of Medical Electricity in Eighteenth-Century England," in *The Uses of Humans in Experiment*, eds. Dyck and Stewart, 111–38; Larry Stewart, "Pneumatic Chemistry: Self-Experimentation and the Burden of Revolution, 1780–1805," in *The Uses of Humans in Experiment*, eds. Dyck and Stewart, 139–69.

8. Schiebinger, "Human Experimentation in the Eighteenth Century," 394. Enslaved people, one of the most vulnerable populations of the early modern period, were a notable exception to this rule. Mostly, their bodies were deemed too economically valuable to their owners to be used for scientific experimentation. See Londa Schiebinger,

"Medical Experimentation and Race in the Eighteenth-Century Atlantic World," *Social History of Medicine* 26 (2013): 364–82.

9. Anita Guerrini, "The Human Experimental Subject," in *A Companion to the History of Science*, ed. Bernard Lightman (West Sussex: John Wiley & Sons Ltd, 2016), 126–38.

10. John Rosser Matthews, *Quantification and the Quest for Medical Certainty* (Princeton, NJ: Princeton University Press, 1995); Theodore M. Porter, *The Rise of Statistical Thinking, 1820–1900* (Princeton, NJ: Princeton University Press, 1986).

11. Andrew R. Cunningham and Perry Williams, eds., *The Laboratory Revolution in Medicine* (Cambridge: Cambridge University Press, 1992); Ilana Löwy, "The Experimental Body," in *Medicine in the Twentieth Century*, eds. John V. Pickstone and Roger Cooter (Amsterdam: Harwood Academic Press, 2000): 435–49.

12. Claude Bernard, *An Introduction to the Study of Experimental Medicine* (1865; trans. 1927; reprint, New York: Dover, 1957): 102.

13. Ronald L. Numbers, "William Beaumont and the Ethics of Human Experimentation," *Journal of the History of Biology* 12, no. 1 (Spring 1979): 113–35, at 134.

14. William F. Bynum, "Reflections on the History of Human Experimentation," in *The Use of Human Beings in Research: With Special Reference to Clinical Trials*, eds. Stuart F. Spicker et al. (Dordrecht: Kluwer Academic Publishers, 1988): 29–46; Erwin H. Ackerknecht, *Medicine at the Paris Hospital, 1794–1848* (Baltimore, MD: Johns Hopkins University Press, 1967).

15. Mary E. Fissell, "The Medical Marketplace, the Patient, and the Absence of Medical Ethics in Early Modern Europe and North America," in *The Cambridge World History of Medical Ethics*, eds. Baker and McCullough, 533–39; John Harley Warner, *The Therapeutic Perspective: Medical Practice, Knowledge, and Identity in America, 1820–1885* (Princeton, NJ: Princeton University Press, 1997); Annet Mooij, "Roddels, ruzie, achterklap: Veranderende omgangsvormen in de medische beroepsgroep," *Gewina* 21 (1998): 30–37.

16. Roger Cooter, "Medicine and Modernity," in *The Oxford Handbook of the History of Medicine*, ed. Mark Jackson (Oxford: Oxford University Press, 2011): 100–16.

17. M. J. van Lieburg, "De tweede geneeskundige stand (1818–1865): Een bijdrage tot de geschiedenis van het medisch beroep in Nederland," *Tijdschrift voor Geschiedenis* 96 (1983): 433–53.

18. Henri Festen, *125 jaar geneeskunst en maatschappij* (Utrecht: Koninklijke Nederlandsche Maatschappij tot Bevordering der Geneeskunst, 1974).

19. Ulrich Tröhler, "'To Improve the Evidence of Medicine: Arithmetic Observation in Clinical Medicine in the Eighteenth and Early Nineteenth Centuries," *History and Philosophy of the Life Sciences* 10, supplement (1988): 31–40; Andrea A. Rusnock, "The Weight of Evidence and the Burden of Authority: Case Histories, Medical Statistics and Smallpox Inoculation," *Clio Medica* 29 (1995): 289–315.

20. See John Harley Warner, *Against the Spirit of System: The French Impulse in*

Nineteenth-Century American Medicine (Princeton, NJ: Princeton University Press, 1998).

21. Cunningham and Williams, eds., *The Laboratory Revolution in Medicine*; William F. Bynum et al., *The Western Medical Tradition, 1800–2000* (Cambridge: Cambridge University Press, 2006).

22. Annet Mooij, *De polsslag van de stad: 350 jaar academische geneeskunde in Amsterdam* (Amsterdam: Uitgeverij De Arbeiderspers, 1999).

23. Eduard Simon Houwaart, *De hygiënisten: Artsen, staat en volksgezondheid in Nederland, 1840–1890* (Groningen: Historische Uitgeverij Groningen, 1991); Klasien Horstman and Gerard de Vries, "Experimenten met mensen: De constitutie van een medisch-wetenschappelijke praktijk en een ethisch probleem (Nederland, 1870–1915)," *Kennis en Methode* 1 (1989): 62–83; H. Beukers, "Een nieuwe werkplaats in de geneeskunde. De opkomst van laboratoria in de geneeskundige faculteiten," *Tijdschrift voor de Geschiedenis van de Geneeskunde, Natuurkunde, Wiskunde en Techniek* 9 (1986): 266–77; M. J. van Lieburg, "De ontwikkeling van het klinisch-diagnostisch laboratorium in Nederland tot omstreeks 1925," *Tijdschrift voor de Geschiedenis van de Geneeskunde, Natuurkunde, Wiskunde en Techniek* 9 (1986): 278–318.

24. Mooij, *De polsslag van de stad*, 270; Annemieke Klein, *Verlangen naar verbetering: 375 jaar academische geneeskunde in Utrecht* (Amsterdam: Boom, 2010): 116.

25. Erika Dyck and Larry Stewart, eds., "Introduction," in *The Uses of Humans in Experiment*, 1–27, at 14.

26. Dyck and Stewart, eds., "Introduction," in *The Uses of Humans in Experiment*, 15. See also Simon Schaffer, "Regeneration: The Body of Natural Philosophers in Restoration England," in *Science Incarnate: Historical Embodiments of Natural Knowledge*, eds. Christopher Lawrence and Steven Shapin (Chicago: University of Chicago Press, 1998): 83–120; Peter Moore, *Blood and Justice: The Seventeenth-Century Parisian Doctor Who Made Blood Transfusion History* (London: John Wiley, 2003); Andreas-Holger Maehle, *Drugs on Trial: Experimental Pharmacology and Therapeutic Innovation in the Eighteenth Century* (Amsterdam: Rodopi, 1999).

27. Sydney Halpern, *Lesser Harms: The Morality of Risk in Medical Research* (Chicago: University of Chicago Press, 2004).

28. Martin S. Pernick, *A Calculus of Suffering: Pain, Professionalism, and Anesthesia in Nineteenth-Century America* (New York: Columbia University Press, 1985).

29. See also Martin S. Pernick, "The Calculus of Suffering in Nineteenth-Century Surgery," *The Hastings Center Report* 13 (1983): 26–36.

30. Halpern, *Lesser Harms*, 5.

31. Amanda Kluveld, "Felix Ortt: De kleine geloven als brug tussen wetenschap en geloof," *De Negentiende Eeuw* 25 (2001): 137–46.

32. Nicolaas A. Rupke, "Introduction," in *Vivisection in Historical Perspective*, ed. Rupke, 8. Also: Jan Romein, *Op het breukvlak van twee eeuwen*, 2nd ed. (Amsterdam: Em. Querido's Uitgeverij, 1976): 631–51.

33. Susan E. Lederer, *Subjected to Science: Human Experimentation in America before the Second World War* (Baltimore, MD: Johns Hopkins University Press, 1995).

34. Amanda Kluveld, *Reis door de hel der onschuldigen: De expressieve politiek van de Nederlandse anti-vivisectionisten, 1890–1940* (Amsterdam: Amsterdam University Press, 2000).

35. Handelingen Tweede Kamer (Acts of the House of Representatives) 1903–1904, December 12, 1903: 865–66.

36. Hendrik Burger, "Proefnemingen op menschen," *Nederlandsch Tijdschrift voor Geneeskunde* part I (1904): 317–20, at 318.

37. W. Koster, "Nog eens proefnemingen op menschen," *Nederlandsch Tijdschrift voor Geneeskunde* part I. (1904): 378–79; Hendrik Burger, "Nog eens proefnemingen op menschen," *Nederlandsch Tijdschrift voor Geneeskunde* part I (1904): 379–80; J. C. Kindermann, "Proefnemingen op menschen," *Nederlandsch Tijdschrift voor Geneeskunde* part I (1904): 414–15; Hendrik Burger, "Proefnemingen op menschen," *Nederlandsch Tijdschrift voor Geneeskunde* part I (1904): 415–16; W. Koster, "De bewijsvoering van Dr. Burger," *Nederlandsch Tijdschrift voor Geneeskunde* part I (1904): 463–65; Hendrik Burger, "De bewijsvoering van Dr. Burger," *Nederlandsch Tijdschrift voor Geneeskunde* part I (1904): 466–67; M. A. Brants, "Proefnemingen op menschen," *Nederlandsch Tijdschrift voor Geneeskunde* part I (1904): 520–22; Hendrik Burger, "Proefnemingen op menschen," *Nederlandsch Tijdschrift voor Geneeskunde* part I (1904): 522–24.

38. For more on the notion of the old gentleman-physician, see Edward Shorter, *Bedside Manners: The Troubled History of Doctors and Patients* (New York: Simon and Schuster, 1985).

39. Mattheus Colenbrander, C. Fehmers, and Theodoor Hammes, *Medische ethiek* (Amsterdam: Nederlandsche Maatschappij tot Bevordering der Geneeskunst, 1936); Hector Treub, *Medische fatsoensleer: Drie colleges* (Amsterdam: Scheltema & Holkema, 1903).

40. In 1930, these organs were augmented by an official medical court in which jurists and "colleagues" held seats.

41. Colenbrander, Fehmers, and Hammes, *Medische ethiek.*

42. A notable exception was Germany. Already in 1900, the Prussian government had issued official instructions advising surgeons and physicians to obtain informed consent. In 1931, the Reich's Ministry of the Interior sent around *Richtlinien* [guidelines] to each of the German federal states, strictly condemning nontherapeutic experiments on patients and emphasizing the importance of what is now called "informed consent" for any intervention other than diagnostic or therapeutic ones. At the time, these types of formal state measures were internationally without precedent. See Barbara Elkeles, "The German Debate on Human Experimentation between 1880 and 1914," in *Twentieth Century Ethics of Human Subjects Research: Historical Perspectives on Values, Practices, and Regulations*, eds. Volker Roelcke and Giovanni Maio (Stuttgart: Franz Steiner Verlag, 2004): 19–33; Daniel S. Nadav, "The 'Death Dance of Lübeck':

Julius Moses and the German Guidelines for Human Experimentation, 1930," in *Twentieth Century Ethics of Human Subjects Research,* eds. Roelcke and Maio, 129–35.

43. The experiments on Chinese prisoners by their Japanese oppressors during World War II should certainly not be forgotten. Yet in the immediate postwar decade, little was known in the Netherlands about these experiments and they therefore had little impact on public policy. Dutch physicians and antivivisectionists referred solely in publications to "Nazi" or "German" concentration-camp experiments. For more information on the Japanese experiments, see Takashi Tsuchiya, "The Imperial Japanese Experiments in China," in *The Oxford Textbook of Clinical Research Ethics,* eds. Ezekiel J. Emanuel et al. (Oxford: Oxford University Press, 2008): 31–45.

44. See Paul J. Weindling, "The Nazi Medical Experiments," in *The Oxford Textbook of Clinical Research Ethics,* eds. Emanuel et al., 18–30; Ulf Schmidt, "Medical Ethics and Nazism," in *The Cambridge World History of Medical Ethics,* eds. Baker and McCullough, 595–608; Michael R. Marrus, "The Nuremberg Doctors' Trial in Historical Context," *Bulletin for the History of Medicine* 73 (1999): 106–23.

45. See for instance "De nieuwe procesronde in Neurenberg: Experimenten op mensen worden berecht: Gruwelijke details," *Het Vrije Volk,* December 10, 1946: 3; "Het proces tegen de fabeltjes: Medici staan terecht te Neurenberg," *De Tijd,* December 10, 1946: 3; "Kinderen werden gesteriliseerd in Ravensbrück," *De Waarheid,* December 21, 1946: front page; "Gevangenen werden met mosterdgas bewerkt: Gruwelijke bijzonderheden voor het hof te Neurenberg," *De Waarheid,* January 4, 1947: front page.

46. F. Dekking, "'Medische' experimenten in Duitsche concentratiekampen," *Nederlandsch Tijdschrift voor Geneeskunde* 90 (1946): 1011; F. Dekking, "Het proces der Duitse artsen," *Nederlandsch Tijdschrift voor Geneeskunde* 91 (1947): 1830–33.

47. D. K. de Jongh, "Medische ethiek: Antwoord aan Prof.dr. G.C. Heringa," *Medisch Contact* 4 (1949): 600–04, at 602–03.

48. J. J. van Loghem, "Geneeskundige proefnemingen bij mensen," *Nederlands Tijdschrift voor Geneeskunde* 97 (1953): 518–20, at 518. This dissociation of medical science from the Nazi crimes was an active strategy of the prosecution at Nuremberg, which sought to prove that the experiments "revealed nothing which civilized medicine can use." See Telford Taylor, "Opening Statement of the Prosecution: December 9, 1946," reprinted in *The Nazi Doctors and the Nuremberg Code: Human Rights in Human Experimentation,* eds. George J. Annas and Michael A. Grodin (Oxford: Oxford University Press, 1992): 67–93, at 91. Also: Jenny Hazelgrove, "The Old Faith and the New Science: The Nuremberg Code and Human Experimentation Ethics in Britain, 1946–73," *Social History of Medicine* 15 (2002): 109–35; Gonzalo Herranz, "The Inclusion of the Ten Principles of Nuremberg in Professional Codes of Ethics: An International Comparison," in *Ethics Codes in Medicine: Foundations and Achievements of Codification since 1947,* eds. Ulrich Tröhler and Stella Reiter-Theil (Aldershot: Ashgate, 1998): 127–39; George J. Annas and Michael A. Grodin, "The Nuremberg Code," in *The Oxford Textbook of Clinical Research Ethics,* eds. Emanuel et al., 136–40.

49. Van Loghem, "Geneeskundige proefnemingen bij mensen," 518; emphasis original.

50. Ibid., 518. During the Doctors' Trial, the defense had offered evidence that also American researchers had conducted dangerous experiments on prisoners during World War II. See Ulf Schmidt, "The Nuremberg Doctors' Trial and the Nuremberg Code," in *History and Theory of Human Experimentation*, eds. Frewer and Schmidt, 71–116; Jon M. Harkness, "Nuremberg and the Issue of Wartime Experiments on U.S. Prisoners: The Green Committee," *Journal of the American Medical Association* 276 (1996): 1672–75. For an example of a Dutch newspaper report, see: "Amerikaanse artsen nemen proeven op mensen," *De Waarheid*, February 11, 1947: 2.

51. Van Loghem, "Geneeskundige proefnemingen bij mensen," 520. See also J. J. van Loghem, "Geneeskundige proefnemingen bij mensen (II) & (III)," in *Nederlandsch Tijdschrift voor Geneeskunde* 98 (1954): 2266–67, 3038–39.

52. G. C. Heringa, "Medische Ethiek, Practische Geneeskunde en Wetenschap," *Medisch Contact* 4 (1949): 539–45, at 540. In response to: D. K. de Jongh, "Over medische ethiek," *Medisch Contact* 4 (1949): 526–32.

53. Jongh, "Medische ethiek," 602.

54. F. Wibaut to P. A. van Luijt, February 11, 1954, National Archive, The Hague, Gezondheidsraad 1920–1956, access no. 2.15.33, inv. no. 549.

55. "Dr. J.J. Brutel de la Rivière 60 jaar arts," *Nederlands Tijdschrift voor Geneeskunde* 116 (1972): 585–86. See also Gerrit Arie Lindeboom, *Dutch Medical Biography: A Biographical Dictionary of Dutch Physicians and Surgeons 1475–1975* (Amsterdam: Rodopi, 1984): 1642–43. On the Dutch medical resistance, see the issue "Artsen en hun oorlog," *Medisch Contact* 64 (2009), and Hanna van den Ende, *'Vergeet niet dat je arts bent': Joodse artsen in Nederland, 1940–1945* (Amsterdam: Boom, 2015).

56. R. B. M. Rigter, *Met raad en daad: De geschiedenis van de Gezondheidsraad, 1902–1985* (Rotterdam: Erasmus Publishing, 1992).

57. "Amerikaanse onderscheidingen voor twintig Nederlanders: Medal of Freedom o.a. voor de minister-president," *De Tijd*, April 7, 1953: 4.

58. Jean Jacques Brutel de la Rivière, "Uitoefening der Geneeskunst in Vrij Beroep tegenover deze Uitoefening in Dienstverband," *Medisch Contact* 2 (1947): 189–97, at 191.

59. Brutel de la Rivière, "Uitoefening der Geneeskunst in Vrij Beroep," 194, 197.

60. Brutel de la Rivière, "Uitoefening der Geneeskunst in Vrij Beroep," 197.

61. F. Wibaut, "Reorganisatie der Maatschappij, betekenis der te stichten secties," *Medisch Contact* 2 (1947): 1–4, at 1–2.

62. Heringa, "Medische Ethiek, Practische Geneeskunde en Wetenschap," 539.

63. L. van der Drift, "Medische Ethiek anno 1970: Inleiding van de voorzitter der Maatschappij, Dr. L. van der Drift, ter Algemene Vergadering op 18 april 1970 te Utrecht," *Medisch Contact* 25 (1970): 413–17.

64. Andreas Frewer, "Human Rights from the Nuremberg Doctors Trial to the Geneva Declaration," *Medicine, Health Care and Philosophy* 13 (2010): 259–68.

65. "Kort verslag van de 99ste algemene vergadering," *Medisch Contact* 4 (1949): 246–66, at 253–54.

66. "Kort verslag van de 99ste algemene vergadering," 254; F. Wibaut, "Notulen vergadering 5 februari 1949," *Medisch Contact* 4 (1949): 22–27.

67. Roel J. Hamburger and H. Beukenhorst, "De belofte bij het toetreden der Mij," *Medisch Contact* 6 (1951): 15–16, at 15.

68. Roel J. Hamburger, "RAPPORT uitgebracht door Dr. R.J. Hamburger […] inzake experimenten met mensen," April 11, 1953, National Archive, The Hague, Gezondheidsraad 1920–1956, access no. 2.15.33, inv. no. 549; L. A. Hulst, "Experiments on Human Beings, 10 April 1953," National Archive, The Hague, Gezondheidsraad 1920–1956, access no. 2.15.33, inv. no. 549.

69. L. A. Hulst, "Van het Hoofdbestuur: De World Medical Association," *Medisch Contact* 8 (1953): 504–08. See also Susan E. Lederer, "Research Without Borders: The Origins of the Declaration of Helsinki," in *History and Theory of Human Experimentation*, eds. Frewer and Schmidt, 145–64.

70. G. C. Heringa, "De verantwoordelijkheid van medische redacties voor de instandhouding der medische ethiek," *Medisch Contact* 9 (1954): 554–57.

71. G. C. Heringa, "Prof. Dr. L.A. Hulst. Lid van de Council der W.M.A.," *Medisch Contact* 10 (1955): 789.

72. Roel J. Hamburger, "Proeven op mensen," *Medisch Contact* 10 (1955): 333–34, at 334.

73. Appendix to secretary of the Dutch Health Council to the minister of social affairs, July 17, 1947, National Archive, The Hague, Afdeling Volksgezondheid, access no. 2.15.37, inv. no. 2357.

74. M. Stuart to the minister of social affairs, September 16, 1947, National Archive, The Hague, access no. 2.15.37, inv. no. 2357.

75. Appendix to M. Stuart to the minister of social affairs, September 16, 1947, 1, National Archive, The Hague, access no. 2.15.37, inv. no. 2357.

76. Appendix to M. Stuart to the minister of social affairs, September 16, 1947, 1, National Archive, The Hague, access no. 2.15.37, inv. no. 2357, 2–3.

77. M. Stuart to the minister of social affairs, September 16, 1947, National Archive, The Hague, access no. 2.15.37, inv. no. 2357.

78. Anti-Vivisectie-Stichting, "Aan de leden van de 1ste en 2de Kamer der Staten Generaal," date unknown, National Archive, The Hague, Gezondheidsraad 1920–1956, access no. 2.15.33, inv. no. 547.

79. This letter was published by the Association for Homeopathic Healers as "Homoeopathie," *Medisch Contact* 5 (1950): 438–40.

80. Handelingen Tweede Kamer 1949–1950, December 16, 1949: 1097–98.

81. Anti-Vivisectie-Stichting, "Aan de leden van de 1ste en 2de Kamer der Staten Generaal," 1.

82. Rigter, *Met raad en daad*; Roland Bal, Wiebe E. Bijker, and Ruud Hendriks, *Par-*

adox van wetenschappelijk gezag: over de maatschappelijke invloed van adviezen van de Gezondheidsraad (The Hague: Gezondheidsraad, 2002).

83. Jean Jacques Brutel de la Rivière, *Over allergische huidreacties bij niet-allergische personen* (PhD diss., Leiden University, 1932).

84. Appendix to M. Stuart to the minister of social affairs, September 16, 1947, 6, National Archive, The Hague, access no. 2.15.37, inv. no. 2357.

85. "Betreffende: leerstoelen vivisectie-vrije geneeskunde," brief, May 28, 1948, National Archive, The Hague, Gezondheidsraad 1920–1956, access no. 2.15.33, inv. no. 547.

86. Handelingen Tweede Kamer 1949–1950, December 16, 1949: 1099.

87. Handelingen Tweede Kamer 1949–1950, December 16, 1949: 1100.

88. See also J. J. van Loghem, "De Vivisectievrije Geneeskunde in de Tweede Kamer," *Nederlandsch Tijdschrift voor Geneeskunde* 94 (1950): 18–19.

89. G. C. Heringa, "Een leerstoel voor de homoeopathie?," *Medisch Contact* 5 (1950): 191–93, at 193.

90. Published as "Leerstoel voor de homoeopathie?," *Medisch Contact* 5 (1950): 303–06.

91. A. M. Joekes, "Leerstoel homoeopathische geneeskunde," Minister of Social Affairs A. M. Joekes to the minister of education, arts, and sciences, April 13, 1950, National Archive, The Hague, Gezondheidsraad 1920–1956, access no. 2.15.33, inv. no. 547.

92. Jean Jacques Brutel de la Rivière, "Bericht op schrijven 14 April 1953 No. 5148, Directie Volksgezondheid, Afd. M. Z. B, Betreffende: vivisectie," 11–12, National Archive, The Hague, Gezondheidsraad 1920–1956, access no. 2.15.33, inv. no. 546.

93. Rigter, *Met raad en daad*, 209.

94. J. R. Prakken, "A.A. Botter: 'Over de aetiologie van de strophulus infantum,'" *Nederlands Tijdschrift voor Geneeskunde* 94 (1950): 2766.

95. "Ernstige beschuldiging tegen Leids ziekenhuis," *Het Vrije Volk*, May 9, 1953: 5.

96. L. Schalm, "Prof. Dr. C.D. de Langen 75 jaar," *Nederlands Tijdschrift der Geneeskunde* 106 (1962): 1825–26; N. H. Swellengrebel, "Levensbericht C.D. de Langen," in *Jaarboek KNAW 1966–1967* (Amsterdam: KNAW, 1967): 353–57; Lindeboom, *Dutch Medical Biography*, 1139–41.

97. J. B. Scholten, "J.H. Pannekoek 50 jaar arts," *Nederlands Tijdschrift voor Geneeskunde* 123 (1979): 1359–60; M. J. van Lieburg, "Vergeten helden," *Medisch Contact* 64 (2009): 812–15.

98. P. J. Gaillard, "Levensbericht S.E. De Jongh," in *Jaarboek Huygens Institute–KNAW* (Amsterdam: KNAW, 1976): 200–02; E. L. Noach, "In memoriam Prof.Dr. S.E. de Jongh," *Nederlands Tijdschrift voor Geneeskunde* 120 (1976): 1226–28.

99. F. Th. van Genderen, "In Memoriam Prof. Dr. W.K. Dicke," *Nederlands Tijdschrift voor Geneeskunde* 106 (1962): 1108.

100. P. G. Hart, "In memoriam Prof. Dr. W.P. Plate," *Nederlands Tijdschrift voor Geneeskunde* 127 (1983): 1269–70.

101. Also installed were professor in bacteriology and serology A. B. F.A. Pondman, professor of internal medicine and physician-director of the Nijmegen Canisius Hospital J. A. M. J. Enneking, professor of psychiatry and experimental physiology L. Van der Horst, pediatrician H. P. J. Koenen, lung specialist H. C. Hallo, and medical statistician M. G. Neurdenburg. In the final report, State Secretary Piet Muntendam was listed as a committee member, as was physician Pieter Adrianus van Luijt, President of the Health Council from 1951 to 1954. In 1955, van Luijt was replaced by physician Jan Wester. The secretary of the committee was physician V. M. J. Kettlitz.

102. Notulen van de vergadering van de commissie, December 14, 1953, 1, National Archive, The Hague, Gezondheidsraad 1920–1956, access no. 2.15.33, inv. no. 548.

103. Notulen van de vergadering van de commissie, December 14, 1953, 1, 2.

104. On this, see also C. D. de Langen, "Proeven op mensen en de verschuiving van te stellen normen," *Nederlands Tijdschrift voor Geneeskunde* 102 (1958): 25–27, at 27.

105. Notulen van de vergadering van de commissie, February 9, 1954, 7, National Archive, The Hague, Gezondheidsraad 1920–1956, access no. 2.15.33, inv. no. 548.

106. Notulen van de vergadering van de commissie, September 22, 1955, 5, National Archive, The Hague, Gezondheidsraad 1920–1956, access no. 2.15.33, inv. no. 548.

107. Notulen van de vergadering van de commissie, January 27, 1955, 8, National Archive, The Hague, Gezondheidsraad 1920–1956, access no. 2.15.33, inv. no. 548.

108. Wester, "Advies van de Voorzitter van de Gezondheidsraad," 7.

109. Wester, "Advies van de Voorzitter van de Gezondheidsraad," 5.

110. "Concept betreffende: vivisectie," October 8, 1948, 1–2, National Archive, The Hague, Gezondheidsraad 1920–1956, access no. 2.15.33, inv. no. 547.

111. "Concept betreffende: vivisectie," October 8, 1948, 1–2.

112. Notulen van de vergadering van de commissie, March 11, 1954, 2, National Archive, The Hague, Gezondheidsraad 1920–1956, access no. 2.15.33, inv. no. 548.

113. Notulen van de vergadering van de commissie: December 23, 1954, 7, National Archive, The Hague, Gezondheidsraad 1920–1956, access no. 2.15.33, inv. no. 548.

114. Notulen van de vergadering van de commissie, December 23, 1954, 13.

115. Notulen van de vergadering van de commissie, December 23, 1954, 12.

116. Notulen van de vergadering van de commissie, December 23, 1954, 12.

117. Notulen van de vergadering van de commissie, December 23, 1954, 14.

118. Wester, "Advies van de Voorzitter van der Gezondheidsraad," 10.

119. Wester, "Advies van de Voorzitter van der Gezondheidsraad," 7.

120. Wester, "Advies van de Voorzitter van der Gezondheidsraad," 7.

121. Notulen van de vergadering van de commissie, April 5, 1955, 7–8, National Archive, The Hague, Gezondheidsraad 1920–1956, access no. 2.15.33, inv. no. 548.

122. Wester, "Advies van de Voorzitter van der Gezondheidsraad," 10.

123. Wester, "Advies van de Voorzitter van der Gezondheidsraad," 11.

124. Wester, "Advies van de Voorzitter van der Gezondheidsraad," 11.

125. Wester, "Advies van de Voorzitter van der Gezondheidsraad," 12.

CHAPTER TWO

1. O. Fokkens, "Oordeelsvorming in de geneeskunde," *Nederlands Tijdschrift voor Geneeskunde* 106 (1962): 1896–99. All quotes in this paragraph are from page 1896.

2. Harry M. Marks, *The Progress of Experiment: Science and Therapeutic Reform in the United States, 1900–1990* (Cambridge: Cambridge University Press, 1997): 4.

3. Also: Peter Temin, *Taking Your Medicine: Drug Regulation in the United States* (Cambridge, MA: Harvard University Press, 1980); Joseph M. Gabriel, *Medical Monopoly: Intellectual Property Rights and the Origins of the Modern Pharmaceutical Industry* (Chicago: University of Chicago Press, 2015): 103–06.

4. Gabriel, *Medical Monopoly*, 19–20.

5. See also Desiree Cox-Maksimov, "The Making of the Clinical Trial in Britain, 1910–1945: Expertise, the State and the Public" (PhD diss., University of Cambridge, 1997); Martin Edwards, *Control and the Therapeutic Trial: Rhetoric and Experimentation in Britain, 1918–1948* (Amsterdam: Rodopi, 2007); Linda Bryder, "The Medical Research Council and Clinical Trial Methodologies before the 1940s: The Failure to Develop a 'Scientific' Approach," *JLL Bulletin: Commentaries on the History of Treatment Evaluation* (2010), https://www.jameslindlibrary.org/articles/the-medical-research -council-and-clinical-trial-methodologies-before-the-1940s-the-failure-to-develop -a-scientific-approach/.

6. Also: Daniel J. Kevles, *The Physicists: The History of a Scientific Community in Modern America* (New York: Vintage Books, 1979): 296–301; Jon Agar, *Science in the Twentieth Century and Beyond* (Cambridge: Polity Press, 2012): 264–68.

7. Henry K. Beecher, "Ethics and Clinical Research," *New England Journal of Medicine* 74 (1966): 1354–60.

8. David J. Rothman, *Strangers at the Bedside: A History of How Law and Bioethics Transformed Medical Decision Making*, 3rd ed. (New Brunswick, NJ: AldineTransaction, 1991/2003): 53.

9. "Streptomycin Treatment of Pulmonary Tuberculosis: A Medical Research Council Investigation," *British Medical Journal* 2, 4582 (1948): 769–82; Alan Yoshioka, "Use of Randomisation in the Medical Research Council's Clinical Trial of Streptomycin in Pulmonary Tuberculosis in the 1940s," *British Medical Journal* 317 (1998): 1120–223.

10. Marcia L. Meldrum, "A Brief History of the Randomized Controlled Trial: From Oranges and Lemons to the Gold Standard," *Hematology/Oncology Clinics of North America* 14 (2000): 745–60.

11. Peter Temin, "Government Actions in Times of Crisis: Lessons from the History of Drug Regulation," *Journal of Social History* 18 (1985): 433–38.

12. Rothman, *Strangers at the Bedside*, 51.

13. Rothman, *Strangers at the Bedside*, 51–69. This remark has since been repeated by Robert Baker in *Before Bioethics: A History of American Medical Ethics from the Colonial Period to the Bioethics Revolution* (Oxford: Oxford University Press, 2013).

14. Marks, *The Progress of Experiment*, 157.

15. Anne Hardy and E. M. Tansey, "Medical Enterprise and Global Response, 1945–2000," in William F. Bynum et al., *The Western Medical Tradition, 1800–2000* (Cambridge: Cambridge University Press, 2006): 405–534, at 471–87.

16. Marks, *The Progress of Experiment*, 157–58; Bradford Hill, quoted in Donald Mainland, "The Modern Method of the Clinical Trial," *Methods of Medical Research* 6 (1954): 157.

17. W. Lammers, "Bij het afscheid van Professor Gaarenstroom," *Nederlands Tijdschrift voor Geneeskunde* 109 (1965): 1889.

18. In the early 1920s, German pharmacologist Rudolf Magnus acquired funds from the Rockefeller Foundation to build a pharmacological laboratory in Utrecht. In 1923, German pharmacologist Ernst Laqueur co-founded the Dutch pharmaceutical company Organon, which provided the funds for his famous research into the industrial production of hormones. This influx of finances contributed to the emergence of a well-known generation of Dutch pharmacologists in the mid-twentieth century. See E. L. Noach, "The History of Pharmacology in the Netherlands," *Trends in Pharmacological Sciences* 11 (1990): 236–39; J. H. Gaarenstroom, "Het aandeel van Nederland in de vooruitgang der geneeskundige wetenschap van 1900 tot 1950," *Nederlandsch Tijdschrift voor Geneeskunde* 95 (1951): 762–67; Annet Mooij, "Laqueur, Ernst (1880–1947)," *Biografisch Woordenboek van Nederland* (November 12, 2013), http://resources .huygens.knaw.nl/bwn/BWN/lemmata/bwn6/laqueur; R. H. Vermij, *David de Wied: Toponderzoeker in polderland* (Utrecht: Universiteit van Utrecht, 2008); H. Timmermans and D. D. Breimer, "Levensbericht Everhardus Jacobus Ariëns," in *Levensberichten en Herdenkingen 2007* (Amsterdam: Koninklijke Nederlandse Akademie van Wetenschappen, 2007): 6–17.

19. Nelly Oudshoorn, "Laqueur en Organon: Het universitaire laboratorium en de farmaceutische industrie in Nederland," *Gewina* 22 (1999): 12–22.

20. Peter Jan Knegtmans, *Geld, ijdelheid en hormonen: Ernst Laqueur, hoogleraar en ondernemer* (Amsterdam: Boom, 2014).

21. P. J. Gaillard, "Levensbericht S.E. De Jongh," in *Jaarboek Huygens Institute–KNAW* (Amsterdam: KNAW, 1976): 200–02.

22. S. E. de Jongh, *De Ontwikkeling der farmacotherapie: Rede ter herdenking van de 383ste verjaardag der Rijksuniversiteit te Leiden op 8 februari 1958* (Leiden: Universitaire Pers, 1958): 4.

23. De Jongh, *De Ontwikkeling der farmacotherapie*, 14.

24. De Jongh, *De Ontwikkeling der farmacotherapie*, 10. De Jongh borrowed this argument from Gerrit Arie Lindeboom, "Ethiek in de medische wetenschap," *Universiteit en Hogeschool* 3 (1957): 131–41.

25. F. A. Nelemans, *Klinische Farmacologie: Openbare les gehouden aan de Rijksuniversiteit te Utrecht op dinsdag 13 November 1956* (Utrecht, 1956). The status of *privatdozent* was an unsalaried position, typically used to teach classes in a new academic subject not yet part of the standard curriculum.

26. The quote is from the English abstract of Rümke's inaugural lecture, reprinted as Chr. L. Rümke, "De taak van de medische ethiek," *Statistica Neerlandica*, 12 (1958).

27. De Jongh, *De Ontwikkeling der farmacotherapie*, 14.

28. Harry Lintzen et al., *Tachtig jaar TNO* (Delft: TNO, 2012).

29. J. H. Gaarenstroom, "Nota Dr. J. H. Gaarenstroom betreffende gecoördineerde geneesmiddelen research," December 6, 1951, National Archive, The Hague, Nederlandse Organisatie voor Toegepast Natuurwetenschappelijk Onderzoek (TNO): Gezondheidsorganisatie, access no. 2.14.36.06, inv. no. 608.

30. See also T. van Helvoort, "De publieke functie van universitaire wetenschapsbeoefening: Amerikanisering als leidmotief bij de scheikunde aan de Groningse universiteit," in *Onderzoek in opdracht: De publieke functie van het universitaire onderzoek in Nederland sedert 1876*, eds. L. J. Dorsman and P. J. Knegtmans (Hilversum: Verloren, 2007): 67–92.

31. Bestuursnotulen. December 6, 1951, National Archive, The Hague, TNO: Gezondheidsorganisatie, access no. 2.14.36.06, inv. no. 608.

32. Nota Dr. J.H. Gaarenstroom, December 6, 1951, National Archive, The Hague, TNO: Gezondheidsorganisatie, access no. 2.14.36.06, inv. no. 608.

33. Bestuursnotulen, December 6, 1951, National Archive, The Hague, TNO: Gezondheidsorganisatie, access no. 2.14.36.06, inv. no. 608.

34. Nota Dr. J.H. Gaarenstroom, December 6, 1951, National Archive, The Hague, TNO: Gezondheidsorganisatie, access no. 2.14.36.06, inv. no. 608.

35. Eerste vergadering, November 19, 1952, National Archive, The Hague, TNO: Gezondheidsorganisatie, access no. 2.14.36.06, inv. no. 608.

36. M. M. Hilfman, "Mededelingen adviescommissie klinisch geneesmiddelenonderzoek," *Nederlands Tijdschrift voor Geneeskunde* 100 (1956): 1671.

37. "Opheffing Werkgroep Klinisch Geneesmiddelenonderzoek TNO," *Nederlands Tijdschrift voor Geneeskunde* 119 (1975): 418.

38. F. A. Nelemans, "Klinische farmacologie," *Algemene farmacotherapie. Het geneesmiddel in theorie en praktijk*, eds. W. Lammers, F. A. Nelemans, and P. Siderius (Leiden: L. Stafleu & Zoon, 1961): 19–20, at 20.

39. "Veiligheid van Nieuwe Geneesmiddelen," *Medisch Contact* 18 (1963): 359–61.

40. "Veilig gebruik nieuwe geneesmiddelen," *Friese Koerier*, November 30, 1963: 21; "Onderzoek nieuw medicijn eist experiment op mens," *De Tijd-Maasbode*, May 10, 1963: 4; "Risico's zijn in farmacologie onvermijdelijk," *De Telegraaf*, May 10, 1963: 3; "De Mens is het Beste Proefdier," *De Waarheid*, November 30, 1963: 4.

41. F. A. Nelemans and W. G. Zelvelder, *Therapeutische evaluatie van geneesmiddelen* (Leiden: Stafleu's Wetenschappelijke Uitgeversmaatschappij, 1970): 5, 9, 5.

42. Nelemans and Zelvelder, *Therapeutische evaluatie van geneesmiddelen*, 140.

43. Nelemans and Zelvelder, *Therapeutische evaluatie van geneesmiddelen*, 139.

44. Aanhangsel tot het Verslag van de Handelingen der Tweede Kamer (Appendix of the Report of the Acts of the House of Representatives) 1967–1968, no. 119: 241–42; "Dr. R.J.H. Kruisinga beantwoordt vragen inzake 'dubbelblinde' farmacologische onderzoeken," *Medisch Contact* 22 (1967): 1125–26.

45. Wet van 28 juli 1958, houdende nieuwe regelen nopens de geneesmiddelenvoorziening en de uitoefening der artsenijbereidkunst (Wet op de geneesmiddelenvoorziening) (Law of July 28, 1958, containing new regulations with regard to the supply of medicines and the practice of pharmaceutical preparation [Law on the Supply of Medicines]), Article 3.

46. M. Cluysenaer and L. Breeveld, *50 Jaar College ter Beoordeling van Geneesmiddelen* (Haarlem: self-published, 2013): 10.

47. Cluysenaer and Breeveld, 3. In 1961, Siderius and Lammers had also formed the editorial board of the Dutch Pharmacotherapy Handbook with Nelemans, whom they appointed as a board member of the MEB in 1963.

48. For how thalidomide influenced the regulation of pharmaceutical drugs in the twentieth century, see Jean-Paul Gaudillière and Volker Hess, eds., *Ways of Regulating Drugs in the 19th and 20th Centuries* (Basingstoke: Palgrave Macmillan, 2013); Temin, "Government Actions in Times of Crisis," 433–38.

49. Whereas in Germany approximately four thousand babies with teratogenic deformities were born because of thalidomide, this number amounted to only twenty-five in the Netherlands. See "Ouders van softenon-kinderen geen kans op schadevergoeding," *De Telegraaf*, February 21, 1968: 9; "Thalidomide eiste ook in Nederland slachtoffers," *Limburgsch Dagblad*, January 2, 1969: 7.

50. "Wij slikken duizenden pilletjes per dag," *De Waarheid*, September 13, 1962: 4; "Talloze problemen voor Veldkamp," *Limburgsch Dagblad*, November 22, 1962: 5; "Wanneer controle op verpakte geneesmiddelen?," *De Waarheid*, November 22, 1962: 3.

51. See also Temin, "Government Actions in Times of Crisis," 433–38.

52. For all, see: 19e vergadering, June 12, 1959, National Archive, The Hague, TNO / Gezondheidsorganisatie, access no. 2.14.36.06, inv. no. 608.

53. Aanhangsel tot het Verslag van de Tweede Kamer 1967–1968, no. 119: 241.

54. Aanhangsel tot het Verslag van de Tweede Kamer 1967–1968, no. 119: 242.

55. Handelingen Tweede Kamer (Acts of the House of Representatives) 1967–1968, Vaste Commissie voor de volksgezondheid, November 2, 1967: T50. See also "Wat hebben ze gezegd," in *Limburgsch Dagblad*, August 29, 1967: 12; "Geen proefkonijnen," *Leeuwarder Courant*, August 26, 1967: 3; "Levens van hartpatiënten door fopmedicijn gered: Onderzoek na vragen Kamerlid," *Nieuwsblad van het Noorden*, August 29, 1967: 3.

56. Handelingen Tweede Kamer 1967–1968: T50.

57. Handelingen Tweede Kamer 1967–1968: T51.

58. Gezondheidsraad, *Advies inzake klinische farmacologie* (The Hague: Staatsuit-geverij, 1982): 111.

59. Rapport inzake klinisch onderzoek van geneesmiddelen, 1971, National Archive, The Hague, Gezondheidsraad 1957–1990, access no. 2.15.36, inv. no. 1476. See also Gezondheidsraad, *Klinische farmacologie*, 111–35.

60. E. L. Noach, *Tweeërlei farmacologie. Inaugurele rede Leiden* (Amsterdam: N.V. Noord-Hollandsche Uitgevers Maatschapij, 1964); David de Wied, "Erik Noach, col-lega en vriend," in *Geneeskunde en ethiek in harmonie: Liber amicorum voor Prof.Dr E.L. Noach bij diens 80ste verjaardag op 21 November 2001*, ed. F. A. Wolff, 11–18 (The Hague: Pasmans Offset Drukkerij BV, 2001).

61. E. L. Noach to Health Council president A. J. Ch. Haex, July 2, 1968, National Archive, The Hague, Gezondheidsraad 1957–1990, access no. 2.15.36, inv. no. 1478.

62. See T. Rinsema, "Brocades & Stheeman. Van apotheker-fabrikant tot farmaceu-tische industrie," *Gewina* 22 (1999): 23–33.

63. Noach to Health Council president A. J. Ch. Haex, 2–3.

64. Rapport inzake klinisch onderzoek van geneesmiddelen, 5. Also: "Principles for the Clinical Evaluation of Drugs," *World Health Organization Technical Report Series* 403 (Geneva, 1968): 6.

65. Rapport inzake klinisch onderzoek van geneesmiddelen, 6–7.

66. Rapport inzake klinisch onderzoek van geneesmiddelen, 5.

67. Rapport inzake klinisch onderzoek van geneesmiddelen, 7.

68. Rapport inzake klinisch onderzoek van geneesmiddelen, 12.

69. Nelemans and Zelvelder, *Therapeutische evaluatie van geneesmiddelen*, 51.

70. Nelemans and Zelvelder, *Therapeutische evaluatie van geneesmiddelen*, 142.

71. Nelemans, *Klinische Farmacologie*, 10.

72. Nelemans, *Klinische Farmacologie*, 11. Italics original.

73. Nelemans and Zelvelder, *Therapeutische evaluatie van geneesmiddelen*.

74. Rapport inzake klinisch onderzoek van geneesmiddelen, 13.

75. Rapport inzake klinisch onderzoek van geneesmiddelen, 13.

76. Rapport inzake klinisch onderzoek van geneesmiddelen, 18.

77. Rapport inzake klinisch onderzoek van geneesmiddelen, 13. For more on the historical practice of "refereeing" by scientific journals and grant organizations, see Melinda Baldwin, *Making Nature: The History of a Scientific Journal* (Chicago: University of Chicago Press, 2015); Alex Csiszar, *The Scientific Journal: Authorship and the Politics of Knowledge in the Nineteenth Century* (Chicago: University of Chicago Press, 2018); Aileen Fyfe, "Journals and Periodicals," in *A Companion to the History of Science*, ed. Bernard Lightman (West Sussex: John Wiley & Sons Ltd., 2016): 387–99; Mark Solovey, *Shaky Foundations: The Politics-Patronage-Social Science Nexus in Cold War America* (New Brunswick, NJ: Rutgers University Press, 2013); Robert E. Kohler, *Partners in Science: Foundations and Natural Scientists, 1900–1945* (Chicago: University of Chicago Press, 1991).

78. "Principles for the Clinical Evaluation of Drugs," 31.

79. Rapport inzake klinisch onderzoek van geneesmiddelen, 13.

80. Rapport inzake klinisch onderzoek van geneesmiddelen, 12.

81. Discussie nota M25-2, 7, National Archive, The Hague, Gezondheidsraad, access no. 2.15.36, inv. no. 1478.

82. Rapport inzake klinisch onderzoek van geneesmiddelen, 10.

83. Rapport inzake klinisch onderzoek van geneesmiddelen, 14.

84. Rapport inzake klinisch onderzoek van geneesmiddelen, 14–15.

85. Rapport inzake klinisch onderzoek van geneesmiddelen, 16.

86. Rapport inzake klinisch onderzoek van geneesmiddelen, 13.

87. In 1976, the committee was joined by another committee tasked to consider the permissibility of experiments with radioactive material. By that time, the Health Council was working on its fourth piece of policy advice on the governance of human experimentation in a period of only twenty years. Commissie experimenten met radioactieve stoffen op proefpersonen, 120, National Archive, The Hague, Gezondheidsraad 1957–1990, access no. 2.15.36, inv. no. 3.3.101.

88. Gezondheidsraad, *Advies inzake normen voor het toedienen van radioactieve stoffen aan vrijwilligers* (The Hague: Staatsuitgeverij, 1981); Gezondheidsraad, *Advies inzake klinische Farmacologie.*

89. Gezondheidsraad, *Advies inzake klinische farmacologie*, 36.

90. Gezondheidsraad, *Advies inzake klinische farmacologie*, 57.

91. Gezondheidsraad, *Advies inzake klinische farmacologie*, 98.

92. Gezondheidsraad, *Advies inzake klinische farmacologie*, 99. E. L. Noach and P. J. W. M. de Kroon, "Medische ethiek: patiënten en proeven: De Commissie Medische Ethiek in het Academisch Ziekenhuis en de Faculteit der Geneeskunde te Leiden," *Medisch Contact* 34 (1979): 1575–83.

93. Gezondheidsraad, *Advies inzake klinische farmacologie*, 57.

CHAPTER THREE

1. See J. M. Coetzee, *Landscape with Rowers: Poetry from the Netherlands* (Princeton, NJ: Princeton University Press, 2003).

2. K. Tamboer, "Groningse zenuwarts R.H. van den Hoofdakker: 'Artsenstand-sleepanker dat vooruitgang afremt,'" *Het Vrije Volk*, August 30, 1969: 5.

3. R. H. van den Hoofdakker, "Het bolwerk der beterweters," *Wijsgerig Perspectief op Maatschappij en Samenleving* 9 (1968–1969): 292–301.

4. R. H. van den Hoofdakker, *Het bolwerk van de beterweters: Over de medische ethiek en de status quo* (Amsterdam: Kritiese Bibliotheek, 1970): 33.

5. Centrale Raad voor de Volksgezondheid, *Deeladvies inzake medische experimenten* (The Hague: Staatsuitgeverij, 1982): 7, 15.

6. Robert Baker, *Before Bioethics: A History of American Medical Ethics from the Colonial Period to the Bioethics Revolution* (Oxford: Oxford University Press, 2013): 317.

7. Draft chapters were regularly printed in *Medisch Contact* between 1954 and 1958. See, for instance, "Het overdoen van de praktijk," *Medisch Contact* 9 (1954): 298–99; "De pers en de geneeskunde," *Medisch Contact* 10 (1955): 242–45; "Assistentie, waarneming en associatie," *Medisch Contact* 11 (1956): 16–21; "Honorarium," *Medisch Contact* 12 (1957): 546–51; "Het ziekenfondswezen," *Medisch Contact* 13 (1958): 105–08.

8. KNMG, *Medische ethiek en gedragsleer* (Amsterdam: Koninklijke Nederlandse Maatschappij tot Bevordering der Geneeskunst, 1959).

9. One chapter addressed the ethics of medical experiments on human beings and contained the ethical guidelines of the 1955 Health Council report. For the publication of the draft chapter in *Medisch Contact*, see "Proeven op mensen," *Medisch Contact* 13 (1958): 108–09.

10. "Commissies," in *Medisch Contact* 13 (1958): 335; Dekker, "De derde druk van het boekje 'Medische Ethiek en Gedragsleer,'" *Medisch Contact* 15 (1960): 162.

11. "'Medische Ethiek' opnieuw gedrukt," *Medisch Contact* 15 (1960): 169–70, at 169.

12. "'Medische Ethiek' opnieuw gedrukt," 170.

13. Gerrit Arie Lindeboom, *Opstellen over medische ethiek* (Kampen: J. H. Kok N. V., 1960). In Catholic circles, discussion of medical ethics was more common. Pope Pius XII, for instance, frequently addressed the subject and spoke at conferences such as that of the World Medical Association. See Darrel W. Amundsen, "The Discourses of Roman Catholic Medical Ethics," in *The Cambridge World History of Medical Ethics*, edited by Robert B. Baker and Laurence B. McCullough (Cambridge: Cambridge University Press, 2009): 218–54.

14. C. L. de Jong, "G.A. Lindeboom, *Opstellen over medische ethiek*," *Nederlands Tijdschrift voor Geneeskunde* 104 (1960): 1897.

15. See, for instance, "Leemte in medische opleiding," *Leeuwarder Courant*, September 13, 1960: 2; "Nieuwe uitgaven," *Nieuwsblad van het Noorden*, June 2, 1960: 27; "Gesprek aan het ziekbed," *Gereformeerd Gezinsblad*, July 16, 1960.

16. "Over medische ethiek: Twee nieuwe uitgaven," *De Tijd-Maasbode*, May 19, 1960: 7.

17. W. Metz, "Over de crisis in de medische ethiek," *Medisch Contact* 25 (1970): 330–32.

18. "Kort verslag H.B.-vergadering," *Medisch Contact* 21 (1966): 210–11, at 210; G. Dekker, "Jaarverslag 1967 der Maatschappij," *Medisch Contact* 23 (1968): 718–23, at 721.

19. "Inleiding 154ste Algemene Vergadering," *Medisch Contact* 25 (1970): 5–6, at 5.

20. Metz, "Over de crisis in de medische ethiek," 330.

21. "Medische Ethiek," *Medisch Contact* 16 (1961): 190–91, at 190. For Johannes (Hannes) de Graaf, who was a pastor as well as the leader of the Pacifist Socialist Party (PSP), see: E. D. J. de Jongh, *Hannes de Graaf: Een leven van bevrijding* (Kampen: Ten Have, 2004).

22. For a similar analysis in this period, see I. Boerema, "De Keerzijde van de Vooruitgang in de Geneeskunde," in W. Peremans et al., *Acht voordrachten over de keer-*

zijde van de vooruitgang in de natuur- en geneeskundige wetenschappen (The Hague: Mar-tinus Nijhoff, 1962): 3955.

23. "Medische Ethiek," *Medisch Contact* 16 (1961): 190.

24. All quotes in this paragraph: "Medische Ethiek," *Medisch Contact* 16 (1961): 191.

25. *Medisch Contact* editors, "Ethische problemen voor de arts," in *Medisch Contact* 17 (1962): 237–38, at 238.

26. *Medisch Contact* editors, "Ethische problemen voor de arts," 238.

27. "Discussie over: rapport kunstmatige inseminatie," *Medisch Contact* 17 (1962): 239–41.

28. "Varia," *Medisch Contact* 20 (1965): 278. Around the same time, *Medisch Contact* started frequently advertising lectures on the topic of medical ethics and any ongoing problems therewith. See, for instance: M. W. Jongsma, "Medische ethiek," *Medisch Contact* 21 (1966): 311–16; "Dr. J.C. Schultsz over Medische Ethiek," *Medisch Contact* 21 (1966): 782–83; "Voordrachten: internist C.L.C. Nieuwenhuizen, onderwerp 'De ethische consequenties van de moderne ontwikkeling in de geneeskunde en biolo-gie,'" *Medisch Contact* 22 (1967): 377; C. Paul Sporken, "Katholieke moraal en abor-tus," *Medisch Contact* 22 (1967): 385–89; "Voordrachten: Dr. H. Hamminga, onder-werp 'Enige medisch-ethische problemen,'" *Medisch Contact* 22 (1967): 469; "Varia: Het dogma in de medische ethiek," *Medisch Contact* 22 (1967): 1163.

29. "Kort verslag H.B.-vergadering," 210; Dekker, "Jaarverslag 1967 der Maatschap-pij," 721.

30. "Korte verslagen vergaderingen hoofdbestuur," *Medisch Contact* 23 (1968): 337–38, at 338; W. B. van der Mijn, "Het takenpakket der maatschappij," *Medisch Contact* 23 (1968): 631–37, at 632.

31. Thus, in addition to the official KNMG journals, Catholic and Protestant medi-cal journals also existed, while hospitals and health funds often operated within these frameworks as well. See Friso Wielenga, *Nederland in de twintigste eeuw* (Amster-dam: Boom, 2009); Peter van Dam, *Staat van verzuiling: Over een Nederlandse mythe* (Amsterdam: Wereldbibliotheek, 2011).

32. J. J. C. Marlet, M. F. J. Marlet, and L. N. Marlet, *Schuld en verontschuldiging in de medische praktijk* (Roermond: J. J. Romen & Zonen, 1966).

33. J. J. C. Marlet, "De in rechten vervolgde arts," in Marlet, Marlet, and Marlet, *Schuld en verontschuldiging,* 57–82.

34. L. N. Marlet, "Enige raakpunten tussen de medische praktijk en het leerstuk der aansprakelijkheid," in Marlet, Marlet, and Marlet, *Schuld en Verontschuldiging,* 5–65, at 7.

35. Marlet, "De in rechten vervolgde arts," 65. See also J. M. F. Phaff, "Toepassing medische psychologie door de huisarts," *Medisch Contact* 18 (1963): 480–83.

36. Dutch historians Stephen Snelders and Frans Meijsman have investigated the history of "de mondige patient" and have concluded that the supposed emergence of the mature patient in the 1960s is largely a historical myth. Dutch patients, they argue, were well capable of voicing their opinions about the treatments they desired long

before the 1960s. See Stephen Snelders and Frans Meijsman, *De mondige patiënt: Historische kijk op een mythe* (Amsterdam: Bert Bakker, 2009).

37. For a contemporary analysis of the emergence of "the mature patient," see A. Querido, "De mondigheid van de patient: I. Diagnose," *Metamedica* 49 (1970): 205–08.

38. "De dokter is God niet," *Algemeen Handelsblad*, May 13, 1967: supplement, 1.

39. The *Algemeen Handelsblad* based its claim that medical misconduct did take place in the Netherlands on an article published in the *Dutch Journal of Medicine* in 1963 that had hardly received any coverage in the general press. See P. J. Kuijer, J. F. van Rhede van der Kloot, and J. Logeman, "Sterfte, medische tekortkomingen en foutenbronnen," *Nederlands Tijdschrift voor Geneeskunde* 107 (1963): 1268–70. In 1967, the editors of *Medisch Contact* responded very angrily to what they called a "sensationalist publication" in the *Algemeen Handelsblad*: "Massamedia en Medici: Het Handelsblad constateert 'de muur van geheimzinnigheid, die de medische wereld om zich heeft opgebouwd, doorbroken,'" *Medisch Contact* 22 (1967): 527–28.

40. See P. Th. Hugenholtz, "Wijziging rechtspraak," *Medisch Contact* 13 (1958): 785.

41. G. Dekker, "Rapport van de commissie herziening rechtspraak: Pre-advies van het hoofdbestuur," *Medisch Contact* 23 (1968): 84–104; W. B. van der Mijn, "De rechtspraak van de maatschappij," *Medisch Contact* 24 (1969): 1029–31; "De 150ste Algemene Vergadering der Maatschappij," *Medisch Contact* 23 (1968): 453–63, at 453.

42. F. F. X. Cerutti et al., *De Geneesheer en het recht* (Deventer: Kluwer, 1968); "Congres te Nijmegen: De geneesheer en het recht," *Medisch Contact* 23 (1968): 315–17; *Medisch Contact* editors, "Aesculapius en Themis: Een nuttige ontmoeting," *Medisch Contact* 23 (1968): 313–14.

43. J. Maeijer, "Juridische relatie geneesheer en patiënt," in Cerutti et al., *De Geneesheer en het Recht*, 9–23, at 9.

44. L. H. Th. S. Kortbeek et al., eds., *Recent medisch ethisch denken I* (De Nederlandse Bibliotheek der Geneeskunde, Editorial Series no. 40) (Leiden: Stafleu's Wetenschappelijke Uitgeversmaatschappij, 1968): 5.

45. A. G. M. van Melsen et al., *Recent medisch ethisch denken II* (De Nederlandse Bibliotheek der Geneeskunde, Editorial Series no. 60) (Leiden: Stafleu's Wetenschappelijke Uitgeversmaatschappij, 1970).

46. J. P. Calff, *Medische ethiek vandaag* (Amsterdam: Agon Elsevier, 1969): back flap.

47. "Medische ethiek tussen natuurwetenschap en samenleving," *Wetenschap en Samenleving* 23, no. 5–6 (1969); Herman J. Heering, *Ethiek der voorlopigheid* (Nijkerk: Callenbach, 1969); C. Paul Sporken, *Voorlopige diagnose: inleiding tot een medische ethiek* (Utrecht: Ambo, 1969).

48. L. van der Drift, "Medische Ethiek anno 1970: Inleiding van de voorzitter der Maatschappij, Dr. L. van der Drift, ter Algemene Vergadering op 18 april 1970 te Utrecht," *Medisch Contact* 25 (1970): 413–17.

49. Drift, 413.

50. Drift, 414.

51. Drift, 415.

52. For an overview of Catholic and Protestant thinking about medical ethics in the Netherlands in 1970, see C. Paul Sporken, "Vijftig jaar medische ethiek in het Katholiek Artsenblad," *Metamedica* 49 (1970): 395–411; Gerrit Arie Lindeboom, "Medisch-ethische bezinning in Protestantse kring," *Metamedica* 49 (1970): 411–16.

53. All quotes in this paragraph are from Drift, "Medische Ethiek anno 1970," 417.

54. Handelingen Tweede Kamer (Acts of the House of Representatives) 1969–1970, February 3, 1970: 1939–98.

55. Handelingen Tweede Kamer 1969–1970, February 3, 1970: 1952.

56. Handelingen Tweede Kamer 1969–1970, February 3, 1970: 1954.

57. Jan Hendrik van den Berg, *Medische Macht en Medische Ethiek* (Nijkerk: Callenbach, 1969). The specialty of "zenuwarts," which understood psychiatric illnesses as nervous disorders, was abolished in 1984.

58. Berg, *Medische Macht en Medische Ethiek*, 47. For more on Berg, see H. Zwart, *Boude Bewoordingen: De historische fenomenologie ("metabletica") van Jan Hendrik van den Berg* (Kampen: Uitgeverij Klement, 2002).

59. The booklet stayed on Dutch bestseller lists until the spring of 1970. See "Het meest verkochte boek," *De Telegraaf*, August 9, 1969: 7; "Succes voor 'Help! De dokter verzuipt . . . ,'" *De Telegraaf*, September 27, 1969: XIII; "Meest verkocht," *De Tijd*, March 9, 1970: 5. By 1985, *Medische Macht en Medische Ethiek* had gone through its twenty-fifth reprint.

60. For similar Dutch essays on euthanasia in this period, see J. J. Prick, "Discussie over: de medische ethiek met betrekking tot de nieuwste ontwikkelingen in de geneeskunde," *Medisch Contact* 24 (1969): 83–85; C. J. Goudsmit, "Discussie over: de medische ethiek met betrekking tot de nieuwste ontwikkelingen in de geneeskunde," *Medisch Contact* 24 (1969): 386.

61. C. Paul Sporken, "Medische ethiek als cultuurkritiek: Naar aanleiding van revalidatie, levensverlenging en euthanasia," *Medisch Contact* 24 (1969): 1431–34, at 1432.

62. "Macht en ethiek," *Nederlands Dagblad*, February 24, 1972: 6.

63. C. Wennen-Van der Mey, "Medische ethiek ter discussie," *De Groene Amsterdammer*, October 4, 1969: 10.

64. Handelingen Tweede Kamer 1969–1970, February 3, 1970: 1954.

65. Handelingen Tweede Kamer 1969–1970, February 3, 1970: 1983.

66. Henri Festen, *Spanningen in de gezondheidszorg: 25 jaar Centrale Raad voor de Volksgezondheid* (Zoetermeer: Nationale Raad voor de Volksgezondheid, 1985).

67. Handelingen Tweede Kamer 1969–1970, February 3, 1970: 1987.

68. Handelingen Tweede Kamer 1969–1970, February 3, 1970: 1993. Emphasis added.

69. Notulen van de Commissie Medische Ethiek, April 20, 1971, 11, National Archive, The Hague, Gezondheidsraad 1957–1990, access no. 2.15.36, inv. no. 1374.

70. Gezondheidsraad, *Interim-advies inzake euthanasie* (The Hague: Staatsuitgeverij, 1972): 3–4.

71. Notulen van de Commissie Medische Ethiek, January 23, 1973, 2, National Archive, The Hague, Gezondheidsraad 1957–1990, access no. 2.15.36, inv. no. 1374.

72. Notulen van de Commissie Medische Ethiek, April 20, 1971, 7.

73. Notulen van de Commissie Medische Ethiek, December 13, 1973, National Archive, The Hague, Gezondheidsraad 1957–1990, access no. 2.15.36, inv. no. 1374.

74. Notulen van de Commissie Medische Ethiek, December 13, 1973, 2.

75. Notulen van de Commissie Medische Ethiek, February 14, 1972, 10, National Archive, The Hague, Gezondheidsraad 1957–1990, access no. 2.15.36, inv. no. 1374.

76. Gezondheidsraad, *Interim-advies inzake euthanasie*, 10.

77. Gezondheidsraad, *Interim-advies inzake euthanasie*, 10.

78. Gezondheidsraad, *Interim-advies inzake euthanasie*, 6.

79. Gezondheidsraad, *Interim-advies inzake euthanasie*, 16.

80. Notulen van de Commissie Medische Ethiek, April 20, 1971, 6.

81. H. L., "De rechten van de patiënt," *Katholiek Artsenblad* 47 (1968): 162–64.

82. Hans Righart, *De eindeloze jaren zestig: Geschiedenis van een generatieconflict* (Amsterdam: De Arbeiderspers, 1995); James Kennedy, *Nieuw Babylon in aanbouw: Nederland in de jaren zestig* (Amsterdam: Boom, 1995).

83. E. H. Tonkens, *Het zelfontplooiingsregime: De actualiteit van Dennendal en de jaren zestig* (Amsterdam: Bakker, 1999). Also: Commissie van advies inzake het democratisch en doelmatig functioneren van gesubsidieerde instellingen, *Discussie-nota, September 1975* (Rijswijk: Secretariaat, 1975): 8.

84. Duco Hellema, *Nederland en de jaren zeventig* (Amsterdam: Boom, 2012).

85. Handelingen Tweede Kamer 1969–1970, February 3, 1970: 1952.

86. See Sporken, "Medische ethiek als cultuurkritiek," 1431–34; "Stervensbegeleiding: Medisch-ethische plicht? Door Dr. C.P. Sporken, ethicus, directeur van het Mgr. Bekkers Centrum, Katholieke Universiteit Nijmegen," *Medisch Contact* 25 (1970): 418–24. For a similar understanding of medical ethics, see W. Metz, "Wijsgerige heroriëntatie in de medische ethiek," *Algemeen Nederlands Tijdschrift voor Wijsbegeerte en Psychologie* 61 (1969): 1–18.

87. Berg, *Medische Macht en Medische Ethiek*, 48.

88. For all quotations in this paragraph, see Notulen van de Commissie Medische Ethiek, April 20, 1971, 6–7.

89. Gezondheidsraad, *Interim-advies inzake euthanasie*, 8, 15.

90. See Loes Kater, *Disciplines met dadendrang: Gezondheidsrecht en gezondheidsethiek in het Nederlandse euthanasiedebat 1960–1994* (Amsterdam: Aksant, 2004).

91. Henk J. J. Leenen, *Sociale grondrechten en gezondheidszorg* (PhD diss., Utrecht University, 1966); Henk J. J. Leenen, "Vereniging voor Gezondheidsrecht 25 jaar: geschiedenis van de start," *Tijdschrift voor Gezondheidsrecht* 16 (1992): 128–34; Henk J. J. Leenen, "De geschiedenis van de Vereniging voor Gezondheidsrecht," *Tijdschrift*

voor *Gezondheidsrecht* 2 (1978): 184–89. Leenen also founded the Dutch Journal for Health Law and wrote two handbooks on health law. He is often regarded as the father of Dutch health law. For more on Leenen, see J. K. M. Gevers and J. H. Hubben, eds., *Grenzen aan de zorg, zorgen aan de grens: Liber amicorum voor Prof.dr. H.J.J. Leenen* (Alphen aan den Rijn: Samsom H. D. Tjeenk Willink, 1990).

92. Henk J. J. Leenen, "Gezondheidsrecht: Een poging tot plaatsbepaling," *Tijdschrift voor Sociale Geneeskunde* 46 (1968): 778–85, at 784.

93. Jacob F. Rang, *Patiëntenrecht* (Leiden: Stafleu's Wetenschappelijke Uitgeversmaatschappij, 1973). It should be noted that Leenen had by then already taken up a professorial chair at the University of Amsterdam, but his appointment was officially to study "the social backgrounds of health and health care." See Henk J. J. Leenen, *Systeem-denken in de gezondheidszorg* (Alphen aan den Rijn: Samson, 1971).

94. Rang, *Patiëntenrecht*, 11.

95. Rang, *Patiëntenrecht*, 33. Rang lists H. H. Eyck and A. J. Verstegen, *Arts en wet: Rechtskundige handleiding voor geneeskundigen*, 2nd ed. (Haarlem: De Erven Bohn, 1929); W. Schuurmans Stekhoven, *Jurisprudentia Medica* (Groningen: Wolters-Noordhoff, 1972).

96. Rang, *Patiëntenrecht*, 33.

97. See also H. Nys, "Van Leenen tot Legemaate: 40 jaar Nederlands gezondheidsrecht in een twintigtal oraties," in *Oratiebundel gezondheidsrecht: Verzamelde redes 1971–2011*, ed. Vereniging voor Gezondheidsrecht (The Hague: SDU Uitgevers, 2012).

98. In 1982, Rang also became the first national Dutch ombudsman: a government official tasked to investigate complaints by citizens against any violation of their rights by the government.

99. Commissie van advies, *Discussie-nota, September 1975*, 8.

100. For a few examples, see "Dokter kijkt uit naar mondige patiënt," *Limburgsch Dagblad*, May 2, 1970: 40; "Heeft zieke recht op volwassen behandeling?," *Leeuwarder Courant*, January 29, 1971: 2; "Cruijf lichtend voorbeeld van mondige patiënt," *De Tijd*, April 13, 1972: front page; "Patiënten betuttelen . . . hoe lang duurt dat nog?," *Het Vrije Volk*, February 7, 1973: 4; "Arts moet uitleggen wat hij voorschrijft," *Nieuwsblad van het Noorden*, April 24, 1974: 3; H. S. Terburgh, "Groeiende mondigheid patiënt door overheid weer afgenomen?," *NRC Handelsblad*, October 4, 1975: 4.

101. See J. B. Ahlers, *Meer mensen mondig maken* (The Hague: Staatsuitgeverij, 1975).

102. Handelingen Tweede Kamer 1974–1975, May 6, 1975: 4257.

103. Kamerstuk Tweede Kamer (parliamentary document of the House of Representatives) 1974–1975, no. 13012 sec. 11, Structuurnota Gezondheidszorg, motie van het lid Dees c.s., proposed May 7, 1975.

104. Handelingen Tweede Kamer 1974–1975, May 13, 1975: 4241.

105. W. B. van der Mijn, "De wetgever en het medisch handelen," *Medisch Contact* 27 (1972): 1165–71.

106. Adviesaanvrage inzake patiëntenrecht, October 26, 1977, National Archive, The Hague, Centrale Raad voor de Volksgezondheid, access no. 2.27.16, inv. no. 803.

107. 8006 6, Nota voor het C. v. G., 7, National Archive, The Hague, Centrale Raad voor de Volksgezondheid, access no. 2.27.16, inv. no. 803.

108. 8006 6, Nota voor het C. v. G., 14.

109. 1002 135, Zakelijk verslag van de 135e Raadsvergadering op maandag 13 maart 1978, March 13, 1978, 2–10, at 7, National Archive, The Hague, Centrale Raad voor de Volksgezondheid, access no. 2.27.16, inv. no. 22.

110. 1002 135, Zakelijk verslag van de 135e Raadsvergadering op maandag 13 maart 1978, 8.

111. G. M. J. van der Haak-Tielens, brief van Drs. G. M. J. Van der Haak-Tielens, namens Vereniging Patiëntenbelangen aan de Voorzitter van de CRV, October 16, 1978, National Archive, The Hague, Centrale Raad voor de Volksgezondheid, access no. 2.27.16, inv. no. 803.

112. T. J. van Goelst Meijer, brief van T. J. Van Goelst Meijer, sekretaris Gezamenlijk Overleg Beroepsverenigingen in de Gezondheidszorg, October 16, 1978, National Archive, The Hague, Centrale Raad voor de Volksgezondheid, access no. 2.27.16, inv. no. 803.

113. J. Brouwer, brief van J. Brouwer, voorzitter vereniging gelijke rechten voor alle geneeswijzen aan de Voorzitter van de Gezondheidsraad, October 13, 1978, National Archive, The Hague, Centrale Raad voor de Volksgezondheid, access no. 2.27.16, inv. no. 803.

114. Brief aan de Algemeen Secretaris van de CRV van Dr. Sanders, Nefarma, July 17, 1978, National Archive, The Hague, Centrale Raad voor de Volksgezondheid, access no, 2.27.16, inv. no. 803.

115. 8006 80, February 19, 1979, National Archive, The Hague, Centrale Raad voor de Volksgezondheid, access no. 2.27.16, inv. no. 803; J. W. Engelkes, brief van J. W. Engelkes aan de Stichting Nederlandse Gehandicaptenraad, National Archive, The Hague, Centrale Raad voor de Volksgezondheid, access no. 2.27.16, inv. no. 803.

116. 1004 228, Zakelijk verslag van de 209e C. v. G.-vergadering gehouden op maandag 11 juni 1979, June 11, 1979, 11–12, National Archive, The Hague, Centrale Raad voor de Volksgezondheid, access no. 2.27.16, inv. no. 52; Zakelijk verslag van de 147ste Raadsvergadering gehouden op maandag 13 augustus 1979, August 13, 1979, 13, National Archive, The Hague, Centrale Raad voor de Volksgezondheid, access no. 2.27.16, inv. no. 23.

117. Centrale Raad voor de Volksgezondheid, *Deeladvies betreffende de juridische relatie tussen patiënt en arts, het recht van de patiënt op informatie en het toestemmingsvereiste* (The Hague: Staatsuitgeverij, 1980); Centrale Raad voor de Volksgezondheid, *Deeladvies inzake de bescherming van de privacy van de patiënt* (The Hague: Staatsuitgeverij, 1981); Centrale Raad voor de Volksgezondheid, *Deelsadvies inzake bemiddeling van klachten van patiënten* (Rijswijk: Centrale Raad voor de Volksgezondheid, 1982); Cen-

trale Raad voor de Volksgezondheid, *Deeladvies inzake kernbepalingen voor der regeling van de relatie tussen patiënt en arts* (The Hague: Staatsuitgeverij, 1982).

118. 1004 239, Zakelijk verslag van de 239e C. v. G.-vergadering gehouden op donderdag 1 mei 1980, May 1, 1980, 9, National Archive, The Hague, Centrale Raad voor de Volksgezondheid, access no. 2.27.16, inv. no. 54.

CHAPTER FOUR

1. M. B. H. Visser, "Ethische aspecten van medische experimenten op de mens (I) & (II)," *Medisch Contact* 34 (1979): 1351–58 and 1386–90, at 1351, 1352, and 1390.

2. David J. Rothman, *Strangers at the Bedside: A History of How Law and Bioethics Transformed Medical Decision Making*, 3rd ed. (New Brunswick, NJ: AldineTransaction, 1991/2003): 10.

3. Henry K. Beecher, "Ethics and Clinical Research," *New England Journal of Medicine* 74 (1966): 1354–60.

4. Walter M. Robinson and Brandon T. Unruh, "The Hepatitis Experiments at the Willowbrook State School," in *The Oxford Textbook of Clinical Research Ethics*, eds. Ezekiel J. Emanuel et al. (Oxford: Oxford University Press, 2008): 80–85.

5. John D. Arras, "The Jewish Chronic Disease Hospital Case," in *The Oxford Textbook of Clinical Research Ethics*, eds. Emanuel et al., 73–79.

6. D. S. Jones, C. Grady, and S. E. Lederer, "'Ethics and Clinical Research'—The 50th Anniversary of Beecher's Bombshell," *The New England Journal of Medicine* 374 (2016): 2393–98, at 2395.

7. Beecher, "Ethics and Clinical Research."

8. Rothman, *Strangers at the Bedside*, 80.

9. Jones, Grady, and Lederer, "'Ethics and Clinical Research,'" 2396, citing Henry K. Beecher, papers, 1948–1976, Harvard Medical Library, Francis A. Countway Library of Medicine, Boston, MA.

10. Rothman, *Strangers at the Bedside*, 10.

11. James Jones, *Bad Blood: The Tuskegee Syphilis Experiment* (New York: Free Press, 1981); Susan M. Reverby, *Examining Tuskegee: The Infamous Syphilis Study and its Legacy* (Chapel Hill: University of North Carolina Press, 2009).

12. Rothman, *Strangers at the Bedside*, 10. See also Ruth R. Faden and Tom L. Beauchamp, *A History and Theory of Informed Consent* (Oxford: Oxford University Press, 1986).

13. Laura Stark, *Behind Closed Doors: IRBs and the Making of Ethical Research* (Chicago: University of Chicago Press, 2012): 154, citing Memo to the Heads of Institutions Conducting Research with Public Health Service Grants from the Surgeon General, February 8, 1966, folder 2, Ethical, Moral and Legal Aspects, CC, ONIHH, National Institutes of Health.

14. Tom L. Beauchamp, "The Belmont Report," in *The Oxford Textbook of Clinical Research Ethics*, eds. Emanuel et al., 149–55; Joan P. Porter and Greg Koski, "Regula-

tions for the Protection of Humans in Research in the United States," in *The Oxford Textbook of Clinical Research Ethics*, eds. Emanuel et al., 156–67.

15. Duncan Wilson, *The Making of British Bioethics* (Manchester: Manchester University Press, 2014): 45. Original source: Maurice H. Pappworth, "Human Guinea Pigs: A Warning," *Twentieth Century* 171 (1962–1963): 66–75, at 75.

16. Wilson, *The Making of British Bioethics*, 45. See also Jenny Hazelgrove, "The Old Faith and the New Science: The Nuremberg Code and Human Experimentation Ethics in Britain, 1946–73," *Social History of Medicine* 15 (2002): 109–35; A. Mold, "Patient Groups and the Construction of the Patient-Consumer in Britain. An Historical Overview," *Journal of Social Policy* 39 (2010): 505–21.

17. Maurice H. Pappworth, *Human Guinea Pigs: Experiments on Man* (London: Routledge and Kegan Paul, 1967).

18. Pappworth, *Human Guinea Pigs: Experiments on Man*, ix.

19. Wilson, *The Making of British Bioethics*, 48.

20. Wilson, *The Making of British Bioethics*, 44, 43.

21. See "Anti-griepmiddel op krankzinnigen beproefd," *De Waarheid*, September 17, 1966: front page; "Directeur psychiatrische instelling: 'Patiënten geen proefkonijn," *De Waarheid*, September 20, 1966: 2; "Proeven op verpleegden: Prof. Querido: van toestemming kan geen sprake zijn," *Leeuwarder Courant*, September 17, 1966: 7.

22. "Nieuw anti-griep preparaat toegepast in psychiatrische inrichting," *Algemeen Dagblad*, September 19, 1966: 4.

23. Aanhangsel tot het Verslag van de Handelingen der Eerste Kamer (Appendix of the Report of the Acts of the Senate) 1966–1967, 19: 39.

24. "Boek van specialist veroorzaakt storm: Engelse zieken werden als proefkonijnen gebruikt," *Nieuwsblad van het Noorden*, May 18, 1967: front page; "Ernstige beschuldigingen Britse arts: Experimenten op onwetende patiënten: Binnenkort vragen in Lagerhuis," *De Waarheid*, May 18, 1967: 2; "Dr. Maurice Pappworth: In Engeland en VS experimenten op patiënten," *Leeuwarder Courant*, May 18, 1967: front page; "Opwinding in Engeland: Proeven op mensen in ziekenhuizen," *De Tijd*, May 19, 1967: 9.

25. "Bekende Londense arts onthult: Britse zieken zijn vaak 'proefkonijn,'" *De Telegraaf*, October 12, 1971: 9; "Arts beschuldigt: Britse 'fonds'-patiënten als proefkonijnen," *Het Vrije Volk*, October 11, 1971: front page; "Schandaal in Engeland en VS: Fondspatiënten als proefkonijnen: Experimenten met kernstraling," *De Tijd*, October 11, 1971: 5; "Britten bang voor rol van proefkonijn," *Limburgsch Dagblad*, October 12 1971: 3; "Brit blind na experiment in ziekenhuis," *De Telegraaf*, October 13, 1971: 9.

26. "Onthulling na experiment van 40 jaar: Amerikaanse negers waren proefkonijnen voor syfilisonderzoek," *Leeuwarder Courant*, July 26, 1972: 6; "Rumoer om experiment met negers," *Nederlands Dagblad*, July 27, 1972: 3; "Syfilislijders als proefkonijn: Medisch schandaal in VS," *De Tijd*, July 26, 1972: front page; "Proefkonijnen . . . ," *Limburgsch Dagblad*, July 27, 1972: 3. Beecher's accusations seem to have been hardly men-

tioned in Dutch newspapers at all. The only article I could find was "Patiënten gebruikt als proefkonijnen," *Limburgsch Dagblad*, June 17, 1966: 3.

27. C. D. de Langen, "Proeven op mensen en de verschuiving van te stellen normen," *Nederlands Tijdschrift voor Geneeskunde* 102 (1958): 25–27; Gerrit Arie Lindeboom, *Geneeskundige proeven op mensen: Referaat voor de negendertigste wetenschappelijke samenkomst op 3 juli 1957* (Assen: G. F. Hummelen's Boekhandel en Eletrische Drukkerij N. V., 1957); I. Boerema, "De Keerzijde van de Vooruitgang in de Geneeskunde," in W. Peremans et al., *Acht voordrachten over de keerzijde van de vooruitgang in de natuur–en geneeskundige wetenschappen* (The Hague: Martinus Nijhoff, 1962).

28. Thus, when the government asked the Health Council to reconsider Dutch medical ethics in 1970, the topic of tests upon human beings was one on which the committee did not want to spend more than a single meeting.

29. Jacob F. Rang, "Medisch experiment op de mens en strafrecht," in A. G. M. van Melsen et al., *Recent medisch ethisch denken II* (De Nederlandse Bibliotheek der Geneeskunde, Editorial Series no. 60) (Leiden: Stafleu's Wetenschappelijke Uitgeversmaatschappij, 1970): 33–87. See also C. Paul Sporken, "Ethische reflexies: Experimenten met de mens," *Katholieke Gezondheidszorg* 37 (1968): 190–94.

30. Henk J. J. Leenen, "Juridische aspecten van medische experimenten op de mens (I) & (II)," *Medisch Contact* 30 (1975): 746–50 and 753–67.

31. Leenen, "Juridische aspecten van medische experimenten op de mens (I) & (II)," 767.

32. Aanhangsel tot het Verslag van de Handelingen der Tweede Kamer (Appendix of the Report of the Acts of the House of Representatives) 1974–1975, no. 1690: 1307.

33. Aanhangsel tot het Verslag van de Handelingen der Tweede Kamer 1974–1975, no. 1690: 1307.

34. None of the politicians present in this exchange seemed to remember that parliament member Henk Vonhoff had already asked the government in 1968 how it sought to guarantee the rights of patients participating in clinical research, nor that this request had led the government to request a Health Council report on the regulation of clinical drug research.

35. Adviesaanvrage inzake patiëntenrecht, October 26, 1977, National Archive, The Hague, Centrale Raad voor de Volksgezondheid, access no. 2.27.16, inv. no. 803. Emphasis added.

36. See, for example: Frits Gongrijp, "Eis van nieuwe hoogleraar in Leiden: Hersenonderzoek bij delinquenten," *De Telegraaf*, April 20, 1978: 3; "Volgens reclasseringsblad KRI: Dr. R. Buikhuisen wil onderzoek biologische kenmerken delinquent," *Leeuwarder Courant*, April 20, 1978: 15; "Dr. Buikhuisen: hersenonderzoek delinquenten," *Het Vrije Volk*, April 20, 1978: 9; "Eis voor aanvaarden hoogleraarschap in Leiden: Criminoloog dr. Buikhuisen wil onderzoek hersenen misdadigers," *Nieuwsblad van het Noorden*, April 20, 1978: 3.

37. "Opvattingen uit de negentiende eeuw dreigen terug te keren: Buikhuisen wil hersenonderzoek bij gevangenen," *De Waarheid,* April 20, 1978: front page.

38. For the theory that criminals can be identified through inborn degenerative traits, see M. E. Chavennes, "Criminologie met Buikhuisen: terug om beter te springen," *NRC Handelsblad,* April 22, 1978. See also "Dr. W. Buikhuisen: 'Geen sprake van hersenonderzoek bij delinquenten,'" *Nederlands Dagblad,* April 21, 1978: 5. For the comparison with Lombroso, see K. Wiese, "Buikhuisen volhardt in gevaarlijke denkfouten," *Nieuwsblad van het Noorden,* October 10, 1978: 4; "Plannen Buikhuisen oude wijn in nieuwe zakken," *Leeuwarder Courant,* June 27, 1981; "Omstreden geleerde vertrekt," *Limburgsch Dagblad,* March 2, 1989: 5. See also W. Dekker, *De affaire Buikhuisen: het ontstaan en de achtergronden rondom zijn biosociale onderzoek* (PhD diss., Erasmus University Rotterdam, 2009).

39. Fifteen of these columns were published later that year under the title *Buikhuisen: dom én slecht (Buikhuisen: Stupid and Evil).* Piet Grijs, *Buikhuisen: dom én slecht* (Amsterdam: Vrij Nederland, 1978). (Hugo Brandt Corstius published his columns under the pseudonym Piet Grijs.)

40. C. J. M. Schuyt, "Reflex of reflectie: Antwoord aan Buikhuisen en Van Dijk," *Nederlands Juristenblad* 53 (1978): 517–26, at 526. For Buikhuisen's reply, see Wouter Buikhuisen, "De 'regressies' van Schuyt," *Nederlands Juristenblad* 53 (1978): 526–30.

41. C. J. M. Schuyt, "Veroordeeld tot criminaliteit?: Een wetenschapsfilosofische en ethische reflectie op het voorgenomen onderzoek van Prof.dr. W. Buikhuisen." *Nederlands Juristenblad* 53 (1978): 389–99, at 396–97. Schuyt recommended Jay Katz's famous 1972 book *Experimentation with Human Beings* as an "excellent guide" for these discussions. Physician and Yale Law School professor Jay Katz played a defining role in the fledgling bioethics movement in the United States in the 1970s. See J. Katz, *Experimentation with Human Beings* (New York: Russell Sage Foundation, 1972).

42. See "Door CPN'er Wolff: Interpellatie over onderzoek dr. Buikhuisen," *Nieuwsblad van het Noorden,* April 21, 1978: 2; "Joop Wolff interpelleert," *De Waarheid,* April 21, 1978: front page.

43. Handelingen Tweede Kamer (Acts of the House of Representatives) 1977–1978, April 26, 1978: 2199–218.

44. Handelingen Tweede Kamer 1977–1978, April 26, 1978: 2208.

45. Handelingen Tweede Kamer 1977–1978, April 26, 1978: 2205–13. Some politicians also lauded Buikhuisen. The representative of the progressive liberal party D66, for instance, called Buikhuisen an excellent researcher and spoke critically of "those so-called structuralists [. . .] who believe that, when the structure of society changes, criminal behavior will disappear naturally." A member of the Orthodox Calvinist party SGP felt that Buikhuisen's ideas were like a breath of fresh air in an era in which everything was perceived to be caused by societal injustice.

46. All quotes in this paragraph from Handelingen Tweede Kamer 1977–1978, April 26, 1978: 2207.

47. Handelingen Tweede Kamer 1977–1978, April 26, 1978: 2214.

48. Handelingen Tweede Kamer 1977–1978, April 26, 1978: 2215.

49. Handelingen Tweede Kamer 1978–1979, October 18, 1978: 584.

50. "Voorschriften omtrent onderzoek voor wetenschappelijke doeleinden ten aanzien van hen die rechtens vrijheidsbeneming ondergaan," *Staatscourant*, June 9, 1980.

51. Frits Gonggrijp, "Inrichting in Udenhout in opspraak: Ingrepen op zwakzinnigen in onderzoek," *De Telegraaf*, December 13, 1978: 6.

52. A clear overview of the initial breaking of the scandal is provided by D. P. Engberts, "Het verhaal achter het schandaal: Medische proeven met verstandelijke gehandicapten in een Noord-Brabantse inrichting in de jaren zestig en zeventig," in *Geneeskunde en ethiek in harmonie: Liber amicorum voor Prof.Dr E.L. Noach bij diens 80ste verjaardag op 21 November 2001*, ed. F. A. Wolff, 125–53 (The Hague: Pasmans Offset Drukkerij BV, 2001).

53. See "Nieuwe onthullingen over zwakzinnigeninrichting," *De Telegraaf*, December 19, 1978: 7; "Zwakzinnigeninrichting proefterrein: Operaties door niet-deskundigen," *De Waarheid*, December 16, 1978: 7; "Rapport: Verboden operaties in zwakzinnigentehuis," *Nieuwsblad van het Noorden*, December 19, 1978: 3; "Schedelmetende arts voor tuchtcollege," *Het Vrije Volk*, December 28, 1978: 5.

54. Verhoeven, brief van Verhoeven aan Van Soest, Udenhout, January 10, 1979, National Archive, The Hague, Ministerie van Volksgezondheid, Welzijn en Sport: Geneeskundige Hoofdinspectie voor de Geestelijke Volksgezondheid., access no. 2.27.5035, inv. no. 638. See also "Zwakzinnigeninrichting proefterrein: Operaties door niet-deskundigen," 7; "Huisarts en röntgenassistent verdacht: Onderzoek medische experimenten in tehuis," *Leeuwarder Courant*, December 19, 1978: 3.

55. The report in the inspection can be found here: "Onderzoek in de zwakzinnigeninrichting Huize Assisië te Udenhout (1978–1979)," National Archive, The Hague, Tweede Kamer der Staten-Generaal, access no. 2.02.28, inv. no. 11683: 15470–2.

56. "Enkele beschouwingen over de uitspraken van het college voor medisch tuchtrecht te Eindhoven in de zaken tegen artsen Huijsmans en Van Dongen," National Archive, The Hague, Hoofdinspectie Geestelijke Volksgezondheid, access no. 2.27.5035, inv. no. 638.

57. Willem Kloppert, "Dokter Huijsmans werkte in Assisië als in de rimboe," *Het Vrije Volk*, December 20, 1978: 9.

58. Visser, "Ethische aspecten van medische experimenten op de mens," 1351.

59. Visser, "Ethische aspecten van medische experimenten op de mens," 1387.

60. Visser, "Ethische aspecten van medische experimenten op de mens," 1390.

61. L. B. W. Jongkees, "Ethische aspecten van medische experimenten op de mens," *Medisch Contact* 35 (1980): 80–81.

62. Jongkees, "Ethische aspecten van medische experimenten op de mens," 81.

63. See, for instance, A.W. Moll van Charante, "Ethische aspecten van medische experimenten op de mens," *Medisch Contact* 35 (1980): 101.

64. See B. Löwenberg, "Dirk Willem van Bekkum: 30 juli 1925–17 juli 2015," in KNAW, *Levensberichten en Herdenkingen 2015* (Amsterdam: Koninklijke Nederlandse Akademie van Wetenschappen, 2015): 13–22. In 2007, the *Dutch Journal of Medicine* named van Bekkum as one of the Dutch biomedical researchers who might have gotten a Nobel prize for their work: "Wie had de Nobelprijs moeten krijgen?," *Nederlands Tijdschrift voor Geneeskunde* 151 (2007): 73–77.

65. D. W. van Bekkum, "Medische experimenten en proeven op mensen: De rechten van patiënten in het medisch-wetenschappelijk onderzoek," *Medisch Contact* 35 (1980): 115–18, at 115.

66. Handelingen Tweede Kamer 1979–1980, May 28, 1980: 4953.

67. Handelingen Tweede Kamer 1978–1979, June 25, 1979: 5678.

68. 1004 215, Notulen van de 215e C. v. G. bijeenkomst, August 3, 1978, 9, National Archive, The Hague, Centrale Raad voor de Volksgezondheid, access no. 2.27.16, inv. no. 51.

69. 8008 19, Notulen van de werkgroep, May 8, 1979, 2, National Archive, The Hague, Centrale Raad voor de Volksgezondheid, access no. 2.27.16, inv. no. 554.

70. Henk J. J. Leenen, brief van H. J. J. Leenen aan Johan Engelkens, January 2, 1979, National Archive, The Hague, Centrale Raad voor de Volksgezondheid, access no. 2.27.16, inv. no. 549.

71. 8008 2, National Archive, The Hague, Centrale Raad voor de Volksgezondheid, access no. 2.27.16, inv. no. 803; M. J. Aghina, *Patiëntenrecht: Een kwestie van gewicht* (Assen: Van Gorcum, 1978).

72. Centrale Raad voor de Volksgezondheid, *Deeladvies inzake medische experimenten* (The Hague: Staatsuitgeverij, 1982): 38.

73. Centrale Raad voor de Volksgezondheid, *Deeladvies inzake medische experimenten*, 27–31.

74. Centrale Raad voor de Volksgezondheid, *Deeladvies inzake medische experimenten*, 38. The Central Council included minors, detainees, handicapped individuals, patients, and the mentally ill in this category.

75. Centrale Raad voor de Volksgezondheid, *Deeladvies inzake medische experimenten*, 6.

76. Centrale Raad voor de Volksgezondheid, *Deeladvies inzake medische experimenten*, 8.

77. Centrale Raad voor de Volksgezondheid, *Deeladvies inzake medische experimenten*, 15.

78. Centrale Raad voor de Volksgezondheid, *Deeladvies inzake medische experimenten*, 45.

79. Centrale Raad voor de Volksgezondheid, *Deeladvies inzake medische experimenten*, 49–50.

80. Centrale Raad voor de Volksgezondheid, *Deeladvies inzake medische experimenten*, 50.

81. Centrale Raad voor de Volksgezondheid, *Deeladvies inzake medische experimenten*, 47.

82. 8008 100, Notulen van de werkgroep, November 24, 1980, 7, National Archive, The Hague, Centrale Raad voor de Volksgezondheid, access no. 2.27.16, inv. no. 554.

83. Centrale Raad voor de Volksgezondheid, *Deeladvies inzake medische experimenten*, 47.

84. 8008 78, Notulen van de werkgroep, June 23, 1980, National Archive, The Hague, Centrale Raad voor de Volksgezondheid, access no. 2.27.16, inv. no. 554.

85. Centrale Raad voor de Volksgezondheid, *Deeladvies inzake medische experimenten*, 46.

86. M. B. H. Visser, "Medische experimenten: Van experimenten *op* mensen naar experimenten *met* mensen," *Medisch Contact* 37 (1982): 711–13, at 711. Italics original.

87. Centrale Raad voor de Volksgezondheid, *Deeladvies inzake medische experimenten*, 14. See also 8008 24, Notulen van de werkgroep, June 8, 1979, National Archive, The Hague, Centrale Raad voor de Volksgezondheid, access no. 2.27.16, inv. no. 554; 8008 39, Notulen van de werkgroep, August 27, 1979, National Archive, The Hague, Centrale Raad voor de Volksgezondheid, access no. 2.27.16, inv. no. 554.

88. 8008 22, brief van D. W. van Bekkum aan H. T. M. Linssen, June 18, 1979, 1–2, National Archive, The Hague, Centrale Raad voor de Volksgezondheid, access no. 2.27.16, inv. no. 554; underscore original.

89. 8008 45, Notulen van de werkgroep, October 22, 1979, 6, National Archive, The Hague, Centrale Raad voor de Volksgezondheid, access no. 2.27.16, inv. no. 554.

90. 8008 39, Notulen van de werkgroep, August 27, 1979, 2, National Archive, The Hague, Centrale Raad voor de Volksgezondheid, access no. 2.27.16, inv. no. 554.

91. 8008 45, Notulen van de werkgroep, October 22, 1979, 3.

92. 8008 45, Notulen van de werkgroep, October 22, 1979, 7.

93. 8008 51, Notulen van de werkgroep, November 19, 1979, 2, National Archive, The Hague, Centrale Raad voor de Volksgezondheid, access no. 2.27.16, inv. no. 554.

94. 8008 45, Notulen van de werkgroep, October 22, 1979.

95. 8008 45, Notulen van de werkgroep, October 22, 1979, 5.

96. 8008 24, Notulen van de werkgroep, June 8, 1979, 11.

97. Centrale Raad voor de Volksgezondheid, *Deeladvies inzake medische experimenten*, 14. See also van Bekkum, "Medische experimenten en proeven op mensen," 116–17.

98. Centrale Raad voor de Volksgezondheid, *Deeladvies inzake medische experimenten*, 46.

99. 8008 100, Notulen van de werkgroep, November 4, 1980, 7, National Archive, The Hague, Centrale Raad voor de Volksgezondheid, access no. 2.27.16, inv. no. 554.

100. Centrale Raad voor de Volksgezondheid, *Deeladvies inzake medische experimenten*, 27–31.

101. 8008 100, Notulen van de werkgroep, November 4, 1980, 5.

102. 8008 86, Notulen van de werkgroep, September 15, 1980, 7, National Archive, The Hague, Centrale Raad voor de Volksgezondheid, access no. 2.27.16, inv. no. 554.

103. 8008 51, Notulen van de werkgroep, November 19, 1979, 11.

104. Centrale Raad voor de Volksgezondheid, *Deeladvies inzake medische experimenten*, 42.

105. "Bijlage IV: Proeve van werkwijze van een toetsingscommissie," in Centrale Raad voor de Volksgezondheid, *Deeladvies inzake medische experimenten*, 6.

106. 8008 103, Notulen van de werkgroep, January 26, 1981, National Archive, The Hague, Centrale Raad voor de Volksgezondheid, access no. 2.27.16, inv. no. 554.

107. All quotes in the last two paragraphs: 1004 259, Notulen van de 259e C. v. G. bijeenkomst, February 5, 1982, 3–6, National Archive, The Hague, Centrale Raad voor de Volksgezondheid, access no. 2.27.16, inv. no. 51.

108. For the responses, see 8008 139–8008 145, National Archive, The Hague, Centrale Raad voor de Volksgezondheid, access no. 2.27.16, inv. no. 811. For the meeting, see 1002 165, Notulen van de 259e C. v. G. bijeenkomst, February 4, 1979, 4–6, National Archive, The Hague, Centrale Raad voor de Volksgezondheid, access no. 2.27.16, inv. no. 24.

109. Visser, "Medische experimenten," 713.

110. 1002 165, Notulen van de 259e C. v. G. bijeenkomst, February 4, 1979, 10.

111. 1002 165, Notulen van de 259e C. v. G. bijeenkomst, February 4, 1979, 5.

112. 1002 165, Notulen van de 259e C. v. G. bijeenkomst, February 4, 1979, 11.

CHAPTER FIVE

1. "Bijdragende auteurs," in Inez de Beaufort and Heleen M. Dupuis, eds., *Handboek gezondheidsethiek* (Assen: Van Gorcum, 1988): v–vii.

2. Heleen M. Dupuis and Inez de Beaufort, "Ethiek–wat is het en wat kan men er mee," in *Handboek gezondheidsethiek*, eds. Beaufort and Dupuis, 7–20, at 18.

3. Dupuis and Beaufort, "Ethiek–wat is het en wat kan men er mee," 7.

4. Stephen Toulmin, "How Medicine Saved the Life of Ethics," *Perspectives in Biology and Medicine* 25 (1982): 736–50.

5. See also Robert M. Veatch, "The Birth of Bioethics: Autobiographical Reflections of a Patient Person," *Cambridge Quarterly of Health Ethics* 11 (2002): 344–52, at 344; Toulmin, "How Medicine Saved the Life of Ethics."

6. "Introduction," in *The Codification of Medical Morality: Historical and Philosophical Studies of the Formalization of Western Medical Morality in the Eighteenth and Nineteenth Centuries*, eds. Robert Baker, Dorothy Porter and Roy Porter (Dordrecht: Kluwer Academic Publishers, 1993), 1–14, at 2.

7. M. L. Tina Stevens, *Bioethics in America: Origins and Cultural Politics* (Baltimore, MD: Johns Hopkins University Press, 2000): x.

8. Andrew Abbott, *The System of Professions: An Essay on the Division of Expert Labor*

(Chicago: University of Chicago Press, 1988); Duncan Wilson, *The Making of British Bioethics* (Manchester: Manchester University Press, 2014): 12.

9. Patricia Jaspers, "Controversial Issues in the History of Dutch Research Ethics Governance," *Journal of Policy History* 23 (2011): 74–93; Loes Kater, *Disciplines met Dadendrang: Gezondheidsrecht en gezondheidsethiek in het Nederlandse euthanasiedebat 1960–1994* (Amsterdam: Aksant, 2004); Medard Hilhorst, "Klimaatverandering in de medische ethiek," in *Ethiek in Nederland: Van 1900 tot 1970 en daarna*, eds. Bert Musschenga et al. (Budel: Damon, 2010): 181–205; Medard Hilhorst, "Medische ethiek: onnodige misverstanden," *Tijdschrift voor Beleid, Politiek en Maatschappij* 26 (1999): 292–300.

10. Heleen M. Dupuis, "Ontwikkelingen in de medische ethiek: Van artsencode naar ethiek in de gezondheidszorg," in *Handboek gezondheidsethiek*, eds. Beaufort and Dupuis, 21–28, at 25.

11. See Inez de Beaufort, *Ethiek en medische experimenten met mensen* (Assen: Van Gorcum, 1985); Hans Achterhuis, "Schaarste en moraal," *Intermediair* 25 (1989): 41–43, at 41; Henk ten Have, *Een hippocratische erfenis: Ethiek in de medische praktijk* (Lochem: Uitgeversmaatschappij De Tijdstroom, 1990); H. A. M. J. ten Have, R. H. J. ter Meulen, and E. Van Leeuwen, *Medische Ethiek* (Houten: Bohn Stafleu van Loghum, 2003).

12. Jaspers, "Controversial Issues"; Kater, *Disciplines met Dadendrang*; Hilhorst, "Klimaatverandering in de medische ethiek"; Hilhorst, "Medische ethiek: onnodige misverstanden."

13. Beaufort, *Ethiek en medische experimenten met mensen*, 6, 11.

14. See Henri A. Krop, "De babylonische ballingschap der ethiek: C.W. Opzoomer (1821–1892) en Spinoza," in *Filosofie, ethiek en praktijk: Liber amicorum voor Koo van der Wal*, ed. M. Verkerk (Rotterdam: Erasmus Universiteit Rotterdam, Faculteit der Wijsbegeerte, 2000): 43–54; Henri A. Krop, "Laat de universiteit meer dan een vakschool zijn: Het pleidooi voor de Centrale Interfaculteit," in *Universitaire vormingsidealen: De Nederlandse universiteiten sedert 1876*, eds. L. J. Dorsman and P. J. Knegtmans (Hilversum: Verloren, 2006): 39–53.

15. Frits de Lange, "Tweeërlei ethiek: Of: hoe de gereformeerde ethiek zichzelf overbodig maakte," in *Ethiek in Nederland*, eds. Musschenga et al., 77–104; Henri A. Krop and Koo van der Wal, "Een eeuw wijsgerige ethiek in Nederland," in *Ethiek in Nederland*, eds. Musschenga et al., 105–40.

16. Frans Vosman and Carlo Leget, "Rooms-katholieke moraaltheologie in Nederland," in *Ethiek in Nederland*, eds. Musschenga et al., 13–40.

17. See Krop and van der Wal, "Een eeuw wijsgerige ethiek in Nederland," 120–24.

18. Bert Musschenga, "Nederlandse ethiek na 1970: De wending naar de praktijk, het beleid en het internationale forum," in *Ethiek in Nederland*, 143–80, at 143–47; Krop, "Laat de universiteit meer dan een vakschool zijn," 49.

19. Musschenga, "Nederlandse ethiek na 1970," 148.

20. Musschenga, "Nederlandse ethiek na 1970," 158.

21. Krop and van der Wal, "Een eeuw wijsgerige ethiek in Nederland." To make their point, Krop and van der Wal refer to Toulmin, "How Medicine Saved the Life of Ethics."

22. Musschenga, "Nederlandse ethiek na 1970."

23. L. W. Nauta, *Argumenten voor een kritische ethiek* (Amsterdam: Van Gennep, 1971); Herman J. Heering, *Ethiek der voorlopigheid* (Nijkerk: Callenbach, 1969).

24. Heering, *Ethiek der voorlopigheid*, 10.

25. C. Paul Sporken, *Voorlopige diagnose: inleiding tot een medische ethiek* (Utrecht: Ambo, 1969): 16.

26. Sporken, *Voorlopige diagnose*, 21–22.

27. Sporken, *Voorlopige diagnose*, 25.

28. Heering favored a *situation ethics*. See Joseph Fletcher, *Situation Ethics: The New Morality* (Philadelphia: Westminster Press, 1966).

29. C. Paul Sporken, "Medisch-ethische vragen in verband met anesthesie," *Medisch Contact* 25 (1970): 669–73, at 669.

30. Bert Musschenga, "Voorwoord," in *Ethiek in Nederland*, 7–9, at 7.

31. Musschenga, "Voorwoord," 7.

32. Musschenga, "Voorwoord," 8. See also Musschenga, "Nederlandse ethiek na 1970."

33. Paul Schotmans, "In Memoriam Prof. Dr. Paul Sporken," *Ethische Perspectieven* 2 (1992): 13–16, at 13.

34. C. Paul Sporken, *Ethiek en gezondheidszorg*, 4th ed. (Baarn: Amboboeken, 1979): 62.

35. A. J. Ch. Haex to Prof. Dr. Henk J. J. Leenen, March 28, 1977, 2, National Archive, The Hague, Gezondheidsraad, access no. 2.15.36, inv. no. 1692.

36. 125 19, Notulen van de eerste Beraadsgroep Gezondheidsethiek, December 1, 1977, 7, National Archive, The Hague, Gezondheidsraad, access no. 2.15.36, inv. no. 1705.

37. A. J. Ch. Haex to all standing committee members, July 18, 1977, National Archive, The Hague, Gezondheidsraad, access no. 2.15.36, inv. no. 1692; H. Terborgh-Dupuis, *Medische ethiek in perspectief: Een onderzoek naar normen en argumentaties in de (medische) ethiek* (Leiden: Stafleu, 1976).

38. C. M. Voermans-Neleman and H. J. De Roy van Zuydewijn, 125 6, "De Beraads-groep Gezondheidsethiek," November 24, 1977, National Archive, The Hague, Gezond-heidsraad, access no. 2.15.36, inv. no. 1692.

39. 125 294, Notulen van de Beraadsgroep Gezondheidsethiek, May 8–9, 1981, 67, National Archive, The Hague, Gezondheidsraad, access no. 2.15.36, inv. no. 1707.

40. L. B. J. Stuyt, Toespraak door de Voorzitter L. B. J. Stuyt, National Archive, The Hague, L. B. J. Stuyt [levensjaren 1914–2000], access no. 2.21.340, inv. no. 321. The term "bioethics" as it is used today was coined by Hellegers in 1971. Hellegers, who was born in Venlo in 1926 and raised in Flemish Belgium, fled to England when World War II

broke out. In 1953, he migrated to the United States. See John Collins Harvey, "André Hellegers, the Kennedy Institute, and the Development of Bioethics: The American-European Connection," in *The Development of Bioethics in the United States*, eds. Jeremy R. Garrett, Fabrice Jotterand, and D. Christopher Ralston (Dordrecht: Springer, 2013): 37–54.

41. L. B. J. Stuyt and M. A. M. de Wachter. Het instituut voor gezondheidsethiek, voordrachten gehouden bij de plechtige ingebruikneming van het Instituutsgebouw door L. B. J. Stuyt en M. A. M. de Wachter, 8, National Archive, The Hague, access no. 2.21.340, inv. no. 321.

42. H. Tristram Engelhardt Jr., *The Foundations of Bioethics* (Oxford: Oxford University Press, 1986). The quote is from H. Tristram Engelhardt Jr. and Lisa M. Rasmussen, "Secular Humanism," *Encyclopedia of Life Sciences* (September 15, 2006): 1.

43. Het instituut voor gezondheidsethiek, 4, National Archive, The Hague, access no. 2.21.340, inv. no. 321.

44. Musschenga, "Nederlandse ethiek na 1970," 156.

45. "Lectori Salutem," *Tijdschrift voor geneeskunde en ethiek* 1 (1991): 1–2.

46. Musschenga, "Nederlandse ethiek na 1970," 150.

47. See, for instance: "Reageerbuisbaby: hoe ver mag je gaan?," *Limburgsch Dagblad*, March 13, 1982: 19; "Professor Heleen Dupuis: 'Medische beoordeling kan tot massale discriminatie leiden,'" *De Telegraaf*, February 6, 1988: T25; "Welke mensen willen we? Ethiek van biomedisch onderzoek," *NRC Handelsblad*, May 25, 1988: science section, front page; "Medische ethici: Discussie over genetische kennis nog in pril stadium," *De Waarheid*, December 20, 1988: 8; "Prof. Dupuis: dood te negatief gewaardeerd," *Nederlands Dagblad*, November 1, 1986: 2; "Verplicht inenten," *Het Vrije Volk*, February 1, 1988: 3.

48. "Heleen Dupuis (44), Medisch Ethica: 'Misdadig om leven van uitzichtloze comapatiënt eindeloos te rekken,'" *De Telegraaf*, December 30, 1989: TA-3.

49. "Ethicus: aidstest kan ook zonder fiat van patient," *NRC Handelsblad*, August 15, 1987: 3.

50. "Prof. H. Dupuis tegen kunstgrepen op onvruchtbare vrouwen: 'Deze drievoudige abortus was humaan en verstandig,'" *Het Vrije Volk*, June 26, 1986: 5.

51. For her role as chairperson of the NVVE, see "Nieuwe voorzitter NVVE: Wettelijke regeling van euthanasie wellicht als mosterd na de maaltijd," *Leeuwarder Courant*, April 5, 1982: 4.

52. "Voorwoord," in *Handboek gezondheidsethiek*, eds. Beaufort and Dupuis, 1–2, at 1.

53. See, for instance: J. P. Vandenbroucke, "Medische ethiek en gezondheidsrecht: hinderpalen voor de verdere toename van kennis in de geneeskunde?," *Nederlands Tijdschrift voor Geneeskunde* 134 (1990): 5–6.

54. These principles were originally developed in Tom L. Beauchamp and James F. Childress, *Principles of Biomedical Ethics* (New York: Oxford University Press, 1979).

55. Harry M. Kuitert, "Morele consensus: mogelijkheden en grenzen," in *Handboek*

gezondheidsethiek, eds. Beaufort and Dupuis, 29–40, at 31. In Dutch, the terms "smalle en brede moral" (narrow and broad morals) were used to denote this distinction.

56. Kuitert, "Morele consensus: mogelijkheden en grenzen," 31–32.

57. Paul van Tongeren, "Ethiek en Praktijk," *Filosofie en praktijk* 9 (1988): 113–27, at 114.

58. Achterhuis, "Schaarste en moraal," 41.

59. Hans Achterhuis, *Het rijk van de schaarste: Van Thomas Hobbes tot Michel Foucault* (Baarn: Ambo, 1988).

60. Henk ten Have, *Ethiek tussen alliantie en dissidentie* (Maastricht: Rijksuniversiteit Limburg, 1990); Ten Have, *Een hippocratische erfenis*; Henk ten Have and Gerrit Kimsma, *Geneeskunde tussen droom en drama: Voortplanting, ethiek en vooruitgang* (Kampen: Kok Agora, 1987).

61. Ten Have, *Een hippocratische erfenis*, preface.

62. See Arthur Caplan, "Applying Morality to Advances in Biomedicine: Can and Should This Be Done?," in *New Knowledge in the Biomedical Sciences*, eds. W. B. Bondeson, H. Tristram Engelhardt, S. F. Spicker, and J. M. White (Springer: Dordrecht, 1982): 155–68.

63. Ten Have, *Ethiek tussen alliantie en dissidentie*, 18.

64. Ten Have, *Een hippocratische erfenis*, 20.

65. Ten Have, *Een hippocratische erfenis*, 24–25.

66. Ten Have, *Een hippocratische erfenis*, 88.

67. Hub Zwart, *Ethische consensus in een pluralistische samenleving: De gezondheidsethiek als casus* (Amsterdam: Thesis Publishers, 1993).

68. A typical example of this view, Zwart argued, was Heleen M. Dupuis, *Goed te leven: Reflecties op de moraal* (Baarn: Ten Have, 1980).

69. See also Hub Zwart, "De Intolerantie van een Pluralistische Ethiek: De Engelhardt/Callahan-controverse," *Filosofie en Praktijk* 12 (1991): 113–24.

70. Zwart, *Ethische consensus in een pluralistische samenleving*, 350.

71. See also Paul van Tongeren, "De smalle moraal: pluralisme of uniformiteit?," *Algemeen Nederlands Tijdschrift voor de Wijsbegeerte* 80 (1988): 92–102.

72. Van Tongeren, "De smalle moraal: pluralisme of uniformiteit?," 93.

73. Ten Have and Kimsma, *Geneeskunde tussen droom en drama*, 86–87.

74. Ten Have and Kimsma, *Geneeskunde tussen droom en drama*, 87.

75. Gerard H. de Vries and Sara van Epenhuysen, "Niet de handelingen maar het stuk: ethiek en het experimenten met mensen," *De Gids* 154 (1991): 861–70; G. H. de Vries, "Medische technologie en morele twijfel," in *Redes gehouden op de 16e Dies Natalis van de Rijksuniversiteit Limburg, 10 januari 1992*, eds. M. J. Cohen and G. H. de Vries (Maastricht: Rijksuniversiteit Limburg): 5–13; Gerard de Vries, *Gerede Twijfel: Over de rol van de medische ethiek in Nederland* (Amsterdam: De Balie, 1993).

76. De Vries, *Gerede Twijfel*, 34.

77. De Vries, *Gerede Twijfel*, 37.

78. Van Tongeren, "Ethiek en Praktijk," 126.

79. Heleen M. Dupuis, "Recensie van H. ten Have: *Een hippocratische erfenis*," *Nederlands Tijdschrift voor Geneeskunde* 135 (1991): 1333.

80. Frans C. L. M. Jacobs, "Praktische ethiek: onpraktisch en onfilosofisch?," *Filosofie en Praktijk* 12 (1991): 18–30; Frans C. L. M. Jacobs, "Ten overstaan van allen: Universalisering in de ethiek" (PhD diss., Universiteit van Amsterdam, 1985).

81. Jacobs, "Praktische ethiek," 23.

82. Beaufort, *Ethiek en medische experimenten met mensen*, 11.

83. Frans W. A. Brom, "Ethiek in de praktijk van het overheidsbeleid," *Filosofie en Praktijk* 13 (1992): 79–87.

84. Frans W. A. Brom, B. J. van den Bergh, and A. K. Huibers, "Wie is er bang voor de ethiek," in *Beleid en ethiek*, eds. Frans W. A. Brom, B. J. van den Bergh, and A. K. Huibers (Assen: Van Gorcum, 1993): 5–18, at 18.

85. Jacobs, "Praktische ethiek," 22.

86. Theo van Willigenburg, *Inside the Ethical Expert: Problem Solving in Applied Ethics* (Kampen: Kok Pharos Publishing House, 1991).

87. See "Ik roep walging op: Interview met Theo van Willigenburg," *Trouw*, October 11, 2014.

88. Van Willigenburg, *Inside the Ethical Expert*, 122.

89. Van Willigenburg, *Inside the Ethical Expert*, 111.

90. Van Willigenburg, *Inside the Ethical Expert*, 150, 139. Italics original.

91. Van Willigenburg, *Inside the Ethical Expert*, 149.

92. Van Willigenburg, *Inside the Ethical Expert*, 35.

93. Van Willigenburg, *Inside the Ethical Expert*, 36.

94. Van Willigenburg, *Inside the Ethical Expert*, 39.

95. Theo van Willigenburg, "Inleiding," in *Beleid en ethiek*, eds. Brom, van den Bergh, and Huibers, 187–88, at 187.

96. Theo van Willigenburg, "Ik ben een ethisch ingenieur!," in *Beleid en ethiek*, eds. Brom, van den Bergh, and Huibers, 189–204, at 189.

97. Van Willigenburg, "Ik ben een ethisch ingenieur!," 191.

98. Paul van Tongeren, "De ethicus versus de ingenieur," in *Beleid en ethiek*, eds. Brom, van den Bergh, and Huibers, 205–11, at 207.

99. Van Tongeren, "De ethicus versus de ingenieur," 207.

100. Other gatherings and publications include Hans J. Achterhuis, ed., *Deugt de ethiek? Medische, milieu- en bedrijfsethiek tussen trend en traditie* (Baarn: Gooi en Sticht, 1993); J. A. M. van Boxtel, J. Gruppelaar, Hans J. Achterhuis, and J. Vorstenbosch, eds., *Techniek, voorlopigheid en verlegenheid: Ethiek en technologisch aspectenonderzoek* (The Hague: NOTA, 1993).

101. Musschenga, "Nederlandse ethiek na 1970," 158.

102. For prominent Dutch representatives of this perspective, see H. M. Manschot and M. Verkerk, eds., *Ethiek in de zorg* (Amsterdam: Boom, 1994); M. Verkerk, "Zor-

gethiek: naar een geografie van verantwoordelijkheid," in *In gesprek over goede zorg*, eds. H. M. Manschot and H. van Dartel (Meppel: Boom, 2005): 177–84.

103. J. S. Reinders, "Weg uit de ivoren toren? Kanttekeningen bij de tussentijdse evaluatie van het Centrum voor Ethiek KUN," *Tijdschrift voor Geneeskunde en Ethiek* 7 (1997): 90–92, at 90.

CHAPTER SIX

1. Handelingen Tweede Kamer (Acts of the House of Representatives) 1996–1997, September 3, 1997: 103–7289.

2. Handelingen Tweede Kamer 1996–1997, September 3, 1997: 103–7287. Also: Kamerstuk Tweede Kamer (parliamentary document of the House of Representatives), no. 22588, sec. 10, Eindverslag (final report): 29.

3. Handelingen Tweede Kamer 1996–1997, September 3, 1997: 103–7310.

4. Beraadsgroep Gezondheidsethiek, September 9, 1982, 21, National Archive, The Hague, Gezondheidsraad, access no. 2.15.36, inv. no. 1708.

5. Kamerstuk Tweede Kamer 1981–1982, no. 16771, sec. 9, motie van het lid Wessel-Tuinstra c.s.

6. Kamerstuk Tweede Kamer 1984–1985, no. 18600-XVI, sec. 24, verslag van een mondeling overleg; Handelingen Tweede Kamer 1985–1986, January 29, 1986: 2872; J. C. van Es, "Experimenten met mensen en wetgeving," *Medisch Contact* 40 (1985): 1115.

7. Kamerstuk Tweede Kamer 1991–1992, no. 22588-A, Advies Raad van State, Nader rapport: 6.

8. Kamerstuk Tweede Kamer 1991–1992, no. 22588-A: 3.

9. Handelingen Tweede Kamer OCV/UCV 1988–1989, February 27, 1989: 33–6. Also: Kamerstuk Tweede Kamer 1981–1982, no. 16771, sec. 9; Kamerstuk Tweede Kamer 1985–1986, no. 19200-XVI, sec. 89; Kamerstuk Tweede Kamer 1991–1992, no. 21264, sec. 17, motie van het lid Kohnstamm.

10. H. D. C. Roscam Abbing, "Genetische experimenten met mensen: Wetgever quo vadis?," *Medisch Contact* 41 (1986): 533–35.

11. Emmy G. Scholten, "Wetenschappelijk onderzoek huisartspraktijken," *Medisch Contact* 42 (1987): 1188.

12. J. W. van Ree and B. Bottema, "Wetenschappelijk onderzoek huisartspraktijken," *Medisch Contact* 42 (1987): 953.

13. H. A. van Geuns, "Uit de Geneeskundige Hoofdinspectie: Medische experimenten in de huisartspraktijk," *Medisch Contact* 42 (1987): 694.

14. H. A. van Geuns, "Het Staatstoezicht en medische experimenten met mensen," *Medisch Contact* 40 (1985): 801–02, at 802.

15. D. P. Engberts, "De vroege Jaren: Ontstaan en werkzaamheid van een medisch-ethische (toetsings)commissie in Leiden in de Jaren zestig van de vorige eeuw," in *Dilemma's getoetst: Liber amicorum voor prof. dr. H. M. Dupuis en prof. dr. P. Vermeij*, eds.

D. P. Engberts, Y. M. Reidsma, and A. R. Wintzen (Leiden: UFB Universiteit Leiden, 2003): 9–28, at 9.

16. Engberts, "De vroege Jaren," 19.

17. Engberts, "De vroege Jaren," 15.

18. A detailed overview of this development is provided in Laura Stark, *Behind Closed Doors: IRBs and the Making of Ethical Research* (Chicago: University of Chicago Press, 2012). The quote from the 1966 PHS decree can be found on page 154.

19. Engberts, "De vroege Jaren," 22.

20. Engberts, "De vroege Jaren," 22.

21. Engberts, "De vroege Jaren," 23.

22. Lucas Bergkamp, "American IRBs and Dutch Research Ethics Committees: How They Compare," in *IRB: Ethics & Human Research* 10 (1988): 1–6; see also Chr. L. Rümke, brief van Chr. L. Rümke aan TNO, April 1, 1977, National Archive, The Hague, Nederlandse Organisatie voor Toegepast Natuurwetenschappelijk Onderzoek (TNO): Gezondheidsorganisatie, access no. 2.14.36.06, inv. no. 481.

23. T. Gerritsen, brief van T. Gerritsen aan H. G. van Brummen, April 20, 1977, National Archive, The Hague, TNO / Gezondheidsorganisatie, access no. 2.14.36.06, inv. no. 481. In Groningen, a research ethics committee existed on paper but was inactive in practice.

24. "Medisch Ethische Commissie," *Medisch Contact* 36 (1981): 776.

25. E. L. Noach, "De functie van ethische commissies bij medische experimenten met mensen," *Medisch Contact* 40 (1985): 872–74.

26. Lucas Bergkamp, *Medisch Ethische Commissies en het Toezicht op Experimenten met Mensen: Verslag van de eerste fase van een onderzoek naar de structuur en het functioneren van medisch ethische commissies* (Amsterdam: Universiteit van Amsterdam Instituut voor Sociale Geneeskunde, 1986): 204, 14.

27. E. J. Boer, "Medisch-ethische commissies, taak en functie bij wetenschappelijk onderzoek," *Nederlands Tijdschrift voor Geneeskunde* 133 (1989): 1659–64.

28. Bergkamp, *Medisch Ethische Commissies* [. . .] *Verslag van de eerste fase*, 28–29, at 31.

29. TNO, brief van TNO aan de directies van Academische Ziekenhuizen en besturen van Medische Faculteiten in Nederland, April 1, 1980, National Archive, The Hague, TNO / Gezondheidsorganisatie, access no. 2.14.36.06, inv. no. 481. See also M. B. H. Visser, "Nieuwe richtlijnen voor biomedisch onderzoek," *Medisch Contact* 36 (1981): 23–24.

30. John C. Petricciani, "An Overview of FDA, IRBs and Regulations," in *IRB: Ethics & Human Research* 3 (1981): 1–3.

31. Food and Drug Administration, "Protection of Human Subjects; Informed Consent," 21 CFR parts 50, 71, 171, 180, 310, 312, 314, 320, 330, 361, 430, 431, 601, 630, 812, 813, 1003, 1010, docket no. 78N-0400, 46 FR 8942, January 27, 1981, https://www.fda.gov

/science-research/clinical-trials-and-human-subject-protection/protection-human
-subjects-informed-consent.

32. H. D. C. Roscam Abbing, "EG-aanbevelingen inzake experimenten met genees-middelen bij mensen," *Nederlands Tijdschrift voor Geneeskunde* 134 (1990): 2124–25.

33. Emmy G. Scholten and L. H. B. M. van Benthem, "Medische experimenten in de huisartspraktijk," *Medisch Contact* 42 (1987): 953.

34. Bergkamp, *Medisch Ethische Commissies* [. . .] *Verslag van de eerste fase;* Lucas Bergkamp, *Medisch Ethische Commissies en het Toezicht op Experimenten met Mensen: Verslag van de tweede fase van een onderzoek naar de structuur en het functioneren van medisch ethische commissies* (Amsterdam: Universiteit van Amsterdam Instituut voor Sociale Geneeskunde, 1988).

35. Lucas Bergkamp, "Variatie en inconsistentie in de beoordeling van experimen-ten door medisch ethische commissies," *Nederlands Tijdschrift voor Geneeskunde* 133 (1989): 446–49.

36. Boer, "Medisch-ethische commissies," 1659.

37. Boer, "Medisch-ethische commissies," 1660.

38. Beaufort, *Ethiek en medische experimenten met mensen,* 187.

39. Bergkamp, *Medisch Ethische Commissies* [. . .] *Verslag van de eerste fase,* 166. See also Lucas Bergkamp, *Het proefdier mens: De normering en regulering van medische expe-rimenten met mensen* (Alphen aan den Rijn: Samsom Uitgeverij, 1988).

40. See "Ethische beoordeling van medische experimenten met mensen: Boerhaave-cursus van het PAOG," *Medisch Contact* 38 (1983): 12.

41. "Landelijk steunpunt experimenteel mens/patiëntgebonden onderzoek," *Medisch Contact* 42 (1987): 606.

42. "Nieuwe vereniging wil deskundigheid leden van medisch-ethische commissies vergroten," *Medisch Contact* 46 (1991): 1409–10.

43. Boer, "Medisch-ethische commissies," 1662–63.

44. Mark Kranenburg, "Haar rust was haar wapen: Necrologie Els Borst (1932–2014)," *NRC Handelsblad,* February 11, 2014.

45. Nele Beyens and Timo Bolt, "'A Medical Doctor in Politics': Els Borst-Eilers and the Rise of Evidence-Based Healthcare in the Netherlands," *Low Countries Historical Review* 132, no. 1 (2017): 16–37; Louise J. Gunning-Schepers, "In memoriam: Els Borst (1932–2014)," *Nederlands Tijdschrift voor Geneeskunde* 159 (2014): B1026.

46. On February 10, 2014, at the age of eighty-one years old, Els Borst was murdered in her home by a man who later told the police he had killed her because of "an order from God," holding her responsible for the Dutch euthanasia policy. For an English news piece on this, see Associated Press, "Man Claims Killing Dutch Health Minister Was An 'Order from God,'" *The Guardian,* February 4, 2016.

47. Evert Pronk, "Els Borst: arts, minister, euthanasievoorvechtster," *Medisch Con-tact,* February 11, 2014, https://www.medischcontact.nl/nieuws/laatste-nieuws/artikel /els-borst-arts-minister-euthanasievoorvechtster.htm.

48. Els Borst-Eilers, "Review commissie, fouten, ongevallen en near accidents (FONA) comissie en 'medical audit,'" in *Ethische beoordeling van medische experimenten met mensen*, ed. Boerhaave Commissie voor postacademisch onderwijs in de geneeskunde (Leiden: Rijksuniversiteit, Faculteit der Geneeskunde, 1983): 137–39, at 139.

49. Kamerstuk Tweede Kamer 1989–1990, no. 20620, sec. 16, "Grenzen van de zorg," brief van de Staatssecretaris van Welzijn, Volksgezondheid en Cultuur, 2; Gezondheidsraad, *Kerncommissie Ethiek Medisch Onderzoek (KEMO) 1993–1999* (The Hague: Gezondheidsraad, 2004; publication no. 2004/K01).

50. Menno van der Land, *Tussen ideaal en illusie: De geschiedenis van D66, 1966–2003* (The Hague: Sdu Uitgevers, 2003).

51. Margriet Oostveen, "Ik kan me goed voorstellen dat artsen stervenshulp niet melden," *NRC Handelsblad*, April 14, 2001; Kamerstuk Tweede Kamer 2000–2001, no. 27681, sec. 1, motie van het lid De Hoop Scheffer c.s.

52. Addy de Jong, "Slob (CU): Altijd verbinding zoeken," *Reformatorisch Dagblad*, September 1, 2012, https://www.rd.nl/artikel/462537-slob-cu-altijd-verbinding -zoeken.

53. Kamerstuk Tweede Kamer 1995–1996, no. 22588, sec. 10, 19.

54. See, for example: Handelingen Tweede Kamer 1989–1990, January 30, 1990: 33–1720.

55. "Borst: proef op wilsonbekwamen soms toestaan," *NRC Handelsblad*, October 4, 1995.

56. Koen Greven and Joke Mat, "Overleg met familie verzacht angst voor medisch experiment," *NRC Handelsblad*, October 5, 1995.

57. W. H. L. Hoefnagels and M. G. M. Olde Rikkert, "Van ongebreideld medisch onderzoek op wilsonbekwamen is helemaal geen sprake," *NRC Handelsblad*, October 17, 2015.

58. "Borst: proef op wilsonbekwamen soms toestaan."

59. Kamerstuk Tweede Kamer 1995–1996, no. 22588, sec. 10, 17.

60. Kamerstuk Tweede Kamer 1995–1996, no. 22588, sec. 9, 5, 6.

61. Kamerstuk Tweede Kamer 1995–1996, no. 22588, sec. 7, 52–53.

62. Kamerstuk Tweede Kamer 1992–1993, no. 22588, sec. 5, 49, 51. See also: Kamerstuk Tweede Kamer 1995–1996, no. 22588, sec. 10, 29, 37.

63. Kamerstuk Tweede Kamer 1995–1996, no. 22588, sec. 7, 53.

64. Kamerstuk Tweede Kamer 1995–1996, no. 22588, sec. 53.

65. Kamerstuk Tweede Kamer 1995–1996, no. 22588, sec. 55.

66. Kamerstuk Tweede Kamer 1996–1997, no. 22588, sec. 19.

67. Handelingen Tweede Kamer 1996–1997, September 3, 1997: 104–7330; Kamerstuk Tweede Kamer 1996–1997, no. 22588, sec. 23.

68. Kamerstuk Tweede Kamer 1995–1996, no. 22588, sec. 7, 62.

69. Handelingen Tweede Kamer 1996–1997, September 3, 1997: 103–7308.

70. Handelingen Tweede Kamer 1996–1997, September 9, 1997: 105–7417.

71. Handelingen Eerste Kamer (Acts of the Senate) 1997–1998, April 21, 1998: 28–1475.

72. Handelingen Eerste Kamer 1997–1998, April 21, 1998: 28–1475.

73. See also Loes Kater, *Disciplines met Dadendrang: Gezondheidsrecht en gezondheidsethiek in het Nederlandse euthanasiedebat 1960–1994* (Amsterdam: Aksant, 2004).

74. Kamerstuk Tweede Kamer 1991–1992, no. 22588, sec. 3, 30.

75. Kamerstuk Tweede Kamer 1992–1993, no. 22588, sec. 5, 63.

76. Handelingen Tweede Kamer 1996–1997, September 4, 1997: 104–7328.

77. Benjamin Hurlbut, *Experiments in Democracy: Human Embryo Research and the Politics of Bioethics* (Columbia University Press, 2017): 2.

78. Adam Hedgecoe, F. Carvalho, P. Lobmayer, and F. Raka, "Research Ethics Committees in Europe: Implementing the Directive, Respecting Diversity," Journal of Medical Ethics 32 (2006): 483–86.

79. Hurlbut, *Experiments in Democracy*, 10.

80. Duncan Wilson, *The Making of British Bioethics* (Manchester: Manchester University Press, 2014): 12, 3.

81. John H. Evans, *The History and Future of Bioethics: A Sociological Review* (Oxford: Oxford University Press, 2012): 58.

82. Evans, *The History and Future of Bioethics*, 60.

83. Wilson, *The Making of British Bioethics*, 12; Evans, *The History and Future of Bioethics*.

84. *Grenzen van de zorg: Regeringsstandpunt inzake het Advies van de Ziekenfondsraad, de Nationale Raad voor de Volksgezondheid en de Gezondheidsraad* (The Hague: Tweede Kamer der Staten-Generaal 1987–1988, 20 620, nos. 1–2 [1988]): 15.

85. Given the growing diagnostic and therapeutic possibilities, aging population, and increasing expenditures for health care, these reports all asked what had to be considered the "boundaries" of health care—in respects not just economic, but also sociopolitical and ethical. For a detailed description of these reports, see Timo Bolt, "A Doctor's Order: The Dutch Case of Evidence-Based Medicine (1970–2015)" (PhD diss., Utrecht University, 2015): 315–20.

86. *Grenzen van de zorg*, 4.

87. *Grenzen van de zorg*, 15.

88. *Grenzen van de zorg*, 15.

89. Kamerstuk Tweede Kamer 1987–1988, no. 20200 XVI, sec. 97, brief van de minister en van de Staatssecretaris van Welzijn, Volksgezondheid en Cultuur, 2-4.

90. Kamerstuk Tweede Kamer 1987–1988, no. 20200 XVI, sec. 173, Verslag van een Mondeling Overleg, June 1, 1988: 2–3, 6, 7.

91. Handelingen Tweede Kamer 1988–1989, Vaste Commissie voor de volksgezondheid, January 23, 1989: 27.7.

92. Handelingen Tweede Kamer 1988–1989, Vaste Commissies voor justitie en

voor de volksgezondheid, April 17, 1989: 445.26; Handelingen Eerste Kamer 1988–1989, March 21, 1989: 23.890, 23.892.

93. Friso Wielenga, *Nederland in de twintigste eeuw* (Amsterdam: Boom, 2009); Peter van Dam, *Staat van verzuiling: Over een Nederlandse mythe* (Amsterdam: Wereldbibliotheek, 2011).

94. Sjoerd Keulen, *Monumenten van beleid: De wisselwerking tussen Nederlands rijksoverheidsbeleid, sociale wetenschappen en politieke cultuur, 1945–2002* (Hilversum: Uitgeverij Verloren, 2014); Kees-Jan van Klaveren, *Het onafhankelijkheidsyndroom: Een cultuurgeschiedenis van het naoorlogse Nederlandse zorgstelsel* (Amsterdam: Wereldbibliotheek, 2016).

95. Kamerstuk Tweede Kamer 1987–1988, no. 20200 XVI, sec. 97, 2.

96. Handelingen Eerste Kamer 1988–1989, March 22, 1989: 24.912.

97. Kamerstuk Tweede Kamer 1987–1988, no. 20 200 XVI, sec. 173, 2.

98. Handelingen Eerste Kamer 1988–1989, March 22, 1989: 24.921–24.922.

99. Handelingen Tweede Kamer 1988–1989, Vaste Commissies voor justitie en de volksgezondheid, April 17, 1989: 45.43.

100. W. S. P. Fortuyn, *Ordening door ontvlechting: Een advies over de adviesstructuur in de gezondheidszorg* (Rijswijk: Ministerie van WVC, 1990): 24.

101. Handelingen Tweede Kamer 1991–1992, Vaste Commissie voor het wetenschapsbeleid, November 4, 1991: 6.2.

102. Handelingen Tweede Kamer 1991–1992, Vaste Commissie voor het wetenschapsbeleid, November 4, 1991: 6.6.

103. Handelingen Tweede Kamer 1991–1992, Vaste Commissie voor het wetenschapsbeleid, November 4, 1991: 6.7.

104. Handelingen Tweede Kamer 1991–1992, Vaste Commissie voor de volksgezondheid, January 23, 1989: 27.7; Handelingen Eerste Kamer 1992–1993, April 6, 1993: 24.1081.

105. Handelingen Tweede Kamer 1991–1992, Vaste Commissie voor het wetenschapsbeleid, November 4, 1991: 6.14.

106. Handelingen Eerste Kamer 1992–1993, April 6, 1993: 24.1107.

107. All quotes in this paragraph: Els Borst-Eilers, "Geneeskunde, ethiek en de Gezondheidsraad (Gast aan het woord)," *Tijdschrift voor geneeskunde en ethiek* 1 (1991): 48–49, at 49.

108. J. H. W. Kits Nieuwenkamp, "Wat kan de ethiek voor het beleid betekenen? De rol van de ethiek en van ethici bij het beleid," in *Beleid en ethiek*, eds. Frans W. A. Brom, B. J. van den Bergh, and A. K. Huibers (Assen: Van Gorcum, 1993): 34–42, at 37.

109. Kits Nieuwenkamp, "Wat kan de ethiek voor het beleid betekenen?," 37.

110. Handelingen Eerste Kamer 1992–1993, April 6, 1993: 24.1131.

111. J. Th. J. van den Berg, "Plaats en taak van het parlement bij ethische discussies," in *Techniek, voorlopigheid en verlegenheid*, eds. J. A. M. van Boxtel, J. Gruppelaar, Hans J. Achterhuis, and J. Vorstenbosch (The Hague: NOTA, 1993): 129–36, at 131.

112. Also: L. Sterrenberg, "Ethisch aspectenonderzoek: dans met beleid," in *Beleid en ethiek*, eds. Brom, van den Bergh, and Huibers, 26–33.

113. Jouke de Vries, *Paars en de managementstaat: Het eerste kabinet-Kok (1994–1998)* (Apeldoorn: Garant, 2002); Klaartje Peters, *Een doodgewoon kabinet: Acht jaar Paars, 1994–2002* (Amsterdam: Boom, 2015); Keulen, *Monumenten van Beleid*.

114. See Anthony Giddens, *The Third Way: The Renewal of Social Democracy* (Cambridge: Polity Press, 1998).

115. Mark Kranenburg, "The Political Branch of the Polder Model," *NRC Handelsblad*, July 1, 1999.

116. Van der Land, *Tussen ideaal en illusie*; Paul Lucardie, *Nederland stromenland: Een geschiedenis van de politieke stromingen* (Assen: Koninklijke van Gorcum, 2002): 83–87.

117. These departments were the Ministry of Health, Welfare, and Sports, the Ministry of Education, Cultural Affairs, and Science; the Ministry of Housing, Spatial Planning, and the Environment; and the Ministry of Agriculture, Nature Management, and Fisheries.

118. Bert Musschenga, "Nederlandse ethiek na 1970: De wending naar de praktijk, het beleid en het internationale forum," in *Ethiek in Nederland: Van 1900 tot 1970 en daarna*, eds. Bert Musschenga et al. (Budel: Damon, 2010): 143–80, at 159–60. Early in the first decade of the 2000s, this program was extended in slightly augmented form with €4 million to subsidize another twenty ethics projects.

119. Musschenga, "Nederlandse ethiek na 1970," 160.

120. Jan Vorstenbosch, "Dierethiek in Nederland," in *Ethiek in Nederland*, eds. Musschenga et al., 251–76, at 262.

121. See "CCMO Deskundigheidseisen leden METC's," *Staatscourant* 6804 (February 12, 2016).

122. Similarly, committee members evaluating animal studies cannot a priori reject any form of animal experimentation. They have to accept that, in principle, such experiments are permissible and necessary. See Tsjalling Swierstra, "De commissie Biotechnologie bij Dieren: toets of glijmiddel?," in *Afwegen, hoe doe je dat?*, eds. J. Swart, R. Tramper, and M. Jonker (Budel: Damon, 2009): 154–64.

123. Theo van Willigenburg, *Inside the Ethical Expert: Problem Solving in Applied Ethics* (Kampen: Kok Pharos Publishing House, 1991): 36.

124. Heleen M. Dupuis, "Ethische aspecten van experimenten met mensen," in *Geneeskunde en ethiek in nharmonie: Liber amicorum voor Prof.Dr E.L. Noach bij diens 80ste verjaardag op 21 November 2001*, ed. F. A. Wolff, 155–63 (The Hague: Pasmans Offset Drukkerij BV, 2001): 161.

CONCLUSION

1. Allan Sherman, "Peter and the Commissar," on *Peter and the Commissar*, recorded July 22, 1964, Camden, NJ: RCA Red Seal Records, LP record (mono, dyn).

2. M. Perutz, "The New Marxism," *New Scientist* 123 (1989): 72–73.

3. For the by-now classic study in the history of science on the historically evolving notion of objectivity, see Lorraine Daston and Peter Galison, *Objectivity* (New York: Zone Books, 2007).

4. As Lorraine Daston has argued about the rise of accounting traditions in nineteenth-century knowledge production: "Certain forms of quantification have come to be allied with objectivity not because they necessarily mirror reality more accurately, but because they serve the ideal of communicability, especially across barriers of distance and distrust." Lorraine Daston, "Objectivity and the Escape from Perspective," *Social Studies of Science* 22 (1992): 597–618, at 609. See also Theodore M. Porter, "Quantification and the Accounting Ideal in Science," *Social Studies of Science* 22 (1992): 633–52; Theodore M. Porter, "Objectivity as Standardization: The Rhetoric of Impersonality in Measurement Statistics and Cost Benefit Analysis," *Annals of Scholarship* special issue 9, no. 1–2 (1992): 19–59; Steven Shapin, A Social History of Truth: Civility and Science in Seventeenth-Century England (Chicago: University of Chicago Press, 1994).

5. The term *aperspectival* is derived from Daston, "Objectivity and the Escape from Perspective."

6. Michael Polanyi, *The Tacit Dimension* (New York: Doubleday, 1967); Harry Collins and Robert Evans, *Rethinking Expertise* (Chicago: University of Chicago Press, 2007).

7. Thomas Nagel, *The View From Nowhere* (Oxford: Oxford University Press, 1986).

8. Michael Polanyi, "The Republic of Science: Its Political and Economic Theory," *Minerva* 1 (1962): 54–73; Steve Fuller, *The Governance of Science: Ideology and the Future of the Open Society* (Buckingham: Open University Press, 2000).

9. One of the most recent incarnations of this view has been put forward by Steven Pinker. See Steven Pinker, "The Moral Imperative for Bioethics," *Boston Globe*, August 1, 2015.

10. See also Christian Bonah, "'Experimental Rage': The Development of Medical Ethics and the Genesis of Scientific Facts. Ludwik Fleck: An Answer to the Crisis of Modern Medicine in Interwar Germany?" *Social History of Medicine* 15 (2002): 187–207.

11. For the notion of "elite scientists" acting as gatekeepers in order to shape a discipline's contents, see Imogen Clarke, "The Gatekeepers of Modern Physics: Periodicals and Peer Review in 1920s Britain," *Isis* 106 (2014): 70–93; Alex Csiszar, *The Scientific Journal: Authorship and the Politics of Knowledge in the Nineteenth Century* (Chicago: University of Chicago Press, 2018); Melinda Baldwin, *Making Nature: The History of a Scientific Journal* (Chicago: University of Chicago Press, 2015).

12. For an early, and probably still the most famous, statement in this regard, see Franz J. Ingelfinger, "The Unethical in Medical Ethics," *Annals of Internal Medicine* 83 (1975): 264–69.

13. Theodore M. Porter, *Trust in Numbers: The Pursuit of Academic Objectivity in Science and Public Life.* (Princeton, NJ: Princeton University Press, 1995): 8.

BIBLIOGRAPHY

NATIONAL ARCHIVE, THE HAGUE

2.02.28   Tweede Kamer (1945–1999)

        11683   15470-2 Onderzoek in de zwakzinnigeninrichting Huize Assisië te Udenhout (1978–1979)

2.14.36.06   TNO / Gezondheidsorganisatie (1948–1980)

        481   XH 049 Commissie Ethiek proefdieren

        608   Commissie klinisch geneesmiddelenonderzoek

2.15.33   Gezondheidsraad (1920–1956)

        546   Commissie inzake vivisectie: Stukken betreffende het adviseren aan de minister inzake de wenselijkheid van een wettelijke regeling van de vivisectie (1953–1955)

        547   Commissie van Advies inzake het instellen van leerstoelen voor vivisectie-vrije geneeskunde en voor homeopathie: Stukken betreffende het adviseren aan de minister inzake het instellen van leerstoelen voor vivisectie-vrije geneeskunde en voor homeopathie (1947–1953)

        548   Commissie inzake proeven op mensen: Notulen van de vergaderingen (1953–1955)

        549   Commissie inzake proeven op mensen: Stukken betreffende het adviseren aan de minister inzake proeven op mensen (1953–1956)

2.15.36   Gezondheidsraad (1957–1990)

        1374   Commissie medische ethiek: Agenda's en notulen

        1476   Commissie klinisch onderzoek van geneesmiddelen: Rapport inzake klinisch onderzoek van geneesmiddelen (1971)

        1478   Commissie klinisch onderzoek van geneesmiddelen: Algemene correspondentie (1968–1974): Deel II

        1692   Commissie beraadsgroep gezondheidsethiek: Algemene correspondentie (1976–1977)

        1704   Commissie beraadsgroep gezondheidsethiek: Algemene correspondentie (1984–1985)

        1705   Commissie beraadsgroep gezondheidsethiek: Agenda's en notulen (1977–1979)

        1707   Commissie beraadsgroep gezondheidsethiek: Agenda's en notulen (1981)

1708   Commissie beraadsgroep gezondheidsethiek: Agenda's en notulen (1982–1983)

3.3.101 Commissie experimenten met radioactieve stoffen op proefpersonen

3.3.65 Commissie klinische farmacologie

2.15.37   SZ / Volksgezondheid (1918–1950)

2357   Stukken betreffende het onderzoek naar beschuldigingen van het verrichten van vivisectie op mensen in ziekenhuizen (1947)

2.15.65   DG Volksgezondheid (1946–1982)

1373   Het in- en samenstellen van de Staatscommissie Patiëntenrecht, met bijlagen (1975–1977)

1375   Agenda's en notulen van de vergaderingen van de Werkgroep Patiëntenrecht en Kwaliteitsbewaking, met bijlagen (1976)

2456   Kamervragen inzake op geaborteerde foetussen uitgevoerde medische experimenten, waaronder onderzoek in de Bloemenhovekliniek te Heemstede op foetussen van vijf maanden (1980)

2.21.340 Stuyt, L. B. J. (1951–2000)

321   Stukken betreffende de oprichting en openstelling van een Instituut voor Gezondheidsethiek aan de universiteit van Maastricht (1984–1986)

2.27.16   Centr. Raad Volksgezondheid (1958–1982)

22   Vergaderingen van de Raad: Agenda's en notulen van de raadsvergaderingen (vergaderingen 134 t/m 141, 1978)

23   Vergaderingen van de Raad: Agenda's en notulen van de raadsvergaderingen (vergaderingen 142 t/m 149, 1979)

24   Vergaderingen van de Raad: Agenda's en notulen van de raadsvergaderingen (vergaderingen 150 t/m 155, 1980)

51   Vergaderingen van het Comité van Gedelegeerden: Agenda's en notulen van vergaderingen van het Comité van Gedelegeerden (vergaderingen 210 t/m 219, 1978)

52   Vergaderingen van het Comité van Gedelegeerden: Agenda's en notulen van vergaderingen van het Comité van Gedelegeerden (vergaderingen 220 t/m 230, 1979, deel 1)

53   Vergaderingen van het Comité van Gedelegeerden: Agenda's en notulen van vergaderingen van het Comité van Gedelegeerden (vergaderingen 231 t/m 234, 1979, deel 2)

2.15   803–11: Patiëntenrecht: stukken betreffende het adviseren aan de minister inzake patiëntenrecht (1977–1982)

2.13.2   *549–33*: Medische proeven op mensen: Stukken betreffende
het adviseren aan de minister inzake medische proeven op
mensen (1978–1982)

2.13.2   *554*: Medische proeven op mensen: Agenda's en notulen van
de vergaderingen van de Werkgroep medische proeven op
mensen (1979–1981)

2.27.31   Nat. Raad Volksgezondheid (1982–1995)

2.3.28   *1065*: Medische experimenten: Stukken betreffende het
adviseren aan de Staatssecretaris inzake een wettelijke
regeling voor experimenten met geneesmiddelen (1984–
1985)

2.3.28   *1066–68*: Stukken betreffende het adviseren aan de Minister
inzake een wetsontwerp "Regelen inzake medische
experimenten, met het advies 'Medische experimenten'
(1988)" (1984–1992)

2.3.28   *1069*: Agenda's, notulen en stukken betreffende de
samenstelling, taak en werkwijze van de Commissie
Medische Experimenten later Commissie Regelen inzake
Medische Experimenten (1988)

2.27.5035   Hoofdinsp. Geestelijke Volksgezondheid (1962–1994)

638   Onderzoek van de klachten voer bepaalde medische praktijken
in het zwakzinnigeninstituut "Huize Assisië" in Udenhout

PUBLISHED SOURCES

Aanhangsel tot het Verslag van de Handelingen der Eerste Kamer (Appendix of the
Report of the Acts of the Senate) 1966–1967, no. 19: 39. https://repository.overheid
.nl/frbr/sgd/19661967/0000242757/1/pdf/SGD_19661967_0000038.pdf.

Aanhangsel tot het Verslag van de Handelingen der Tweede Kamer (Appendix of
the Report of the Acts of the House of Representatives) 1967–1968, no. 119: 241–
42. https://repository.overheid.nl/frbr/sgd/19671968/0000237992/1/pdf/SGD
_19671968_0000594.pdf.

Aanhangsel tot het Verslag van de Handelingen der Tweede Kamer (Appendix of
the Report of the Acts of the House of Representatives) 1974–1975, no. 1690:
1307. https://repository.overheid.nl/frbr/sgd/19741975/0000200808/1/pdf/SGD
_19741975_0002031.pdf.

Abbott, Andrew. *The System of Professions: An Essay on the Division of Expert Labor.*
Chicago: University of Chicago Press, 1988.

Abbott, Lura, and Christine Grady. "A Systematic Review of the Empirical Literature
Evaluating IRBs: What We Know and What We Still Need to Learn." *Journal of
Empirical Research on Human Research Ethics* 6 (2011): 3–19.

Achterhuis, Hans J. *De markt van welzijn en geluk: Een kritiek van de andragogie*. Baarn: Ambo, 1979.

Achterhuis, Hans J., ed. *Deugt de ethiek?: Medische, milieu- en bedrijfsethiek tussen trend en traditie*. Baarn: Gooi en Sticht, 1993.

Achterhuis, Hans J. *Het rijk van de schaarste: Van Thomas Hobbes tot Michel Foucault*. Baarn: Ambo, 1988.

Achterhuis, Hans J. "Schaarste en moraal." *Intermediair* 25 (1989): 41–43.

Ackerknecht, Erwin H. *Medicine at the Paris Hospital: 1794–1848*. Baltimore, MD: Johns Hopkins University Press, 1967.

Agar, Jon. *Science in the Twentieth Century and Beyond*. Cambridge: Polity Press, 2012.

Aghina, M. J. *Patiëntenrecht: Een kwestie van gewicht*. Assen: Van Gorcum, 1978.

Ahlers, J. B. *Meer mensen mondig maken*. The Hague: Staatsuitgeverij, 1975.

Algemeen Dagblad. "Nieuw anti-griep preparaat toegepast in psychiatrische inrichting." September 19, 1966: 4.

Algemeen Handelsblad. "De dokter is God niet." May 13, 1967: supplement, 1.

Altman, Lawrence. *Who Goes First?: The Story of Self-Experimentation in Medicine*. New York: Random House, 1986.

Amundsen, Darrel W. "The Discourses of Roman Catholic Medical Ethics." In *The Cambridge World History of Medical Ethics*, edited by Robert B. Baker and Laurence B. McCullough, 218–54. Cambridge: Cambridge University Press, 2009.

Annas, George J., and Michael A. Grodin, eds. *The Nazi Doctors and the Nuremberg Code: Human Rights in Human Experimentation*. Oxford: Oxford University Press, 1992.

Annas, George J., and Michael A. Grodin. "The Nuremberg Code." In *The Oxford Textbook of Clinical Research Ethics*, edited by Ezekiel J. Emanuel et al., 136–40. Oxford: Oxford University Press, 2008.

Arras, John D. "The Jewish Chronic Disease Hospital Case." In *The Oxford Textbook of Clinical Research Ethics*, edited by Ezekiel J. Emanuel et al., 73–79. Oxford: Oxford University Press, 2008.

"Artsen en hun oorlog." *Medisch Contact* 64 (2009).

"Assistentie, waarneming en associatie." *Medisch Contact* 11 (1956): 16–21.

Associated Press. "Man Claims Killing Dutch Health Minister Was An 'Order from God.'" *The Guardian*, February 4, 2016.

Association for Homeopathic Healers. "Homoeopathie." *Medisch Contact* 5 (1950): 438–40.

Austoker, Joan, and Linda Bryder, eds. *Historical Perspectives on the Role of the MRC: Essays on the History of the Medical Research Council of the United Kingdom and Its Predecessor, the Medical Research Committee, 1913–1953*. Oxford: Oxford University Press, 1989.

Baker, Robert B. *Before Bioethics: A History of American Medical Ethics from the Colonial Period to the Bioethics Revolution*. Oxford: Oxford University Press, 2013.

Baker, Robert B. "From Metaethicist to Bioethicist." In *Cambridge Quarterly of Health Ethics* 11 (2002): 369–79.

Baker, Robert B. "Transcultural Medical Ethics and Human Rights." In *Ethics Codes in Medicine: Foundations and Achievements of Codification since 1947*, edited by Ulrich Tröhler and Stella Reiter-Theil, 312–31. Aldershot: Ashgate, 1998.

Baker, Robert B., and Laurence B. McCullough, eds. *The Cambridge World History of Medical Ethics.* Cambridge: Cambridge University Press, 2009.

Baker, Robert B., Dorothy Porter, and Roy Porter, eds. *The Codification of Medical Morality: Historical and Philosophical Studies of the Formalization of Western Medical Morality in the Eighteenth and Nineteenth Centuries.* Dordrecht: Kluwer Academic Publishers, 1993.

Bal, Roland, Wiebe E. Bijker, and Ruud Hendriks. *Paradox van wetenschappelijk gezag: over de maatschappelijke invloed van adviezen van de Gezondheidsraad.* The Hague: Gezondheidsraad, 2002.

Baldwin, Melinda. *Making Nature: The History of a Scientific Journal.* Chicago: University of Chicago Press, 2015.

Beauchamp, Tom L. "The Belmont Report." In *The Oxford Textbook of Clinical Research Ethics*, edited by Ezekiel J. Emanuel et al., 149–55. Oxford: Oxford University Press, 2008.

Beauchamp, Tom L., and James F. Childress. *Principles of Biomedical Ethics.* New York: Oxford University Press, 1979.

Beaufort, Inez de. *Ethiek en medische experimenten met mensen.* Assen: Van Gorcum, 1985.

Beaufort, Inez de. "Niet-therapeutisch wetenschappelijk onderzoek met wilsonbekwame personen." *Nederlands Tijdschrift voor Geneeskunde* 133 (1989): 737–40.

Beaufort, Inez de, and Dupuis, Heleen M., eds. *Handboek gezondheidsethiek.* Assen: Van Gorcum, 1988.

Beecher, Henry K. "Ethics and Clinical Research." *New England Journal of Medicine* 74 (1966): 1354–60.

Beecher, Henry K. Papers. 1948–1976. Harvard Medical Library, Francis A. Countway Library of Medicine, Boston, MA.

Bekkum, D. W. van. "Experimenten met mensen." In *Ethiek.* Cahiers van de Stichting Bio-Wetenschappen en Maatschappij 3, no. 2. Deventer: Van Loghum Slaterus, 1976.

Bekkum, D. W. van. "Medische experimenten en proeven op mensen: De rechten van patiënten in het medisch-wetenschappelijk onderzoek." *Medisch Contact* 35 (1980): 115–18.

Bekkum, D. W. van. "Proeven op patiënten: techniek, ethiek." In *Kanker.* Cahiers van de Stichting Bio-Wetenschappen en Maatschappij 3, no. 4. Deventer: Van Loghum Slaterus, 1976.

Bennebroek Gravenhorst, J. "Medisch-ethische toetsing van wetenschappelijk onderzoek in Nederland." In *Geneeskunde en ethiek in harmonie,* edited by F. A. Wolff, 97–105. The Hague: Pasmans Offset Drukkerij BV, 2001.

Berg, C. van den. "Herinneringen aan de wordingsgeschiedenis van de wet op de geneesmiddelvoorziening." *Tijdschrift voor Sociale Geneeskunde* 42 (1964): 12–15.

Berg, Jan Hendrik van den. *Medische macht en medische ethiek.* Nijkerk: Callenbach, 1969.

Berg, J. Th. J. van den. "Plaats en taak van het parlement bij ethische discussies." In *Techniek, voorlopigheid en verlegenheid,* edited by J. A. M. van Boxtel, J. Gruppelaar, Hans J. Achterhuis, and J. Vorstenbosch, 129–36. The Hague: NOTA, 1993.

Bergkamp, Lucas. "American IRBs and Dutch Research Ethics Committees: How They Compare." *IRB: Ethics & Human Research* 10 (1988): 1–6.

Bergkamp, Lucas. "Een voorstel voor een Wet op de medische experimenten: enkele kanttekeningen." *Tijdschrift voor Gezondheidsrecht* 13 (1989): 190–204.

Bergkamp, Lucas. "Het betrekken van incompetenten bij experimenten." *Nederlands Tijdschrift voor Gezondheidsrecht* 14 (1990): 19–26.

Bergkamp, Lucas. *Het proefdier mens: De normering en regulering van medische experimenten met mensen.* Alphen aan den Rijn: Samsom Uitgeverij, 1988.

Bergkamp, Lucas. *Medisch Ethische Commissies en het Toezicht op Experimenten met Mensen: Verslag van de eerste fase van een onderzoek naar de structuur en het functioneren van medisch ethische commissies.* Amsterdam: Universiteit van Amsterdam Instituut voor Sociale Geneeskunde, 1986.

Bergkamp, Lucas. *Medisch Ethische Commissies en het Toezicht op Experimenten met Mensen: Verslag van de tweede fase van een onderzoek naar de structuur en het functioneren van medisch ethische commissies.* Amsterdam: Universiteit van Amsterdam Instituut voor Sociale Geneeskunde, 1988.

Bergkamp, Lucas. "Variatie en inconsistentie in de beoordeling van experimenten door medisch ethische commissies." *Nederlands Tijdschrift voor Geneeskunde* 133 (1989): 446–49.

Bernard, Claude. *An Introduction to the Study of Experimental Medicine.* 1865. Translated in 1927. Reprint, New York: Dover, 1957.

Bertucci, Paola. "Shocking Subjects: Human Experiments and the Material Culture of Medical Electricity in Eighteenth-Century England." In *The Uses of Humans in Experiment: Perspectives from the 17th to the 20th Century,* edited by Erika Dyck and Larry Stewart, 111–38. Leiden: Brill Rodopi, 2016.

Beukers, H. "Een nieuwe werkplaats in de geneeskunde: De opkomst van laboratoria in de geneeskundige faculteiten." *Tijdschrift voor de Geschiedenis van de Geneeskunde, Natuurkunde, Wiskunde en Techniek* 9 (1986): 266–77.

Bevir, Mark. *Governance: A Very Short Introduction.* Oxford: Oxford University Press, 2012.

Beyens, Nele, and Timo Bolt. "'A Medical Doctor in Politics': Els Borst-Eilers and the

Rise of Evidence-Based Healthcare in the Netherlands." *Low Countries Historical Review* 132, no. 1 (2017): 16–37.

Bezemer, F. "In memoriam P.A. van Luijt." *Nederlandsch Tijdschrift der Geneeskunde* 98 (1954): 3513–14.

Bins, J. W. "Experimenten met mensen: Een verdwenen advies." *Medisch Contact* 38 (1983): 97–98.

Boer, E. J. "Medisch-ethische commissies, taak en functie bij wetenschappelijk onderzoek." *Nederlands Tijdschrift voor Geneeskunde* 133 (1989): 1659–64.

Boerema, I. "De Keerzijde van de Vooruitgang in de Geneeskunde." In *Acht voordrachten over de keerzijde van de vooruitgang in de natuur–en geneeskundige wetenschappen*, edited by W. Peremans et al., 39–55. The Hague: Martinus Nijhoff, 1962.

Boerhaave Commissie voor postacademisch onderwijs in de geneeskunde, ed. *Ethische beoordeling van medische experimenten met mensen*. Leiden: Rijksuniversiteit, Faculteit der Geneeskunde, 1983.

Bolt, Timo. "A Doctor's Order: The Dutch Case of Evidence-Based Medicine (1970–2015)." PhD diss., Utrecht University, 2015. http://dspace.library.uu.nl/handle/1874/318971.

Bonah, Christian. "'Experimental Rage': The Development of Medical Ethics and the Genesis of Scientific Facts. Ludwik Fleck: An Answer to the Crisis of Modern Medicine in Interwar Germany?" *Social History of Medicine* 15 (2002): 187–207.

Bonah, Christian, and Philippe Menut. "BCG-Vaccination around 1930—Dangerous Experiment or Established Prevention?: Practices and Debates in France and Germany." In *Twentieth Century Ethics of Human Subjects Research: Historical Perspectives on Values, Practices, and Regulations*, edited by Volker Roelcke and Giovanni Maio, 111–28. Stuttgart: Franz Steiner Verlag, 2004.

Bondeson, W. B., H. Tristram Engelhardt, S. F. Spicker, and J. M. White, eds. *New Knowledge in the Biomedical Sciences*. Springer: Dordrecht, 1982.

Borst-Eilers, Els. "Review commissie, fouten, ongevallen en near accidents (FONA) commissie en 'medical audit.'" In *Ethische beoordeling van medische experimenten met mensen*, edited by the Boerhaave Commissie voor postacademisch onderwijs in de geneeskunde, 137–39. Leiden: Rijksuniversiteit, Faculteit der Geneeskunde, 1983.

Borst-Eilers, Els. "Geneeskunde, ethiek en de Gezondheidsraad (Gast aan het woord)." *Tijdschrift voor geneeskunde en ethiek* 1 (1991): 48–49.

Bosk, Charles L. Review of Strangers at the Bedside: A History of How Law and Bioethics Transformed Medical Decision Making, by David J. Rothman. *Contemporary Sociology* 20 (1991): 831–33.

Bosk, Charles L., and Raymond De Vries. "Bureaucracies of Mass Deception: Institutional Review Boards and the Ethics of Ethnographic Research." *Annals of the American Academy of Political and Social Sciences* 595 (2004): 249–63.

Botter, A. A. "Over de aetiologie van de strophulus infantum." *Verhandelingen van het Instituut voor Praeventieve Geneeskunde* 16 (1950).

Bovens, Mark. "Public Accountability." In the *Oxford Handbook of Public Management*, edited by Ewan Ferlie, Laurence E. Lynn, Jr., and Christopher Pollitt, 182–208. Oxford: Oxford University Press, 2007.

Boxtel, J. A. M. van, J. Gruppelaar, Hans J. Achterhuis, and J. Vorstenbosch, eds. *Techniek, voorlopigheid en verlegenheid: Ethiek en technologisch aspectenonderzoek*. The Hague: NOTA, 1993.

Brants, M. A. "Proefnemingen op menschen." *Nederlandsch Tijdschrift voor Geneeskunde* part I (1904): 520–22.

Braun, D. "The Role of Funding Agencies in the Cognitive Development of Science." *Research Policy* 27 (1998): 807–21.

Brieger, Gert H. "Human Experimentation: I. History." In vol. 2 of *Encyclopedia of Bioethics*, edited by Warren T. Reich, 684–92. New York: Free Press, 1978.

Brom, Frans W. A. "Ethiek in de praktijk van het overheidsbeleid." *Filosofie en Praktijk* 13 (1992): 79–87.

Brom, Frans W. A., B. J. van den Bergh, and A. K. Huibers. *Beleid en ethiek*. Assen: Van Gorcum, 1993.

Brom, Frans W. A., B. J. van den Bergh, and A. K. Huibers. "Wie is er bang voor de ethiek." In *Beleid en ethiek*, edited by Frans W. A. Brom, B. J. van den Bergh, and A. K. Huibers, 5–18. Assen: Van Gorcum, 1993.

Brutel de la Rivière, Jean Jacques. "Over allergische huidreacties bij niet-allergische personen." PhD diss., Leiden University, 1932.

Brutel de la Rivière, Jean Jacques. "Uitoefening der Geneeskunst in Vrij Beroep tegenover deze Uitoefening in Dienstverband." *Medisch Contact* 2 (1947): 189–97.

Bryder, Linda. "The Medical Research Council and Clinical Trial Methodologies before the 1940s: The Failure to Develop a 'Scientific' Approach." *JLL Bulletin: Commentaries on the History of Treatment Evaluation* (2010). https://www.jameslindlibrary.org/articles/the-medical-research-council-and-clinical-trial-methodologies-before-the-1940s-the-failure-to-develop-a-scientific-approach/.

Buikhuisen, Wouter. "De 'regressies' van Schuyt." *Nederlands Juristenblad* 53 (1978): 526–30.

Buikhuisen, Wouter. "De wetenschapsfilosofische en ethische 'reflexen' van Prof. Schuyt." *Nederlandse Juristenblad* 54 (1978): 477–81.

Burger, Hendrik. "De bewijsvoering van Dr. Burger." *Nederlandsch Tijdschrift voor Geneeskunde* part I (1904): 466–67.

Burger, Hendrik. "Nog eens proefnemingen op menschen." *Nederlandsch Tijdschrift voor Geneeskunde* part I (1904): 379–80.

Burger, Hendrik. "Proefnemingen op menschen." *Nederlandsch Tijdschrift voor Geneeskunde* part I (1904): 317–20, 415–16, 522–24.

Bush, Vannevar. *Science: The Endless Frontier: A Report to the President on a Program for Postwar Scientific Research*. Reprint ed. Washington, DC: National Science Foundation, 1960 [1945]. https://archive.org/details/scienceendlessfr00unit/mode/2up?view=theater.

Bynum, William F. "Reflections on the History of Human Experimentation." In *The Use of Human Beings in Research: With Special Reference to Clinical Trials*, edited by Stuart F. Spicker, Ilai Alon, Andre de Vries, and H. Tristram Engelhardt, Jr., 29–46. Dordrecht: Kluwer Academic Publishers, 1988.

Bynum, William F., Anne Hardy, Stephen Jacyna, Christopher Lawrence, and E. M. Tansey. *The Western Medical Tradition, 1800–2000*. Cambridge: Cambridge University Press, 2006.

Calff, J. P. *Medische ethiek vandaag*. Amsterdam: Agon Elsevier, 1969.

Callon, Michel. "Some Elements of a Sociology of Translation: Domestication of the Scallops and the Fishermen of St. Brieuc Bay." *Sociological Review* 32 (1984): 196–233.

Caplan, Arthur. "Applying Morality to Advances in Biomedicine: Can and Should This Be Done?" In *New Knowledge in the Biomedical Sciences*, edited by W. B. Bondeson, H. Tristram Engelhardt, S. F. Spicker, and J. M. White, 155–68. Springer: Dordrecht, 1982.

Carlson, R. V., K. M. Boyd, and D. J. Webb. "The Revision of the Declaration of Helsinki: Past, Present and Future." *British Journal of Clinical Pharmacology* 57 (2004): 695–713.

"CCMO Deskundigheidseisen leden METC's." *Staatscourant* 6804 (February 12, 2016).

Centrale Raad voor de Volksgezondheid. *Deeladvies betreffende de juridische relatie tussen patiënt en arts, het recht van de patiënt op informatie en het toestemmingsvereiste*. The Hague: Staatsuitgeverij, 1980.

Centrale Raad voor de Volksgezondheid. *Deeladvies inzake de bescherming van de privacy van de patiënt*. The Hague: Staatsuitgeverij, 1981.

Centrale Raad voor de Volksgezondheid. *Deeladvies inzake kernbepalingen voor der regeling van de relatie tussen patiënt en arts*. The Hague: Staatsuitgeverij, 1982.

Centrale Raad voor de Volksgezondheid. *Deeladvies inzake medische experimenten*. The Hague: Staatsuitgeverij, 1982.

Centrale Raad voor de Volksgezondheid. *Deelsadvies inzake bemiddeling van klachten van patiënten*. Rijswijk: Centrale Raad voor de Volksgezondheid, 1982.

Cerutti, F. F. X., J. M. M. Maeijer, G. M. J. Veldkamp, W. C. L. van der Grinten, D. van Eck, F. J. H. M. van der Ven, J. Th. M. de Vreeze, and A. Th. L. M. Mertens. *De Geneesheer en het recht*. Deventer: Kluwer, 1968.

Chalmers, I. "Statistical Theory Was Not the Reason That Randomization Was Used in the British Medical Research Council's Clinical Trial of Streptomycin for Pulmonary Tuberculosis." In *Body Counts: Medical Quantification in Historical & Sociolog-*

ical Perspectives, edited by Gérard Jorland, Annick Opinel, and George Weisz, 309–34. Montreal: McGill-Queen's University Press, 2005.

Chavennes, M. E. "Criminologie met Buikhuisen: terug om beter te springen." *NRC Handelsblad*, April 22, 1978.

Clarke, Imogen. "The Gatekeepers of Modern Physics: Periodicals and Peer Review in 1920s Britain." *Isis* 106 (2014): 70–93.

Cluysenaer, M., and L. Breeveld. *50 Jaar College ter Beoordeling van Geneesmiddelen.* Haarlem, self-published, 2013.

Coetzee, J. M. *Landscape with Rowers: Poetry from the Netherlands.* Princeton, NJ: Princeton University Press, 2003.

Cohen, E. A. *Het Duitse concentratiekamp: Een medische en psychologische studie.* Amsterdam: Uitgeverij H. J. Parijs, 1952.

Cohen, M. J., and Gerard H. de Vries, eds. *Redes gehouden op de 16e Dies Natalis van de Rijksuniversiteit Limburg, 10 januari 1992.* Maastricht: Rijksuniversiteit Limburg, 1992.

Colenbrander, Mattheus, C. Fehmers, and Theodoor Hammes. *Medische ethiek.* Amsterdam: Nederlandsche Maatschappij tot Bevordering der Geneeskunst, 1936.

Collins, Harvey J. "André Hellegers, the Kennedy Institute, and the Development of Bioethics: The American-European Connection." In *The Development of Bioethics in the United States*, edited by Jeremy R. Garrett, Fabrice Jotterand, and D. Christopher Ralston, 37–54. Dordrecht: Springer, 2013.

Collins, Harry, and Robert Evans. *Rethinking Expertise.* Chicago: University of Chicago Press, 2007.

Commissie medische experimenten met wilsonbekwamen. *Advies inzake regeling van medisch-wetenschappelijk onderzoek met minderjarigen en meerderjarige wilsonbekwamen.* Rijswijk: Ministerie van Volksgezondheid, Welzijn en Sport, 1995.

Commissie van advies inzake het democratisch en doelmatig functioneren van gesubsidieerde instellingen. *Discussie-nota, September 1975.* Rijswijk: Secretariaat, 1975.

"Commissies." *Medisch Contact* 13 (1958): 335.

"Congres te Nijmegen: De geneesheer en het recht." *Medisch Contact* 23 (1968): 315–17.

Cook, H. J. "Practical Medicine and the British Armed Forces after the 'Glorious Revolution.'" *Medical History* 34 (1990): 1–26.

Cooper, Melinda, and Catherine Waldby. *Clinical Labor: Tissue Donors and Research Subjects in the Global Bioeconomy.* Durham, NC: Duke University Press, 2014.

Cooter, Roger. "Inside the Whale: Bioethics in History and Discourse." *Social History of Medicine* 23 (2010): 662–73.

Cooter, Roger. "Medicine and Modernity." In *The Oxford Handbook of the History of Medicine*, edited by Mark Jackson, 100–16. Oxford: Oxford University Press, 2011.

Cooter, Roger. "The Ethical Body." In *Medicine in the Twentieth Century*, edited by John V. Pickstone and Roger Cooter, 451–67. Amsterdam: Harwood Academic Press, 2000.

Cooter, Roger. "The Resistible Rise of Medical Ethics." *Social History of Medicine* 8 (1995): 275–88.

Cox-Maksimov, Desiree. "The Making of the Clinical Trial in Britain, 1910–1945: Expertise, the State and the Public." PhD diss., University of Cambridge, 1997.

Crofton, J. "The MRC Randomized Trial of Streptomycin and Its Legacy: A View from the Clinical Front Line." *Journal of the Royal Society of Medicine* 99 (2006): 531–34.

Csiszar, Alex. "Broken Pieces of Fact: The Scientific Periodical and the Politics of Search in Nineteenth-Century France and Britain." PhD diss., Harvard University, 2010.

Csiszar, Alex. *The Scientific Journal: Authorship and the Politics of Knowledge in the Nineteenth Century*. Chicago: University of Chicago Press, 2018.

Cunningham, Andrew R., and Perry Williams, eds. *The Laboratory Revolution in Medicine*. Cambridge: Cambridge University Press, 1992.

Dam, Peter van. *Staat van verzuiling: Over een Nederlandse mythe*. Amsterdam: Wereldbibliotheek, 2011.

Daston, Lorraine. "Objectivity and the Escape from Perspective." *Social Studies of Science* 22 (1992): 597–618.

Daston, Lorraine, and Peter Galison. *Objectivity*. New York: Zone Books, 2007.

Daston, Lorraine, and Fernando Vidal. *The Moral Authority of Nature*. Chicago: University of Chicago Press, 2003.

"De 150ste Algemene Vergadering der Maatschappij." *Medisch Contact* 23 (1968): 453–63.

"De 160ste Algemene Vergadering der K.N.M.G." *Medisch Contact* 27 (1972): 1161–64.

Dekker. "De derde druk van het boekje 'Medische Ethiek en Gedragsleer.'" *Medisch Contact* 15 (1960): 162.

Dekker, G. "Jaarverslag 1967 der Maatschappij." *Medisch Contact* 23 (1968): 718–23.

Dekker, G. "Rapport van de commissie herziening rechtspraak: Pre-advies van het hoofdbestuur." *Medisch Contact* 23 (1968): 84–104.

Dekker, W. *De affaire Buikhuisen: het ontstaan en de achtergronden rondom zijn biosociale onderzoek*. PhD diss., Erasmus University Rotterdam, 2009.

Dekking, F. "Het proces der Duitse artsen." *Nederlandsch Tijdschrift voor Geneeskunde* 91 (1947): 1830–33.

Dekking, F. "'Medische' experimenten in Duitsche concentratiekampen." *Nederlandsch Tijdschrift voor Geneeskunde* 90 (1946): 1011.

"De pers en de geneeskunde." *Medisch Contact* 10 (1955): 242–45.

De Telegraaf. "Bekende Londense arts onthult: Britse zieken zijn vaak 'proefkonijn.'" October 12, 1971: 9.

De Telegraaf. "Brit blind na experiment in ziekenhuis." October 13, 1971: 9.

De Telegraaf. "Heleen Dupuis (44), Medisch Ethica: 'Misdadig om leven van uitzichtloze comapatiënt eindeloos te rekken.'" December 30, 1989: TA-3.

De Telegraaf. "Het meest verkochte boek." August 9, 1969: 7.

De Telegraaf. "Nieuwe onthullingen over zwakzinnigeninrichting." December 19, 1978: 7.

De Telegraaf. "Ouders van softenon-kinderen geen kans op schadevergoeding." February 21, 1968: 9.

De Telegraaf. "Professor Heleen Dupuis: 'Medische beoordeling kan tot massale discriminatie leiden.'" February 6, 1988: T25.

De Telegraaf. "Risico's zijn in farmacologie onvermijdelijk." May 10, 1963: 3.

De Telegraaf. "Succes voor 'Help! De dokter verzuipt . . . .'" September 27, 1969: XIII.

De Tijd. "Amerikaanse onderscheidingen voor twintig Nederlanders: Medal of Freedom o.a. voor de minister-president." April 7, 1953: 4.

De Tijd. "Cruijf lichtend voorbeeld van mondige patient." April 13, 1972: front page.

De Tijd. "Het proces tegen de fabeltjes: Medici staan terecht te Neurenberg." December 10, 1946: 3.

De Tijd. "Meest verkocht." March 9, 1970: 5.

De Tijd. "Opwinding in Engeland: Proeven op mensen in ziekenhuizen." May 19, 1967: 9.

De Tijd. "Schandaal in Engeland en VS: Fondspatiënten als proefkonijnen: Experimenten met kernstraling." October 11, 1971: 5.

De Tijd. "Syfilislijders als proefkonijn: Medisch schandaal in VS." July 26, 1972: front page.

De Tijd-Maasbode. "Onderzoek nieuw medicijn eist experiment op mens." May 10, 1963: 4.

De Tijd-Maasbode. "Over medische ethiek: Twee nieuwe uitgaven." May 19, 1960: 7.

De Waarheid. "Anti-griepmiddel op krankzinnigen beproefd." September 17, 1966: front page.

De Waarheid. "De Mens is het Beste Proefdier." November 30, 1963: 4.

De Waarheid. "Directeur psychiatrische instelling: 'Patiënten geen proefkonijn.'" September 20, 1966: 2.

De Waarheid. "Ernstige beschuldigingen Britse arts: Experimenten op onwetende patiënten: Binnenkort vragen in Lagerhuis." May 18, 1967: 2.

De Waarheid. "Gevangenen werden met mosterdgas bewerkt: Gruwelijke bijzonderheden voor het hof te Neurenberg." January 4, 1947: front page.

De Waarheid. "Joop Wolff interpelleert." April 21, 1978: front page.

De Waarheid. "Kinderen werden gesteriliseerd in Ravensbrück." December 21, 1946: front page.

De Waarheid. "Medische ethici: Discussie over genetische kennis nog in pril stadium." December 20, 1988: 8.

De Waarheid. "Opvattingen uit de negentiende eeuw dreigen terug te keren: Buikhuisen wil hersenonderzoek bij gevangenen." April 20, 1978: front page.

De Waarheid. "Wanneer controle op verpakte geneesmiddelen?" November 22, 1962: 3.

De Waarheid. "Wij slikken duizenden pilletjes per dag." September 13, 1962: 4.

De Waarheid. "Zwakzinnigeninrichting proefterrein: Operaties door niet-deskundigen." December 16, 1978: 7.

Dijk, J. J. M. van. "Weerwoord op het requisitoir van Schuyt." *Nederlandse Juristenblad* 54 (1978): 481–87.

Dillmann, R. J. M., and W. R. Kastelein. "Niet-therapeutisch wetenschappelijk onderzoek met wilsonbekwame patiënten: een gezamenlijk standpunt van Nederlandse medisch-wetenschappelijke organisaties." *Nederlands Tijdschrift voor Geneeskunde* 138 (1994): 1676–80.

DiMaggio, Paul J., and Walter W. Powell. "The Iron Cage Revisited: Institutional Isomorphism and Collective Rationality in Organizational Fields." *American Sociological Review* 48 (1983): 147–60.

"Discussie over: rapport kunstmatige inseminatie." *Medisch Contact* 17 (1962): 239–41.

Does de Willebois, A. E. M. van der. "Kroniek van de artsen actie eerbiediging menselijk leven." *Informatiebulletin van het Nederlands Artsenverbond* 1 (1973): 348.

Does de Willebois, A. E. M. van der. *Het Vaderloze Tijdperk: Een cultuur-psychologische verkenning van de geseculariseerde samenleving*. Brugge: Tabor, 1984.

Does de Willebois, J. A. van der. "Medische ethiek." *Vita Humana* 10 (1983): 34.

Dongen, M. A. van. "Experimenten op mensen." *Medisch Contact* 35 (1980): 170.

Dorsman, L. J., and P. J. Knegtmans. *Onderzoek in opdracht: De publieke functie van het universitaire onderzoek in Nederland sedert 1876*. Hilversum: Verloren, 2007.

Dorsman, L. J., and P. J. Knegtmans. *Universitaire vormingsidealen: De Nederlandse universiteiten sedert 1876*. Hilversum: Verloren, 2006.

Drift, L. van der. "Medische ethiek anno 1970: Inleiding van de voorzitter der Maatschappij, Dr. L. van der Drift, ter Algemene Vergadering op 18 april 1970 te Utrecht." *Medisch Contact* 25 (1970): 413–17.

"Dr. J.C. Schultsz over medische ethiek." *Medisch Contact* 21 (1966): 782–83.

"Dr. J.J. Brutel de la Rivière 60 jaar arts." *Nederlands Tijdschrift voor Geneeskunde* 116 (1972): 585–86.

"Dr. R.J.H. Kruisinga beantwoordt vragen inzake 'dubbelblinde' farmacologische onderzoeken." *Medisch Contact* 22 (1967): 1125–26.

Dunning, A. J. "Afscheid prof.dr. Chr. L. Rümke." *Nederlands Tijdschrift voor Geneeskunde* 136 (1992): 900–01.

Dupuis, Heleen M. "Ethische aspecten van experimenten met mensen." In *Geneeskunde en ethiek in harmonie*, edited by F. A. Wolff, 155–63. The Hague: Pasmans Offset Drukkerij BV, 2001.

Dupuis, Heleen M. *Goed te leven: Reflecties op de moraal*. Baarn: Ten Have, 1980.

Dupuis, Heleen M. "Ontwikkelingen in de medische ethiek: Van artsencode naar ethiek in de gezondheidszorg." In *Handboek gezondheidsethiek*, edited by Inez de Beaufort and Heleen M. Dupuis, 21–28. Assen: Van Gorcum, 1988.

Dupuis, Heleen M. "Recensie van H. ten Have: *Een hippocratische erfenis*." *Nederlands Tijdschrift voor Geneeskunde* 135 (1991): 1333.

Dupuis, Heleen M., and Beaufort, Inez D. de. "Ethiek–wat is het en wat kan men er mee." In *Handboek gezondheidsethiek*, edited by Inez de Beaufort and Heleen M. Dupuis, 7–20. Assen: Van Gorcum, 1988.

Dyck, Erika, and Larry Stewart, eds. *The Uses of Humans in Experiment: Perspectives from the 17th to the 20th Century*. Leiden: Brill Rodopi, 2016.

Edeler, H. A. *De drinkwaterfluoridering: Tandartsen, staat en volksgezondheid in Nederland 1946–1976*. Houten: Bohn Stafleu van Loghum, 2009.

Edwards, Martin. *Control and the Therapeutic Trial: Rhetoric and Experimentation in Britain, 1918–1948*. Amsterdam: Rodopi, 2007.

Eijnatten, Joris van. "Beyond Diversity: The Steady State of Reference Cultures." *International Journal for History, Culture and Modernity* 3 (2015): 1–8.

Elkeles, Barbara. "The German Debate on Human Experimentation between 1880 and 1914." In *Twentieth Century Ethics of Human Subjects Research: Historical Perspectives on Values, Practices, and Regulations*, edited by Volker Roelcke and Giovanni Maio, 19–33. Stuttgart: Franz Steiner Verlag, 2004.

Emanuel, Ezekiel J., Christine C. Grady, Robert A. Crouch, Reidar K. Lie, Franklin G. Miller, and David D. Wendler, eds. *The Oxford Textbook of Clinical Research Ethics*. Oxford: Oxford University Press, 2008.

Ende, Hanna van den. *'Vergeet niet dat je arts bent': Joodse artsen in Nederland, 1940–1945*. Amsterdam: Boom, 2015.

Engberts, D. P. "De vroege Jaren: Ontstaan en werkzaamheid van een medisch-ethische (toetsings)commissie in Leiden in de Jaren zestig van de vorige eeuw." In *Dilemma's getoetst: Liber amicorum voor prof.dr. H.M. Dupuis en prof.dr. P.Vermeij*, edited by D. P. Engberts, Y. M. Reidsma, and A. R. Wintzen, 9–28. Leiden: UFB Universiteit Leiden, 2003.

Engberts, D. P. "Het verhaal achter het schandaal: Medische proeven met verstandelijke gehandicapten in een Noord-Brabantse inrichting in de jaren zestig en zeventig." In *Geneeskunde en ethiek in harmonie*, edited by F. A. Wolff, 125–53. The Hague: Pasmans Offset Drukkerij BV, 2001.

Engberts, D. P., Y. M. Reidsma, and A. R. Wintzen, eds. *Dilemma's getoetst: Liber amicorum voor prof.dr. H.M. Dupuis en prof.dr. P.Vermeij*. Leiden: UFB Universiteit Leiden, 2003.

Engelhardt, H. Tristram, Jr. *The Foundations of Bioethics*. Oxford: Oxford University Press, 1986.

Engelhardt, H. Tristram, Jr., and Lisa M. Rasmussen. "Secular Humanism." *Encyclopedia of Life Sciences*, September 15, 2006. https://doi.org/10.1002/9780470015902.a0005890.

Engels, J. W. M. "Constitutionele observaties bij de minister van Staat." In *De Republiek van Oranje, 1813–2013: Jaarboek Parlementaire Geschiedenis 2013*, edited by C. van Baalen et al. Amsterdam: Boom, 2013.

Es, J. C. van. "Experimenten met mensen en wetgeving." *Medisch Contact* 40 (1985): 1115.

"Ethische beoordeling van medische experimenten met mensen: Boerhaave-cursus van het PAOG." *Medisch Contact* 38 (1983): 12.

Evans, John H. "A Sociological Account of the Growth of Principlism." *Hastings Center Report* 30 (2000): 31–38.

Evans, John H. *The History and Future of Bioethics: A Sociological Review.* Oxford: Oxford University Press, 2012.

Evenepoel, S. *Volmaakt onaf: Over de stijl en thematiek in de vroege poëzie van Rutger Kopland.* Leuven: Universitaire Pers Leuven, 2000.

Eyck, H. H., and A. J. Verstegen. *Arts en wet: Rechtskundige handleiding voor geneeskundigen.* 2nd ed. Haarlem: De Erven Bohn, 1929.

Faden, Ruth R., and Tom L. Beauchamp. *A History and Theory of Informed Consent.* Oxford: Oxford University Press, 1986.

Ferlie, Ewan, Laurence E. Lynn, Jr., and Christopher Pollitt, eds. *Oxford Handbook of Public Management.* Oxford: Oxford University Press, 2007.

Festen, Henri. *125 jaar geneeskunst en maatschappij.* Utrecht: Koninklijke Nederlandsche Maatschappij tot Bevordering der Geneeskunst, 1974.

Festen, Henri. *Spanningen in de gezondheidszorg: 25 jaar Centrale Raad voor de Volksgezondheid.* Zoetermeer: Nationale Raad voor de Volksgezondheid, 1985.

"Fifty Years of Randomized Controlled Trials." *British Medical Journal* 317 (1998): 1167.

Fissell, Mary E. "The Medical Marketplace, the Patient, and the Absence of Medical Ethics in Early Modern Europe and North America." In *The Cambridge World History of Medical Ethics,* edited by Robert B. Baker and Laurence B. McCullough, 533–39. Cambridge: Cambridge University Press, 2009.

Fitzgerald, Maureen H. "Punctuated Equilibrium, Moral Panics and the Ethics Review Process." *Journal of Academic Ethics* 2 (2005): 315–38.

Fletcher, Joseph. *Situation Ethics: The New Morality.* Philadelphia: Westminster Press, 1966.

Fokkens, O. "Oordeelsvorming in de geneeskunde." *Nederlands Tijdschrift voor Geneeskunde* 106 (1962): 1896–99.

Food and Drug Administration. "Protection of Human Subjects; Informed Consent." 21 CFR parts 50, 71, 171, 180, 310, 312, 314, 320, 330, 361, 430, 431, 601, 630, 812, 813, 1003, 1010. Docket no. 78N-0400. 46 FR 8942. January 27, 1981. https://www.fda.gov/science-research/clinical-trials-and-human-subject-protection/protection-human-subjects-informed-consent.

Fortuyn, W. S. P. *Ordening door ontvlechting: Een advies over de adviesstructuur in de gezondheidszorg.* Rijswijk: Ministerie van WVC, 1990.

Foucault, Michel. *The Birth of the Clinic.* Translated by A. M. Sheridan-Smith. London: Tavistock Publications, 1973.

Foucault, Michel. *The Order of Things: An Archaeology of the Human Sciences*. New York: Routledge, 1970.

French, R. D. *Antivivisection and Medical Science in Victorian Society*. Princeton, NJ: Princeton University Press, 1975.

Frewer, Andreas. "Human Rights from the Nuremberg Doctors Trial to the Geneva Declaration." *Medicine, Health Care and Philosophy* 13 (2010): 259–68.

Frewer, Andreas, and Ulf Schmidt, eds. *History and Theory of Human Experimentation: The Declaration of Helsinki and Modern Medical Ethics*. Frankfurt: Steiner, 2007.

Friese Koerier. "Veilig gebruik nieuwe geneesmiddelen." November 30, 1963: 21.

Fuller, Steve. *The Governance of Science: Ideology and the Future of the Open Society*. Buckingham: Open University Press, 2000.

Fyfe, Aileen. "Journals and Periodicals." In *A Companion to the History of Science*, edited by Bernard Lightman, 387–99. West Sussex: John Wiley & Sons Ltd., 2016.

Gaarenstroom, J. H. "Het aandeel van Nederland in de vooruitgang der geneeskundige wetenschap van 1900 tot 1950." *Nederlandsch Tijdschrift voor Geneeskunde* 95 (1951): 762–67.

Gabriel, Joseph M. *Medical Monopoly: Intellectual Property Rights and the Origins of the Modern Pharmaceutical Industry*. Chicago: University of Chicago Press, 2015.

Gaillard, P. J. "Levensbericht S.E. De Jongh." In *Jaarboek Huygens Institute–KNAW*, 200–02. Amsterdam: KNAW, 1976.

Garrett, Jeremy R., Fabrice Jotterand, and D. Christopher Ralston, eds. *The Development of Bioethics in the United States*. Dordrecht: Springer, 2013.

Gaudillière, Jean-Paul, and Volker Hess, eds. *Ways of Regulating Drugs in the 19th and 20th Centuries*. Basingstoke: Palgrave Macmillan, 2013.

Geison, G. L. "Pasteur's Work on Rabies: Reexamining the Ethical Issues." *Hastings Center Report* 8 (1978): 26–33.

Genderen, F. Th. van. "In Memoriam Prof. Dr. W.K. Dicke." *Nederlands Tijdschrift voor Geneeskunde* 106 (1962): 1108.

Gereformeerd Gezinsblad. "Gesprek aan het ziekbed." July 16, 1960.

Geuns, H. A. van. "Uit de Geneeskundige Hoofdinspectie: Medische experimenten in de huisartspraktijk." *Medisch Contact* 42 (1987): 694.

Geuns, H. A. van. "Het Staatstoezicht en medische experimenten met mensen." *Medisch Contact* 40 (1985): 801–02.

Gevers, J. K. M., and J. H. Hubben, eds. *Grenzen aan de zorg, zorgen aan de grens: Liber amicorum voor Prof.dr. H.J.J. Leenen*. Alphen aan den Rijn: Samsom H. D. Tjeenk Willink, 1990.

Gezondheidsraad. *Advies inzake euthanasie bij pasgeborenen*. Rijswijk: Staatsuitgeverij, 1975.

Gezondheidsraad. *Advies inzake klinische farmacologie*. The Hague: Staatsuitgeverij, 1982.

Gezondheidsraad. *Advies inzake normen voor het toedienen van radioactieve stoffen aan vrijwilligers*. The Hague: Staatsuitgeverij, 1981.

Gezondheidsraad. *Interim-advies inzake euthanasie*. The Hague: Staatsuitgeverij, 1972.

Gezondheidsraad. *Kerncommissie Ethiek Medisch Onderzoek (KEMO) 1993–1999*. The Hague: Staatsuitgeverij, 2004; publication no. 2004/K01.

Giddens, Anthony. *The Third Way and its Critics*. Cambridge: Polity Press, 2000.

Giddens, Anthony. *The Third Way: The Renewal of Social Democracy*. Cambridge: Polity Press, 1998.

Gieryn, Thomas F. *Cultural Boundaries of Science: Credibility on the Line*. London: University of Chicago Press, 1999.

Gijswijt-Hofstra, M., G. M. van Heteren, and E. M. Tansey, eds. *Biographies of Remedies: Drugs, Medicines and Contraceptives in Dutch and Anglo-American Healing Cultures*. Amsterdam: Rodopi, 2002.

Gonggrijp, Frits. "Commissies gepasseerd: Bloemenhove liet experimenten toe na late abortus." *De Telegraaf*, December 21, 1979: 7.

Gonggrijp, Frits. "Eis van nieuwe hoogleraar in Leiden: Hersenonderzoek bij delinquenten." *De Telegraaf*, April 20, 1978: 3.

Gonggrijp, Frits. "Inrichting in Udenhout in opspraak: Ingrepen op zwakzinnigen in onderzoek." *De Telegraaf*, December 13, 1978: 6.

Goodman, Jordan. "Pharmaceutical Industry." In *Medicine in the Twentieth Century*, edited by John V. Pickstone and Roger Cooter, 141–54. Amsterdam: Harwood Academic Press, 2000.

Goudsmit, C. J. "Discussie over: de medische ethiek met betrekking tot de nieuwste ontwikkelingen in de geneeskunde." *Medisch Contact* 24 (1969): 386.

Gradmann, C., and J. Simon, eds. *Evaluating and Standardizing Therapeutic Agents, 1890–1950*. Basingstoke: Palgrave Macmillan, 2010.

Gray, Bradford H. *Human Subjects in Medical Experimentation: A Sociological Study of the Conduct and Regulation of Clinical Research*. New York: Wiley-Interscience, 1975.

Grenzen van de zorg: Regeringsstandpunt inzake het Advies van de Ziekenfondsraad, de Nationale Raad voor de Volksgezondheid en de Gezondheidsraad. The Hague: Tweede Kamer der Staten-Generaal 1987–1988, 20 620, nos. 1–2 (1988).

Greven, Koen, and Joke Mat. "Overleg met familie verzacht angst voor medisch experiment." *NRC Handelsblad*, October 5, 1995.

Griffiths, J., A. Bood, and H. Weyers. *Euthanasia and Law in the Netherlands*. Amsterdam: Amsterdam University Press, 1998.

Grijs, Piet. *Buikhuisen: dom én slecht*. Amsterdam: Vrij Nederland, 1978.

Groen, J. J. "Iedere tijd heeft zijn eigen ethiek." *De Groene Amsterdammer*, July 5, 1969: 9–10.

Guerrini, Anita. *Experimenting with Humans and Animals: From Galen to Animal Rights*. Baltimore, MD: Johns Hopkins University Press, 2003.

Guerrini, Anita. "The Human Experimental Subject." In *A Companion to the History of Science*, edited by Bernard Lightman, 126–38. West Sussex: John Wiley & Sons Ltd., 2016.

Gunning, K. F. "Eerbiediging menselijk leven: Voorwoord." *Informatiebulletin van het Nederlands Artsenverbond* 1 (1973): 2.

Gunning-Schepers, Louise J. "In memoriam: Els Borst (1932–2014)." *Nederlands Tijdschrift voor Geneeskunde* 159 (2014): B1026.

Gusfield, Joseph R. *The Culture of Public Problems: Drinking-Driving and the Symbolic Order*. London: University of Chicago Press, 1981.

Haggerty, Kevin D. "Ethics Creep: Governing Social Science Research in the Name of Ethics." *Qualitative Sociology* 27 (2004): 391–414.

Halpern, Sydney. *Lesser Harms: The Morality of Risk in Medical Research*. Chicago: University of Chicago Press, 2004.

Hamburger, Roel J. "Proeven op mensen." *Medisch Contact* 10 (1955): 333–34.

Hamburger, Roel J., and H. Beukenhorst. "De belofte bij het toetreden der Mij." *Medisch Contact* 6 (1951): 15–16.

Handelingen Eerste Kamer (Acts of the Senate) 1988–1989. March 21, 1989. https://repository.overheid.nl/frbr/sgd/19881989/0000089624/1/pdf/SGD_19881989_0000025.pdf.

Handelingen Eerste Kamer (Acts of the Senate) 1988–1989. March 22, 1989. https://repository.overheid.nl/frbr/sgd/19881989/0000089625/1/pdf/SGD_19881989_0000026.pdf.

Handelingen Eerste Kamer (Acts of the Senate) 1992–1993. April 6, 1993. https://repository.overheid.nl/frbr/sgd/19921993/0000010330/1/pdf/SGD_19921993_0000026.pdf.

Handelingen Eerste Kamer (Acts of the Senate) 1997–1998. April 21, 1998. https://zoek.officielebekendmakingen.nl/h-ek-19971998-1469-1483.pdf.

Handelingen Tweede Kamer (Acts of the House of Representatives) 1903–1904. December 12, 1903. https://repository.overheid.nl/frbr/sgd/19031904/0000359995/1/pdf/SGD_19031904_0000159.pdf.

Handelingen Tweede Kamer (Acts of the House of Representatives) 1949–1950. December 16, 1949. https://repository.overheid.nl/frbr/sgd/19491950/0000083711/1/pdf/SGD_19491950_0000357.pdf.

Handelingen Tweede Kamer (Acts of the House of Representatives) 1967–1968. Vaste Commissie voor de volksgezondheid. November 2, 1967. https://repository.overheid.nl/frbr/sgd/19671968/0000237870/1/pdf/SGD_19671968_0000472.pdf.

Handelingen Tweede Kamer (Acts of the House of Representatives) 1969–1970. February 3, 1970. https://repository.overheid.nl/frbr/sgd/19691970/0000228046/1/pdf/SGD_19691970_0000418.pdf.

Handelingen Tweede Kamer (Acts of the House of Representatives) 1974–1975. May 6,

1975. https://repository.overheid.nl/frbr/sgd/19741975/0000199051/1/pdf/SGD_19741975_0000490.pdf.

Handelingen Tweede Kamer (Acts of the House of Representatives) 1974–1975. May 13, 1975. https://repository.overheid.nl/frbr/sgd/19741975/0000199053/1/pdf/SGD_19741975_0000492.pdf.

Handelingen Tweede Kamer (Acts of the House of Representatives) 1978–1979. June 25, 1979. https://repository.overheid.nl/frbr/sgd/19781979/0000174430/1/pdf/SGD_19781979_0000504.pdf.

Handelingen Tweede Kamer (Acts of the House of Representatives) 1979–1980. May 28, 1980. https://repository.overheid.nl/frbr/sgd/19791980/0000166084/1/pdf/SGD_19791980_0000493.pdf.

Handelingen Tweede Kamer (Acts of the House of Representatives) 1985–1986. January 29, 1986. https://repository.overheid.nl/frbr/sgd/19851986/0000114262/1/pdf/SGD_19851986_0000715.pdf.

Handelingen Tweede Kamer (Acts of the House of Representatives) 1988–1989. Vaste Commissie voor de volksgezondheid. January 23, 1989. https://repository.overheid.nl/frbr/sgd/19881989/0000090572/1/pdf/SGD_19881989_0000891.pdf.

Handelingen Tweede Kamer (Acts of the House of Representatives) 1988–1989. Vaste Commissies voor justitie en voor de volksgezondheid. April 17, 1989. https://repository.overheid.nl/frbr/sgd/19881989/0000090590/1/pdf/SGD_19881989_0000909.pdf.

Handelingen Tweede Kamer (Acts of the House of Representatives) OCV/UCV 1988–1989. February 27, 1989. https://repository.overheid.nl/frbr/sgd/19881989/0000090578/1/pdf/SGD_19881989_0000897.pdf.

Handelingen Tweede Kamer (Acts of the House of Representatives) 1989–1990. January 30, 1990. https://repository.overheid.nl/frbr/sgd/19891990/0000035220/1/pdf/SGD_19891990_0000734.pdf.

Handelingen Tweede Kamer (Acts of the House of Representatives) 1991–1992. Vaste Commissie voor het wetenschapsbeleid. November 4, 1991: 6.2. https://repository.overheid.nl/frbr/sgd/19911992/0000019354/1/pdf/SGD_19911992_0000899.pdf.

Handelingen Tweede Kamer (Acts of the House of Representatives) 1996–1997. September 3, 1997. https://zoek.officielebekendmakingen.nl/h-tk-19961997-7288-7315.pdf.

Handelingen Tweede Kamer (Acts of the House of Representatives) 1996–1997. September 4, 1997. https://zoek.officielebekendmakingen.nl/h-tk-19961997-7341-7354.pdf.

Handelingen Tweede Kamer (Acts of the House of Representatives) 1996–1997. September 9, 1997. https://zoek.officielebekendmakingen.nl/h-tk-19961997-105-7405-7430.pdf.

Hardy, Anne, and E. M. Tansey. "Medical Enterprise and Global Response, 1945–

2000." In William F. Bynum et al., *The Western Medical Tradition, 1800–2000*, 405–534. Cambridge: Cambridge University Press, 2006.

Harkness, Jon M. "Nuremberg and the Issue of Wartime Experiments on U.S. Prisoners: The Green Committee." *Journal of the American Medical Association* 276 (1996): 1672–75.

Hart, P. G. "In memoriam Prof. Dr. W.P. Plate." *Nederlands Tijdschrift voor Geneeskunde* 127 (1983): 1269–70.

Have, Henk ten. *Een hippocratische erfenis: Ethiek in de medische praktijk*. Lochem: Uitgeversmaatschappij De Tijdstroom, 1990.

Have, Henk ten. *Ethiek tussen alliantie en dissidentie*. Maastricht: Rijksuniversiteit Limburg, 1990.

Have, Henk ten, and Gerrit Kimsma. *Geneeskunde tussen droom en drama: Voortplanting, ethiek en vooruitgang*. Kampen: Kok Agora, 1987.

Have, H. A. M. J. ten, R. H. J. ter Meulen, and E. van Leeuwen. *Medische ethiek*. Houten: Bohn Stafleu van Loghum, 2003.

Hazelgrove, Jenny. "The Old Faith and the New Science: The Nuremberg Code and Human Experimentation Ethics in Britain, 1946–73." *Social History of Medicine* 15 (2002): 109–35.

Hazelgrove, Jenny. "British Research Ethics after the Second World War: The Controversy at the British Postgraduate Medical School, Hammersmith Hospital." In *Twentieth Century Ethics of Human Subjects Research: Historical Perspectives on Values, Practices, and Regulations*, edited by Volker Roelcke and Giovanni Maio, 181–97. Stuttgart: Franz Steiner Verlag, 2004.

Hedgecoe, Adam. "'A Form of Practical Machinery': The Origins of Research Ethics Committees in the UK, 1967–1972." *Medical History* 53 (2009): 331–50.

Hedgecoe, Adam. "Research Ethics Review and the Sociological Research Relationship." *Sociology* 42 (2008): 873–86.

Hedgecoe, Adam. "Scandals, Ethics, and Regulatory Change in Biomedical Research." *Science, Technology, and Human Values* 42 (2017): 577–99.

Hedgecoe, Adam. *Trust in the System: Research Ethics Committees and the Regulation of Biomedical Research*. Manchester: Manchester University Press, 2020.

Hedgecoe, Adam, F. Carvalho, P. Lobmayer, and F. Raka. "Research Ethics Committees in Europe: Implementing the Directive, Respecting Diversity." *Journal of Medical Ethics* 32 (2006): 483–86.

Heering, Herman J. *Ethiek der voorlopigheid*. Nijkerk: Callenbach, 1969.

Hellema, Duco. *Nederland en de jaren zeventig*. Amsterdam: Boom, 2012.

Helvoort, T. van. "De publieke functie van universitaire wetenschapsbeoefening: Amerikanisering als leidmotief bij de scheikunde aan de Groningse universiteit." In *Onderzoek in opdracht: De publieke functie van het universitaire onderzoek in Nederland sedert 1876*, edited by L. J. Dorsman and P. J. Knegtmans, 67–92. Hilversum: Verloren, 2007.

Heringa, G. C. "De verantwoordelijkheid van medische redacties voor de instandhouding der medische ethiek." *Medisch Contact* 9 (1954): 554–57.

Heringa, G. C. "Een leerstoel voor de homoeopathie?" *Medisch Contact* 5 (1950): 191–93.

Heringa, G. C. "Medische Ethiek, Practische Geneeskunde en Wetenschap." *Medisch Contact* 4 (1949): 539–45.

Heringa, G. C. "Prof. Dr. L.A. Hulst. Lid van de Council der W.M.A." *Medisch Contact* 10 (1955): 789.

Herranz, Gonzalo. "The Inclusion of the Ten Principles of Nuremberg in Professional Codes of Ethics: An International Comparison." In *Ethics Codes in Medicine: Foundations and Achievements of Codification since 1947*, edited by Ulrich Tröhler and Stella Reiter-Theil, 127–39. Aldershot: Ashgate, 1998.

"Het overdoen van de praktijk." *Medisch Contact* 9 (1954): 298–99.

Het Vrije Volk. "Arts beschuldigt: Britse 'fonds'-patiënten als proefkonijnen." October 11, 1971: front page.

Het Vrije Volk. "De nieuwe procesronde in Neurenberg: Experimenten op mensen worden berecht: Gruwelijke details." December 10, 1946: 3.

Het Vrije Volk. "Dr. Buikhuisen: hersenonderzoek delinquenten." April 20, 1978: 9.

Het Vrije Volk. "Ernstige beschuldiging tegen Leids ziekenhuis." May 9, 1953: 5.

Het Vrije Volk. "Patiënten betuttelen . . . hoe lang duurt dat nog?" February 7, 1973: 4.

Het Vrije Volk. "Prof. H. Dupuis tegen kunstgrepen op onvruchtbare vrouwen: 'Deze drievoudige abortus was humaan en verstandig.'" June 26, 1986: 5.

Het Vrije Volk. "Schedelmetende arts voor tuchtcollege." December 28, 1978: 5.

Het Vrije Volk. "Verplicht inenten." February 1, 1988: 3.

"Het ziekenfondswezen." *Medisch Contact* 13 (1958): 105–08.

Hilfman, M. M. "Mededelingen adviescommissie klinisch geneesmiddelenonderzoek." *Nederlands Tijdschrift voor Geneeskunde* 100 (1956): 1671.

Hilhorst, Medard. "Medische ethiek: onnodige misverstanden." *Tijdschrift voor Beleid, Politiek en Maatschappij* 26 (1999): 292–300.

Hilhorst, Medard. "Klimaatverandering in de medische ethiek." In *Ethiek in Nederland*, edited by Bert Musschenga et al., 181–205. Budel: Damon, 2010.

Hoefnagels, W. H. L., and M. G. M. Olde Rikkert. "Van ongebreideld medisch onderzoek op wilsonbekwamen is helemaal geen sprake." *NRC Handelsblad*, October 17, 2015.

Hoffman, H. "Géén experimenten Bloemenhove-kliniek: Bloedmonsters genomen van foetaal weefsel." *Het Vrije Volk*, December 28, 1979: 7.

"Honorarium." *Medisch Contact* 12 (1957): 546–51.

Hoofdakker, R. H. van den. "Het bolwerk der beterweters." *Wijsgerig Perspectief op Maatschappij en Samenleving* 9 (1968–1969): 292–301.

Hoofdakker, R. H. van den. *Het bolwerk van de beterweters: Over de medische ethiek en de status quo*. Amsterdam: Kritiese Bibliotheek, 1970.

Hoonaard, Will C. van den. *The Seduction of Ethics: Transforming the Social Sciences.* Toronto: University of Toronto Press, 2011.

Horstman, Klasien, and Gerard de Vries. "Experimenten met mensen: De constitutie van een medisch-wetenschappelijke praktijk en een ethisch probleem (Nederland, 1870–1915)." *Kennis en Methode* 1 (1989): 62–83.

Houwaart, Eduard Simon. *De hygiënisten: Artsen, staat en volksgezondheid in Nederland, 1840–1890.* Groningen: Historische Uitgeverij Groningen, 1991.

Hoven, M. van der, L. van der Scheer, and D. Willems, eds. *Ethiek in discussie: Praktijkvoorbeelden van ethische expertise.* Assen: Van Gorcum, 2010.

Hugenholtz, P. Th. "Wijziging rechtspraak." *Medisch Contact* 13 (1958): 785.

Huisman, F., and H. te Velde. "Op zoek naar nieuwe vormen in wetenschap en politiek: De 'medische' kleine geloven." *De Negentiende Eeuw* 25 (2001): 129–36.

Hulst, L. A. "Van het Hoofdbestuur: De World Medical Association." *Medisch Contact* 8 (1953): 504–08.

Hurlbut, Benjamin. *Experiments in Democracy: Human Embryo Research and the Politics of Bioethics.* Columbia University Press, 2011.

Illich, I. *Medical Nemesis: The Expropriation of Health.* London: Calder and Boyars, 1975.

Ingelfinger, Franz J. "The Unethical in Medical Ethics." *Annals of Internal Medicine* 83 (1975): 264–69.

"Inleiding 154ste Algemene Vergadering." *Medisch Contact* 25 (1970): 5–6.

Jackson, Mark, ed. *The Oxford Handbook of the History of Medicine.* Oxford: Oxford University Press, 2011.

Jacobs, Frans C. L. M. "Ten overstaan van allen: Universalisering in de ethiek." PhD diss., University of Amsterdam, 1985.

Jacobs, Frans C. L. M. "Praktische ethiek: onpraktisch en onfilosofisch?" *Filosofie en Praktijk* 12 (1991): 18–30.

Jaeger, Jan. "An Ethnographic Analysis of Institutional Review Board Decision-Making." PhD diss., University of Pennsylvania, 2006.

Jasanoff, Sheila. *Designs on Nature: Science and Democracy in Europe and the United States.* Princeton, NJ: Princeton University Press, 2005.

Jasanoff, Sheila. *The Fifth Branch: Science Advisers as Policymakers.* Cambridge, MA: Harvard University Press, 1990.

Jaspers, Patricia. "Controversial Issues in the History of Dutch Research Ethics Governance." *Journal of Policy History* 23 (2011): 74–93.

Jaspers, Patricia, Rob Houtepen, and Klasien Horstman. "Ethical Review: Standardizing Procedures and Local Shaping of Ethical Review Practices." *Social Science & Medicine* 98 (2013): 311–18.

Jones, D. S., C. Grady, and S. E. Lederer. "'Ethics and Clinical Research'—The 50th Anniversary of Beecher's Bombshell." *The New England Journal of Medicine* 374 (2016): 2393–98.

Jones, James. *Bad Blood: The Tuskegee Syphilis Experiment.* New York: Free Press, 1981.

Jong, Addy de. "Slob (CU): Altijd verbinding zoeken." *Reformatorisch Dagblad,* September 1, 2012. https://www.rd.nl/artikel/462537-slob-cu-altijd-verbinding-zoeken.

Jong, C. L. de. "G.A. Lindeboom, *Opstellen over medische ethiek.*" *Nederlands Tijdschrift voor Geneeskunde* 104 (1960): 1897.

Jongh, D. K. de. "Medische ethiek: Antwoord aan Prof.dr. G.C. Heringa." *Medisch Contact* 4 (1949): 600–04.

Jongh, D. K. de. "Over medische ethiek." *Medisch Contact* 4 (1949): 526–32.

Jongh, E. D. J. de. *Hannes de Graaf: Een leven van bevrijding.* Kampen: Ten Have, 2004.

Jongh, S. E. de. *De Ontwikkeling der farmacotherapie*: Rede ter herdenking van de 383ste verjaardag der Rijksuniversiteit te Leiden op 8 februari 1958. Leiden: Universitaire Pers, 1958.

Jongkees, L. B. W. "Ethische aspecten van medische experimenten op de mens." *Medisch Contact* 35 (1980): 80–81.

Jongsma, M. W. "Medische ethiek." *Medisch Contact* 21 (1966): 311–16.

Jonsen, Albert R. *The Birth of Bioethics.* Oxford: Oxford University Press, 1998.

Jorland, Gérard, Annick Opinel, and George Weisz, eds. *Body Counts: Medical Quantification in Historical and Sociological Perspectives.* Montreal: McGill-Queen's University Press, 2005.

Kamerstuk Tweede Kamer (parliamentary document of the House of Representatives) 1974–1975, no. 13012, sec. 11. Structuurnota Gezondheidszorg. Motie van het lid Dees c.s., proposed May 7, 1975. https://repository.overheid.nl/frbr/sgd/19741975/0000201555/1/pdf/SGD_19741975_0002754.pdf.

Kamerstuk Tweede Kamer (parliamentary document of the House of Representatives) 1981–1982, no. 16771, sec. 9. Motie van het lid Wessel-Tuinstra c.s. https://repository.overheid.nl/frbr/sgd/19811982/0000151601/1/pdf/SGD_19811982_0002621.pdf.

Kamerstuk Tweede Kamer (parliamentary document of the House of Representatives) 1984–1985, no. 18600-XVI, sec. 24. Verslag van een mondeling overleg. https://repository.overheid.nl/frbr/sgd/19841985/0000127797/1/pdf/SGD_19841985_0005467.pdf.

Kamerstuk Tweede Kamer (parliamentary document of the House of Representatives) 1985–1986, no. 19200-XVI, sec. 89. https://repository.overheid.nl/frbr/sgd/19851986/0000119006/1/pdf/SGD_19851986_0005249.pdf.

Kamerstuk Tweede Kamer (parliamentary document of the House of Representatives) 1987–1988, no. 20200 XVI, sec. 97 (brief van de minister en van de Staatssecretaris van Welzijn, Volksgezondheid en Cultuur, 2-4), sec. 173 (verslag van een Mondeling Overleg, June 1, 1988). https://repository.overheid.nl/frbr/sgd/19871988/0000102418/1/pdf/SGD_19871988_0004525.pdf.

Kamerstuk Tweede Kamer (parliamentary document of the House of Representatives) 1989–1990, no. 20620, sec. 16, "Grenzen van de zorg," brief van de Staatssecretaris van Welzijn, Volksgezondheid en Cultuur. https://repository.overheid.nl/frbr/sgd/19891990/0000037152/1/pdf/SGD_19891990_0002635.pdf.

Kamerstuk Tweede Kamer (parliamentary document of the House of Representatives) 1991–1992, no. 21264, sec. 17. Motie van het lid Kohnstamm. https://repository.overheid.nl/frbr/sgd/19911992/0000021111/1/pdf/SGD_19911992_0002597.pdf.

Kamerstuk Tweede Kamer (parliamentary document of the House of Representatives) 1991–1992, no. 22588, sec. A, Advies Raad van State, Nader rapport. https://repository.overheid.nl/frbr/sgd/19911992/0000025690/1/pdf/SGD_19911992_0007059.pdf.

Kamerstuk Tweede Kamer (parliamentary document of the House of Representatives) 1991–1992, no. 22588, sec. 3. https://repository.overheid.nl/frbr/sgd/19911992/0000025689/1/pdf/SGD_19911992_0007058.pdf.

Kamerstuk Tweede Kamer (parliamentary document of the House of Representatives) 1992–1993, no. 22588, sec. 5. https://repository.overheid.nl/frbr/sgd/19921993/0000013822/1/pdf/SGD_19921993_0003377.pdf.

Kamerstuk Tweede Kamer (parliamentary document of the House of Representatives) 1996–1997, no. 22588, sec. 19.

Kamerstuk Tweede Kamer (parliamentary document of the House of Representatives) 2000–2001, no. 27681, sec. 1. Motie van het lid De Hoop Scheffer c.s. https://zoek.officielebekendmakingen.nl/kst-27681-1.pdf.

Kater, Loes. *Disciplines met dadendrang: Gezondheidsrecht en gezondheidsethiek in het Nederlandse euthanasiedebat 1960–1994.* Amsterdam: Aksant, 2004.

Katz, Jay. *Experimentation with Human Beings.* New York: Russell Sage Foundation, 1972.

Katz, Jay. "The Consent Principle of the Nuremberg Code: Its Significance Then and Now." In *The Nazi Doctors and the Nuremberg Code: Human Rights in Human Experimentation,* edited by George J. Annas and Michael A. Grodin, 227–39. Oxford: Oxford University Press, 1992.

Kennedy, James. *Een weloverwogen dood: Euthanasie in Nederland.* Amsterdam: Uitgeverij Bert Bakker, 2002.

Kennedy, James. *Nieuw Babylon in aanbouw: Nederland in de jaren zestig.* Amsterdam: Boom, 1995.

Keulen, Sjoerd. *Monumenten van beleid: De wisselwerking tussen Nederlands rijksoverheidsbeleid, sociale wetenschappen en politieke cultuur, 1945–2002.* Hilversum: Uitgeverij Verloren, 2014.

Kevles, Daniel J. *The Physicists: The History of a Scientific Community in Modern America.* New York: Vintage Books, 1979.

Kindermann, J. C. "Proefnemingen op menschen." *Nederlandsch Tijdschrift voor Geneeskunde* part I (1904): 414–15.

Kits Nieuwenkamp, J. H. W. "Wat kan de ethiek voor het beleid betekenen?: De rol van de ethiek en van ethici bij het beleid" In *Beleid en ethiek*, edited by Frans W. A. Brom, B. J. van den Bergh, and A. K. Huibers, 34–42. Assen: Van Gorcum, 1993.

Klaveren, Kees-Jan van. *Het onafhankelijkheidsyndroom: Een cultuurgeschiedenis van het naoorlogse Nederlandse zorgstelsel*. Amsterdam: Wereldbibliotheek, 2016.

Klein, Annemieke. *Verlangen naar verbetering: 375 jaar academische geneeskunde in Utrecht*. Amsterdam: Boom, 2010.

Klitzman, Robert L. *The Ethics Police?: The Struggle to Make Human Research Safe*. Oxford: Oxford University Press, 2015.

Kloppert, Willem. "Dokter Huijsmans werkte in Assisië als in de rimboe." *Het Vrije Volk*, December 20, 1978: 9.

Kluveld, Amanda. "Felix Ortt: De kleine geloven als brug tussen wetenschap en geloof." *De Negentiende Eeuw* 25 (2001): 137–46.

Kluveld, Amanda. *Reis door de hel der onschuldigen: De expressieve politiek van de Nederlandse anti-vivisectionisten, 1890–1940*. Amsterdam: Amsterdam University Press, 2000.

Knegtmans, Peter Jan. *Geld, ijdelheid en hormonen: Ernst Laqueur, hoogleraar en ondernemer*. Amsterdam: Boom, 2014.

KNMG. *Levensberichten en Herdenkingen 2007*. Amsterdam: Koninklijke Nederlandse Akademie van Wetenschappen, 2007.

KNMG. *Levensberichten en Herdenkingen 2015*. Amsterdam: Koninklijke Nederlandse Akademie van Wetenschappen, 2015.

KNMG. *Medische ethiek en gedragsleer*. Amsterdam: Koninklijke Nederlandse Maatschappij tot Bevordering der Geneeskunst, 1959.

Kohler, Robert E. *Partners in Science: Foundations and Natural Scientists, 1900–1945*. Chicago: University of Chicago Press, 1991.

Kortbeek, L. H. Th. S., H. J. Heering, P. E. Treffers, M. W. Jongsma, J. B. Stolte, J. Th. R. Schreuder, J. J. C. Marlet, F. J. M. Hillen, J. F. Rang, and G. A. Lindeboom. *Recent medisch ethisch denken I*. De Nederlandse Bibliotheek der Geneeskunde, Editorial Series no. 40. Leiden: Stafleu's Wetenschappelijke Uitgeversmaatschappij, 1968.

"Korte verslagen vergaderingen hoofdbestuur." *Medisch Contact* 23 (1968): 337–38.

"Kort verslag H.B.-vergadering." *Medisch Contact* 21 (1966): 210–11.

"Kort verslag van de 99ste algemene vergadering." *Medisch Contact* 4 (1949): 246–66.

Koster, W. "De bewijsvoering van Dr. Burger." *Nederlandsch Tijdschrift voor Geneeskunde* part I (1904): 463–65.

Koster, W. "Nog eens proefnemingen op menschen." *Nederlandsch Tijdschrift voor Geneeskunde* part I (1904): 378–79.

Krabbendam, H., and H.-M. T. D. ten Napel. *Regulating Morality: A Comparison of the Role of the States in Mastering the Mores in the Netherlands and the United States*. Apeldoorn: 2000.

Kranenburg, Mark. "Haar rust was haar wapen: Necrologie Els Borst (1932–2014)." *NRC Handelsblad*, February 11, 2014.

Kranenburg, Mark. "The Political Branch of the Polder Model." *NRC Handelsblad,* July 1, 1999.

Kroon, P. J. W. M. de. "De begintijd van de Leidse Commissie voor Medische Ethiek." In *Geneeskunde en ethiek in harmonie,* edited by F. A. Wolff, 93–95. The Hague: Pasmans Offset Drukkerij BV, 2001.

Krop, Henri A. "De babylonische ballingschap der ethiek: C.W. Opzoomer (1821–1892) en Spinoza." In *Filosofie, ethiek en praktijk: Liber amicorum voor Koo van der Wal,* edited by M. Verkerk, 43–54. Rotterdam: Erasmus Universiteit Rotterdam, Faculteit der Wijsbegeerte, 2000.

Krop, Henri A. "Laat de universiteit meer dan een vakschool zijn: Het pleidooi voor de Centrale Interfaculteit." In *Universitaire vormingsidealen: De Nederlandse universiteiten sedert 1876,* edited by L. J. Dorsman and P. J. Knegtmans, 39–53. Hilversum: Verloren, 2006.

Krop, Henri A., and Koo van der Wal. "Een eeuw wijsgerige ethiek in Nederland." In *Ethiek in Nederland,* edited by Bert Musschenga et al., 105–40. Budel: Damon, 2010.

Kruithof, B. "Wetgeving of Marktordening?: Apothekers en Drogisten in het Interbellum." *Gewina* 22 (1999): 34–45.

Kuhn, Thomas S. *The Structure of Scientific Revolutions.* 4th ed. Chicago: University of Chicago Press, 2012.

Kuijer, P. J., J. F. van Rhede van der Kloot, and J. Logeman. "Sterfte, medische tekortkomingen en foutenbronnen." *Nederlands Tijdschrift voor Geneeskunde* 107 (1963): 1268–70.

Kuitert, Harry M. "Morele consensus: mogelijkheden en grenzen." In *Handboek gezondheidsethiek,* edited by Inez de Beaufort and Heleen M. Dupuis, 29–40. Assen: Van Gorcum, 1988.

L., H. "De rechten van de patiënt." *Katholiek Artsenblad* 47 (1968): 162–64.

Lammers, W. "Bij het afscheid van Professor Gaarenstroom." *Nederlands Tijdschrift voor Geneeskunde* 109 (1965): 1889.

Lammers, W., F. A. Nelemans, and P. Siderius, eds. *Algemene farmacotherapie: Het geneesmiddel in theorie en praktijk.* Leiden: L. Stafleu & Zoon, 1961.

Land, Menno van der. *Tussen ideaal en illusie: De geschiedenis van D66, 1966–2003.* The Hague: Sdu Uitgevers, 2003.

"Landelijk steunpunt experimenteel mens/patiëntgebonden onderzoek." *Medisch Contact* 42 (1987): 606.

Lange, Frits de. "Tweeërlei ethiek: Of: hoe de gereformeerde ethiek zichzelf overbodig maakte." In *Ethiek in Nederland,* edited by Bert Musschenga et al., 77–104. Budel: Damon, 2010.

Langen, C. D. de. "Proeven op mensen en de verschuiving van te stellen normen." *Nederlands Tijdschrift voor Geneeskunde* 102 (1958): 25–27.

Latour, Bruno. *Reassembling the Social: An Introduction to Actor-Network-Theory.* Oxford: Oxford University Press, 2005.

Lawrence, Christopher, and Steven Shapin, eds. *Science Incarnate: Historical Embodiments of Natural Knowledge*. Chicago: University of Chicago Press, 1998.

Lears, J. *Fables of Abundance: A Cultural History of Advertising in America*. New York: Basic Books, 1994.

"Lectori Salutem." *Tijdschrift voor geneeskunde en ethiek* 1 (1991): 1–2.

Lederer, Susan E. "Research Without Borders: The Origins of the Declaration of Helsinki." In *History and Theory of Human Experimentation*, edited by Andreas Frewer and Ulf Schmidt, 145–64. Frankfurt: Steiner, 2007.

Lederer, Susan E. *Subjected to Science: Human Experimentation in America before the Second World War*. Baltimore, MD: Johns Hopkins University Press, 1995.

Lederer, Susan E. "The Ethics of Experimenting on Human Beings." In *The Cambridge World History of Medical Ethics*, edited by Robert B. Baker and Laurence B. McCullough, 558–65. Cambridge: Cambridge University Press, 2009.

Leenen, Henk J. J. "Commentaar." *Nederlands Tijdschrift voor Geneeskunde* 134 (1990): 926.

Leenen, Henk J. J. "De geschiedenis van de Vereniging voor Gezondheidsrecht." *Tijdschrift voor Gezondheidsrecht* 2 (1978): 184–89.

Leenen, Henk J. J. "Gezondheidsrecht: Een poging tot plaatsbepaling." *Tijdschrift voor Sociale Geneeskunde* 46 (1968): 778–85.

Leenen, Henk J. J. "Het betrekken van incompetenten bij experimenten." *Nederlands Tijdschrift voor Gezondheidsrecht* 14 (1990): 29–32.

Leenen, Henk J. J. "Juridische aspecten van medische experimenten op de mens (I) & (II)." *Medisch Contact* 30 (1975): 746–50, 753–67.

Leenen, Henk J. J. "Niet-therapeutische experimenten met incompetenten." *Nederlands Juristenblad* 64 (1989): 1501–04.

Leenen, Henk J. J. "Sociale grondrechten en gezondheidszorg." PhD diss., Utrecht University, 1966.

Leenen, Henk J. J. *Systeem-denken in de gezondheidszorg*. Alphen aan den Rijn: Samson, 1971.

Leenen, Henk J. J. "Vereniging voor Gezondheidsrecht 25 jaar: geschiedenis van de start." *Tijdschrift voor Gezondheidsrecht* 16 (1992): 128–34.

"Leerstoel voor de homoeopathie?" *Medisch Contact* 5 (1950): 303–06.

Leeuwarder Courant. "Dr. Maurice Pappworth: In Engeland en VS experimenten op patiënten." May 18, 1967: front page.

Leeuwarder Courant. "Geen proefkonijnen." August 26, 1967: 3.

Leeuwarder Courant. "Heeft zieke recht op volwassen behandeling?" January 29, 1971: 2.

Leeuwarder Courant. "Huisarts en röntgenassistent verdacht: Onderzoek medische experimenten in tehuis." December 19, 1978: 3.

Leeuwarder Courant. "Leemte in medische opleiding." September 13, 1960: 2.

Leeuwarder Courant. "Nieuwe voorzitter NVVE: Wettelijke regeling van euthanasie wellicht als mosterd na de maaltijd." April 5, 1982: 4.

Leeuwarder Courant. "Onthulling na experiment van 40 jaar: Amerikaanse negers waren proefkonijnen voor syfilisonderzoek." July 26, 1972: 6.

Leeuwarder Courant. "Plannen Buikhuisen oude wijn in nieuwe zakken." June 27, 1981.

Leeuwarder Courant. "Proeven op verpleegden: Prof. Querido: van toestemming kan geen sprake zijn." September 17, 1966: 7.

Leeuwarder Courant. "Volgens reclasseringsblad KRI: Dr. R. Buikhuisen wil onderzoek biologische kenmerken delinquent." April 20, 1978: 15.

Leeuwen, S. van. "Medische Ethiek." *Cicero,* November 24, 1989.

Le Fanu, James. *The Rise and Fall of Modern Medicine.* New York: Basic Books, 2012.

Lewis, S. *Arrowsmith.* New York: Grosset and Dunlap, 1925.

Lieburg, M. J. van. "De ontwikkeling van het klinisch-diagnostisch laboratorium in Nederland tot omstreeks 1925." *Tijdschrift voor de Geschiedenis van de Geneeskunde, Natuurkunde, Wiskunde en Techniek* 9 (1986): 278–318.

Lieburg, M. J. van. "De tweede geneeskundige stand (1818–65): Een bijdrage tot de geschiedenis van het medisch beroep in Nederland." *Tijdschrift voor Geschiedenis* 96 (1983): 433–53.

Lieburg, M. J. van. "Vergeten helden." *Medisch Contact* 64 (2009): 812–15.

Lightman, Bernard, ed. *A Companion to the History of Science.* West Sussex: John Wiley & Sons Ltd, 2016.

Limburgsch Dagblad. "Britten bang voor rol van proefkonijn." October 12, 1971: 3.

Limburgsch Dagblad. "Dokter kijkt uit naar mondige patient." May 2, 1970: 40.

Limburgsch Dagblad. "Omstreden geleerde vertrekt." March 2, 1989: 5.

Limburgsch Dagblad. "Patiënten gebruikt als proefkonijnen." June 17, 1966: 3.

Limburgsch Dagblad. "Proefkonijnen . . . ." July 27, 1972: 3.

Limburgsch Dagblad. "Reageerbuisbaby: hoe ver mag je gaan?" March 13, 1982: 19.

Limburgsch Dagblad. "Talloze problemen voor Veldkamp." November 22, 1962: 5.

Limburgsch Dagblad. "Thalidomide eiste ook in Nederland slachtoffers." January 2, 1969: 7.

Limburgsch Dagblad. "Wat hebben ze gezegd." August 29, 1967: 12.

Lindeboom, Gerrit Arie. *Dutch Medical Biography: A Biographical Dictionary of Dutch Physicians and Surgeons 1475–1975.* Amsterdam: Rodopi, 1984.

Lindeboom, Gerrit Arie. "Ethiek in de medische wetenschap." *Universiteit en Hogeschool* 3 (1957): 131–41.

Lindeboom, Gerrit Arie. *Geneeskundige proeven op mensen: Referaat voor de negendertigste wetenschappelijke samenkomst op 3 juli 1957.* Assen: G. F. Hummelen's Boekhandel en Electrische Drukkerij N. V., 1957.

Lindeboom, Gerrit Arie. "Medisch-ethische bezinning in Protestantse kring." *Metamedica* 49 (1970): 411–16.

Lindeboom, Gerrit Arie. *Opstellen over medische ethiek.* Kampen: J. H. Kok N. V., 1960.

Lindeboom, Gerrit Arie. "Tegen de stroom in (Tien jaren Nederlands Artsenverbond)." *Vita Humana* 10 (1983): 5–30.

Lintzen, Harry, H. Schippers, E. Berkers, A. van Rooij, and H. Buiter. *Tachtig jaar TNO.* Delft: TNO, 2013.

Loghem, J. J. van. "De Vivisectievrije Geneeskunde in de Tweede Kamer." *Nederlandsch Tijdschrift voor Geneeskunde* 94 (1950): 18–19.

Loghem, J. J. van. "Geneeskundige proefnemingen bij mensen." *Nederlands Tijdschrift voor Geneeskunde* 97 (1953): 518–20.

Loghem, J. J. van. "Geneeskundige proefnemingen bij mensen (II) & (III)." *Nederlandsch Tijdschrift voor Geneeskunde* 98 (1954): 2266–67, 3038–39.

Löwenberg, B. "Dirk Willem van Bekkum: 30 juli 1925–17 juli 2015." In KNAW, *Levensberichten en Herdenkingen 2015,* 13–22. Amsterdam: Koninklijke Nederlandse Akademie van Wetenschappen, 2015.

Löwy, Ilana. "The Experimental Body." In *Medicine in the Twentieth Century,* edited by John V. Pickstone and Roger Cooter, 435–49. Amsterdam: Harwood Academic Press, 2000.

Lucardie, Paul. *Nederland stromenland: Een geschiedenis van de politieke stromingen.* Assen: Koninklijke van Gorcum, 2002.

Maehle, Andreas-Holger. *Drugs on Trial: Experimental Pharmacology and Therapeutic Innovation in the Eighteenth Century.* Amsterdam: Rodopi, 1999.

Maehle, Andreas-Holger, and Ulrich Tröhler. "Animal Experimentation from Antiquity to the End of the Eighteenth Century. Attitudes and Arguments." In *Vivisection in Historical Perspective,* edited by Nicolaas A. Rupke, 14–47. London: Croom Helm, 1987.

Maeijer, J. "Juridische relatie geneesheer en patiënt." In F. F. X. Cerutti et al., *De Geneesheer en het Recht,* 9–23. Deventer: Kluwer, 1968.

Mainland, Donald. "The Modern Method of the Clinical Trial." *Methods of Medical Research* 6 (1954): 157.

Majoor, C. L. "In memoriam Prof. Jules A.M.J. Enneking." *Folia Medica Neerlandica* 8 (1965): 163–66.

Manschot, H. M., and H. van Dartel, eds. *In gesprek over goede zorg.* Meppel: Boom, 2005.

Manschot, H. M., and M. Verkerk, eds. *Ethiek in de zorg.* Amsterdam: Boom, 1994.

Marks, Harry M. *The Progress of Experiment: Science and Therapeutic Reform in the United States, 1900–1990.* Cambridge: Cambridge University Press, 1997.

Marlet, J. J. C. "De in rechten vervolgde arts." In J. J. C. Marlet, M. F. J. Marlet, and L. N. Marlet, *Schuld en verontschuldiging in de medische praktijk,* 57–82. Roermond: J. J. Romen & Zonen, 1966.

Marlet, J. J. C., M. F. J. Marlet, and L. N. Marlet. *Schuld en verontschuldiging in de medische praktijk.* Roermond: J. J. Romen & Zonen, 1966.

Marlet, L. N. "Enige raakpunten tussen de medische praktijk en het leerstuk der aansprakelijkheid." In J. J. C. Marlet, M. F. J. Marlet, and L. N. Marlet, *Schuld en Verontschuldiging in de medische praktijk,* 5–65. Roermond: J. J. Romen & Zonen, 1966.

Marrus, Michael R. "The Nuremberg Doctors' Trial in Historical Context." *Bulletin for the History of Medicine* 73 (1999): 106–23.

Medisch Contact editors. "Ethische problemen voor de arts." *Medisch Contact* 17 (1962): 237–38.

Medisch Contact editors. "Aesculapius en Themis: Een nuttige ontmoeting." *Medisch Contact* 23 (1968): 313–14.

Medisch Contact editors. "Massamedia en Medici: Het Handelsblad constateert 'de muur van geheimzinnigheid, die de medische wereld om zich heeft opgebouwd, doorbroken.'" *Medisch Contact* 22 (1967): 527–28.

"Medische Ethiek." *Medisch Contact* 16 (1961): 190–91.

"'Medische Ethiek' opnieuw gedrukt." *Medisch Contact* 15 (1960): 169–70.

"Medische ethiek tussen natuurwetenschap en samenleving." *Wetenschap en Samenleving* 23, no. 5–6 (1969).

"Medisch Ethische Commissie." *Medisch Contact* 36 (1981): 776.

Meldrum, Marcia L. "A Brief History of the Randomized Controlled Trial: From Oranges and Lemons to the Gold Standard." *Hematology/Oncology Clinics of North America* 14 (2000): 745–60.

Melsen, A. G. M. van, J. F. Rang, W. F. Tordoir, H. M. van der Vegt, G. J. Kloosterman, A. C. Regensburg, J. H. Plokker, F. J. M. Hillen, M. W. Jongsma, H. van Oyen, J. de Graaf, A. C. Drogendijk, and J. Droogleever Fortuyn. *Recent medisch ethisch denken II.* De Nederlandse Bibliotheek der Geneeskunde, Editorial Series no. 60. Leiden: Stafleu's Wetenschappelijke Uitgeversmaatschappij, 1970.

Metz, W. "Over de crisis in de medische ethiek." *Medisch Contact* 25 (1970): 330–32.

Metz, W. "Wijsgerige heroriëntatie in de medische ethiek." *Algemeen Nederlands Tijdschrift voor Wijsbegeerte en Psychologie* 61 (1969): 1–18.

Mijn, W. B. van der. "De rechtspraak van de maatschappij." *Medisch Contact* 24 (1969): 1029–31.

Mijn, W. B. van der. "De wetgever en het medisch handelen." *Medisch Contact* 27 (1972): 1165–71.

Mijn, W. B. van der. "Het takenpakket der maatschappij." *Medisch Contact* 23 (1968): 631–37.

Mold, A. "Patient Groups and the Construction of the Patient-Consumer in Britain: An Historical Overview." *Journal of Social Policy* 39 (2010): 505–21.

Moll van Charante, A. W. "Ethische aspecten van medische experimenten op de mens." *Medisch Contact* 35 (1980): 101.

Mooij, Annet. *De polsslag van de stad: 350 jaar academische geneeskunde in Amsterdam.* Amsterdam: Uitgeverij De Arbeiderspers, 1999.

Mooij, Annet. "Laqueur, Ernst (1880–1947)." *Biografisch Woordenboek van Nederland.* November 12, 2013. http://resources.huygens.knaw.nl/bwn/BWN/lemmata /bwn6/laqueur.

Mooij, Annet. "Roddels, ruzie, achterklap: Veranderende omgangsvormen in de medische beroepsgroep." *Gewina* 21 (1998): 30–37.

Moore, Peter. *Blood and Justice: The Seventeenth-Century Parisian Doctor Who Made Blood Transfusion History.* London: John Wiley, 2003.

Moran, Michael. *The British Regulatory State: High Modernism and Hyper-Innovation.* Oxford: Oxford University Press, 2003.

Musschenga, Bert. "Nederlandse ethiek na 1970: De wending naar de praktijk, het beleid en het internationale forum." In *Ethiek in Nederland,* edited by Bert Musschenga et al., 143–80. Budel: Damon, 2010.

Musschenga, Bert. "Voorwoord." In *Ethiek in Nederland,* edited by Bert Musschenga et al., 7–9. Budel: Damon, 2010.

Musschenga, Bert et al., eds. *Ethiek in Nederland: Van 1900 tot 1970 en daarna.* Budel: Damon, 2010.

Nadav, Daniel S. "The 'Death Dance of Lübeck': Julius Moses and the German Guidelines for Human Experimentation, 1930." In *Twentieth Century Ethics of Human Subjects Research: Historical Perspectives on Values, Practices, and Regulations,* edited by Volker Roelcke and Giovanni Maio, 129–35. Stuttgart: Franz Steiner Verlag, 2004.

Nagel, Thomas. *The View From Nowhere.* Oxford: Oxford University Press, 1986.

Nauta, L. W. *Argumenten voor een kritische ethiek.* Amsterdam: Van Gennep, 1971.

Nederlands Dagblad. "Bloemenhove experimenteerde al op levend-geaborteerde kinderen." December 22, 1979: 2.

Nederlands Dagblad. "Dr. W. Buikhuisen: 'Geen sprake van hersenonderzoek bij delinquenten.'" April 21, 1978: 5.

Nederlands Dagblad. "Macht en ethiek." February 24, 1972: 6.

Nederlands Dagblad. "Prof. Dupuis: dood te negatief gewaardeerd." November 1, 1986: 2.

Nederlands Dagblad. "Rumoer om experiment met negers." July 27, 1972: 3.

Nelemans, F. A. "De Behandeling van Coronaire Aandoeningen met Orale Anticoagulantia." *Nederlands Tijdschrift voor Geneeskunde* 111 (1967): 510.

Nelemans, F. A. "Klinische farmacologie." In *Algemene farmacotherapie: Het geneesmiddel in theorie en praktijk,* eds. W. Lammers, F. A. Nelemans, and P. Siderius, 19–20. Leiden: L. Stafleu & Zoon, 1961.

Nelemans, F. A. *Klinische farmacologie: Openbare les gehouden aan de Rijksuniversiteit te Utrecht op dinsdag 13 November 1956.* Utrecht, 1956.

Nelemans, F. A., and W. G. Zelvelder. *Therapeutische evaluatie van geneesmiddelen.* Leiden: Stafleu's Wetenschappelijke Uitgeversmaatschappij, 1970.

Niemantverdriet, T. *De vechtpartij: De PvdA van Kok tot Samsom.* Amsterdam: Athenaeum Boekhandel, 2014.

"Nieuwe vereniging wil deskundigheid leden van medisch-ethische commissies vergroten." *Medisch Contact* 46 (1991): 1409–10.

Nieuwsblad van het Noorden. "Arts moet uitleggen wat hij voorschrijft." April 24, 1974: 3.

Nieuwsblad van het Noorden. "Boek van specialist veroorzaakt storm: Engelse zieken werden als proefkonijnen gebruikt." May 18, 1967: front page.

Nieuwsblad van het Noorden. "Door CPN'er Wolff: Interpellatie over onderzoek dr. Buikhuisen." April 21, 1978: 2.

Nieuwsblad van het Noorden. "Eis voor aanvaarden hoogleraarschap in Leiden: Criminoloog dr. Buikhuisen wil onderzoek hersenen misdadigers." April 20, 1978: 3.

Nieuwsblad van het Noorden. "Levens van hartpatiënten door fopmedicijn gered: Onderzoek na vragen Kamerlid." August 29, 1967: 3.

Nieuwsblad van het Noorden. "Nieuwe uitgaven." June 2, 1960: 27.

Nieuwsblad van het Noorden. "Rapport: Verboden operaties in zwakzinnigentehuis." December 19, 1978: 3.

Noach, E. L. "De functie van ethische commissies bij medische experimenten met mensen." *Medisch Contact* 40 (1985): 872–74.

Noach, E. L. "In memoriam Prof.Dr. S.E. de Jongh." *Nederlands Tijdschrift voor Geneeskunde* 120 (1976): 1226–28.

Noach, E. L. "The History of Pharmacology in the Netherlands." *Trends in Pharmacological Sciences* 11 (1990): 236–39.

Noach, E. L. *Tweeërlei farmacologie: Inaugurele rede Leiden.* Amsterdam: N.V. Noord-Hollandsche Uitgevers Maatschapij, 1964.

Noach, E. L. "Verschuivende normen in de Medische Ethiek." Lecture HOVO Courses 1989–99. University of Leiden.

Noach, E. L., and P. J. W. M. de Kroon. "Medische ethiek: patiënten en proeven. De Commissie Medische Ethiek in het Academisch Ziekenhuis en de Faculteit der Geneeskunde te Leiden." *Medisch Contact* 34 (1979): 1575–83.

NRC Handelsblad. "Borst: proef op wilsonbekwamen soms toestaan." October 4, 1995.

NRC Handelsblad. "Ethicus: aidstest kan ook zonder fiat van patient." August 15, 1987: 3.

NRC Handelsblad. "Welke mensen willen we? Ethiek van biomedisch onderzoek." May 25, 1988: science section, front page.

Numbers, Ronald L. "William Beaumont and the Ethics of Human Experimentation." *Journal of the History of Biology* 12, no. 1 (Spring 1979): 113–35.

Nye, Joseph S., Jr. "Soft Power." *Foreign Policy* 80, twentieth anniversary issue (Autumn 1990): 159–71.

Nye, Joseph S., Jr. *Soft Power: The Means to Success in World Politics.* New York: Public-Affairs, 2004.

Nys, H. "Van Leenen tot Legemaate: 40 jaar Nederlands gezondheidsrecht in een twintigtal oraties." In *Oratiebundel gezondheidsrecht: Verzamelde redes 1971–2011*, edited by the Vereniging voor Gezondheidsrecht. The Hague: SDU Uitgevers, 2012.

Olesko, Kathryn M. "Science Pedagogy as a Category of Historical Analysis: Past, Present, and Future." *Science & Education* 15 (2006): 863–80.

Oosterhuis, H., and F. Huisman, eds. *Health and Citizenship*. New York: Routledge, 2014.

Oostveen, Margriet. "Ik kan me goed voorstellen dat artsen stervenshulp niet melden." *NRC Handelsblad*, April 14, 2001.

"Openbare hoorzitting abortus provocatus." *Medisch Contact* 26 (1971): 1031–32.

"Opheffing Werkgroep Klinisch Geneesmiddelenonderzoek TNO." *Nederlands Tijdschrift voor Geneeskunde* 119 (1975): 418.

Otterspeer, Willem. *The Bastion of Liberty: Leiden University Today and Yesterday*. Leiden: Leiden University Press, 2008.

Oudshoorn, Nelly. "Laqueur en Organon: Het universitaire laboratorium en de farmaceutische industrie in Nederland." *Gewina* 22 (1999): 12–22.

Pappworth, Maurice H. "Human Guinea Pigs: A Warning." *Twentieth Century* 171 (1962–1963): 66–75.

Pappworth, Maurice H. *Human Guinea Pigs: Experiments on Man*. London: Routledge and Kegan Paul, 1967.

Peremans, W., G. P. Baerends, I. Boerema, A. H. W. Aten, J. Kok, L. van der Horst, G. T. Hoitink, and A. J. F. Köbben. *Acht voordrachten over de keerzijde van de vooruitgang in de natuur- en geneeskundige wetenschappen*. The Hague: Martinus Nijhoff, 1962.

Perkin, Harold. *The Rise of Professional Society: England since 1800*. London: Routledge, 1990.

Pernick, Martin S. *A Calculus of Suffering: Pain, Professionalism, and Anesthesia in Nineteenth Century America*. New York: Columbia University Press, 1985.

Pernick, Martin S. "The Calculus of Suffering in Nineteenth-Century Surgery." *The Hastings Center Report* 13 (1983): 26–36.

Perutz, M. "The New Marxism." *New Scientist* 123 (1989): 72–73.

Peters, Klaartje. *Een doodgewoon kabinet: Acht jaar Paars, 1994–2002*. Amsterdam: Boom, 2015.

Petricciani, John C. "An Overview of FDA, IRBs and Regulations." *IRB: Ethics & Human Research* 3 (1981): 1–3.

Petryna, Adriana. *When Experiments Travel: Clinical Trials and the Global Search for Human Subjects*. Princeton, NJ: Princeton University Press, 2009.

Petryna, Adriana, Andrew Lakoff, and Arthur Kleinman, eds. *Global Pharmaceuticals: Ethics, Markets, Practices*. Durham, NC: Duke University Press, 2006.

Phaff, J. M. F. "Toepassing medische psychologie door de huisarts." *Medisch Contact* 18 (1963): 480–83.

Pickstone, John V. "Production, Community and Consumption: The Political Economy of Twentieth-Century Medicine." In *Medicine in the Twentieth Century*, edited by John V. Pickstone and Roger Cooter, 1–19. Amsterdam: Harwood Academic Press, 2000.

Pickstone, John V., and Roger Cooter, eds. *Medicine in the Twentieth Century*. Amsterdam: Harwood Academic Press, 2000.

Pieters, T. "Tussen controle op afstand en betrokken begeleiding: Historische trajecten in het staatstoezicht op geneesmiddelen." In *Kennis Cahier*, 49–60. Inspectie voor de Gezondheidszorg, 2010.

Pinker, Steven. "The Moral Imperative for Bioethics." *Boston Globe*, August 1, 2015.

Polanyi, Michael. "The Republic of Science: Its Political and Economic Theory." *Minerva* 1 (1962): 54–73.

Polanyi, Michael. *The Tacit Dimension*. New York: Doubleday, 1967.

Porter, Joan P., and Greg Koski. "Regulations for the Protection of Humans in Research in the United States." In *The Oxford Textbook of Clinical Research Ethics*, edited by Ezekiel J. Emanuel et al., 156–67. Oxford: Oxford University Press, 2008.

Porter, Theodore M. "Medical Quantification: Science, Regulation, and the State." In *Body Counts: Medical Quantification in Historical & Sociological Perspectives*, edited by Gérard Jorland, Annick Opinel, and George Weisz, 394–401. Montreal: McGill-Queen's University Press, 2005.

Porter, Theodore M. "Objectivity as Standardization: The Rhetoric of Impersonality in Measurement Statistics and Cost Benefit Analysis." *Annals of Scholarship* special issue 9, no. 1–2 (1992): 19–59.

Porter, Theodore M. "Quantification and the Accounting Ideal in Science." *Social Studies of Science* 22 (1992): 633–52.

Porter, Theodore M. *The Rise of Statistical Thinking, 1820–1900*. Princeton, NJ: Princeton University Press, 1986.

Porter, Theodore M. *Trust in Numbers: The Pursuit of Academic Objectivity in Science and Public Life*. Princeton, NJ: Princeton University Press, 1995.

Powers, Michael. *The Audit Society: Rituals of Verification*. Oxford: Oxford University Press, 1997.

Prakken, J. R. "A.A. Botter: 'Over de aetiologie van de strophulus infantum.'" *Nederlandsch Tijdschrift voor Geneeskunde* 16 (1950): 2766.

Prakken, J. R. "Dr. J. Wester 65 jaar." *Nederlands Tijdschrift voor Geneeskunde* 110 (1966): 595.

Prakken, J. R. "Tekortkomingen van het klinisch geneesmiddelenonderzoek en gevaren van de industriële propaganda." *Nederlands Tijdschrift voor Geneeskunde* 105 (1961): 1569–71.

Prick, J. J. "Discussie over: de medische ethiek met betrekking tot de nieuwste ontwikkelingen in de geneeskunde." *Medisch Contact* 24 (1969): 83–85.

"Proeven op mensen." *Medisch Contact* 13 (1958): 108–09.

Pronk, Evert. "Els Borst: arts, minister, euthanasievoorvechtster." Medisch Contact, February 11, 2014. https://www.medischcontact.nl/nieuws/laatste-nieuws/artikel /els-borst-arts-minister-euthanasievoorvechtster.htm.

Querido, A. "De mondigheid van de patient: I. Diagnose." *Metamedica* 49 (1970): 205–08.

Querido, A. *Een eeuw staatstoezicht op de volksgezondheid.* The Hague: Staatsuitgeverij, 1965.

Rang, Jacob F. "Medisch experiment op de mens en strafrecht." In A. G. M. van Melsen et al., *Recent medisch ethisch denken II*, De Nederlandse Bibliotheek der Geneeskunde, Editorial Series no. 60, 33–87. Leiden: Stafleu's Wetenschappelijke Uitgeversmaatschappij, 1970.

Rang, Jacob F. *Patiëntenrecht.* Leiden: Stafleu's Wetenschappelijke Uitgeversmaatschappij, 1973.

Ree, J. W. van, and B. Bottema. "Wetenschappelijk onderzoek huisartspraktijken." *Medisch Contact* 42 (1987): 953.

Reich, Warren T., ed. *Encyclopedia of Bioethics* Vol. 2. New York: Free Press, 1978.

Reinders, J. S. "Weg uit de ivoren toren?: Kanttekeningen bij de tussentijdse evaluatie van het Centrum voor Ethiek KUN." *Tijdschrift voor Geneeskunde en Ethiek* 7 (1997): 90–92.

Reubi, David. "The Will to Modernize: A Genealogy of Biomedical Research Ethics in Singapore." *International Political Sociology* 4 (2010): 142–58.

Reverby, Susan M. *Examining Tuskegee: The Infamous Syphilis Study and its Legacy.* Chapel Hill: University of North Carolina Press, 2009.

Righart, Hans. *De eindeloze jaren zestig: Geschiedenis van een generatieconflict.* Amsterdam: De Arbeiderspers, 1995.

Rigter, R. B. M. *Met raad en daad: De geschiedenis van de Gezondheidsraad, 1902–1985.* Rotterdam: Erasmus Publishing, 1992.

Rinsema, T. "Brocades & Stheeman: Van apotheker-fabrikant tot farmaceutische industrie." *Gewina* 22 (1999): 23–33.

Risse, G. B. *Mending Bodies, Saving Souls: A History of Hospitals.* Oxford: Oxford University Press, 1999.

Robinson, Walter M., and Brandon T. Unruh. "The Hepatitis Experiments at the Willowbrook State School." In *The Oxford Textbook of Clinical Research Ethics*, edited by Ezekiel J. Emanuel et al., 80–85. Oxford: Oxford University Press, 2008.

Roelcke, Volker, and Giovanni Maio, eds. *Twentieth Century Ethics of Human Subjects Research: Historical Perspectives on Values, Practices, and Regulations.* Stuttgart: Franz Steiner Verlag, 2004.

Romein, Jan. *Op het breukvlak van twee eeuwen.* 2nd ed. Amsterdam: Em. Querido's Uitgeverij, 1976.

Roscam Abbing, H. D. C. "EG-aanbevelingen inzake experimenten met geneesmiddelen bij mensen." *Nederlands Tijdschrift voor Geneeskunde* 134 (1990): 2124–25.

Roscam Abbing, H. D. C. "Genetische experimenten met mensen: Wetgever quo vadis?" *Medisch Contact* 41 (1986): 533–35.

Rose, Nikolas. *The Politics of Life Itself.* Princeton, NJ: Princeton University Press, 2007.

Rose, Nikolas, and Peter Miller. *Governing the Present: Administering Economic, Social and Personal Life*. Cambridge: Polity Press, 2008.

Rosenberg, Charles E. *The Care of Strangers: The Rise of America's Hospital System*. New York: Basic Books, 1987.

Rosenberg, Charles E. "The Therapeutic Revolution: Medicine, Meaning and Social Change in Nineteenth Century America." In *The Therapeutic Revolution: Essays in the Social History of American Medicine*, edited by Morris J. Vogel and Charles E. Rosenberg, 3–25. Philadelphia: University of Pennsylvania Press, 1979.

Rosenberg, Charles E. "The Tyranny of Diagnosis: Specific Entities and Individual Experience." *Milbank Quarterly* 80 (2002): 237–60.

Rosser Matthews, John. *Quantification and the Quest for Medical Certainty*. Princeton, NJ: Princeton University Press, 1995.

Rothman, David J. *Strangers at the Bedside: A History of How Law and Bioethics Transformed Medical Decision Making*. 3rd ed. New Brunswick, NJ: AldineTransaction, 1991/2003.

Rümke, Chr. L. "De taak van de medische ethiek." *Statistica Neerlandica* 12 (1958).

Rupke, Nicolaas A., ed. *Vivisection in Historical Perspective*. London: Croom Helm, 1987.

Rusnock, Andrea A. "The Weight of Evidence and the Burden of Authority: Case Histories, Medical Statistics and Smallpox Inoculation." *Clio Medica* 29 (1995): 289–315.

Schaffer, Simon. "Regeneration: The Body of Natural Philosophers in Restoration England." In *Science Incarnate: Historical Embodiments of Natural Knowledge*, edited by Christopher Lawrence and Steven Shapin, 83–120. Chicago: University of Chicago Press, 1998.

Schaffer, Simon. "Self Evidence." *Critical Inquiry* 18 (1992): 327–62.

Schalm, L. "Prof. Dr. C.D. de Langen 75 jaar." *Nederlands Tijdschrift der Geneeskunde* 106 (1962): 1825–26.

Schiebinger, Londa. "Human Experimentation in the Eighteenth Century: Natural Boundaries and Valid Testing." In *The Moral Authority of Nature*, edited by Lorraine Daston and Fernando Vidal, 384–408. Chicago: University of Chicago Press, 2003.

Schiebinger, Londa. "Medical Experimentation and Race in the Eighteenth-Century Atlantic World." *Social History of Medicine* 26 (2013): 364–82.

Schmidt, Ulf. "Medical Ethics and Nazism." In *The Cambridge World History of Medical Ethics*, edited by Robert B. Baker and Laurence B. McCullough, 595–608. Cambridge: Cambridge University Press, 2009.

Schmidt, Ulf. "The Nuremberg Doctors' Trial and the Nuremberg Code." In *History and Theory of Human Experimentation*, edited by Andreas Frewer and Ulf Schmidt, 71–116. Frankfurt: Steiner, 2007.

Scholten, Emmy G. "Wetenschappelijk onderzoek huisartspraktijken." *Medisch Contact* 42 (1987): 1188.

Scholten, Emmy G., and L. H. B. M. van Benthem. "Medische experimenten in de huisartspraktijk." *Medisch Contact* 42 (1987): 953.

Scholten, J. B. "J.H. Pannekoek 50 jaar arts." *Nederlands Tijdschrift voor Geneeskunde* 123 (1979): 1359–60.

Schotmans, P. "In Memoriam Prof. Dr. Paul Sporken." *Ethische Perspectieven* 2 (1992): 13–16.

Schrag, Zachary M. *Ethical Imperialism: Institutional Review Boards and the Social Sciences, 1965–2009.* Baltimore, MD: Johns Hopkins University Press, 2010.

Schrag, Zachary M. "Review: Behind Closed Doors: IRBs and the Making of Ethical Research by Laura Stark." *American Journal of Sociology* 118 (2012): 494–96.

Schuurmans Stekhoven, W. *Jurisprudentia Medica.* Groningen: Wolters-Noordhoff, 1972.

Schuyt, C. J. M. "Reflex of reflectie: Antwoord aan Buikhuisen en Van Dijk." *Nederlands Juristenblad* 53 (1978): 517–26.

Schuyt, C. J. M. "Veroordeeld tot criminaliteit?: Een wetenschapsfilosofische en ethische reflectie op het voorgenomen onderzoek van Prof.dr. W. Buikhuisen." *Nederlands Juristenblad* 53 (1978): 389–99.

Shapin, Steven. *A Social History of Truth: Civility and Science in Seventeenth-Century England.* Chicago: University of Chicago Press, 1994.

Shapin, Steven. *The Scientific Life: A Moral History of a Late Modern Vocation.* Chicago: University of Chicago Press, 2008.

Sherman, Allen. "Peter and the Commissar." On Peter and the Commissar. Recorded July 22, 1964. Camden, NJ: RCA Red Seal Records. LP record (mono, dyn).

Shore, Cris, and Susan Wright. "Governing by Numbers: Audit Culture, Rankings and the New World Order." *Social Anthropology* 23 (2015): 22–28.

Shorter, Edward. *Bedside Manners: The Troubled History of Doctors and Patients.* New York: Simon and Schuster, 1985.

Singer, Peter, ed. *Applied Ethics.* Oxford: Oxford University Press, 1986.

Singer, Peter. "Introduction." In *Applied Ethics*, edited by Peter Singer, 1–9. Oxford: Oxford University Press, 1986.

Snelders, Stephen, and Frans Meijsman. *De mondige patiënt: Historische kijk op een mythe.* Amsterdam: Bert Bakker, 2009.

Solovey, Mark. *Shaky Foundations: The Politics-Patronage-Social Science Nexus in Cold War America.* New Brunswick, NJ: Rutgers University Press, 2013.

Spicker, Stuart F., Ilai Alon, Andre de Vries, and H. Tristram Engelhardt, Jr., eds. *The Use of Human Beings in Research: With Special Reference to Clinical Trials.* Dordrecht: Kluwer Academic Publishers, 1988.

Sporken, C. Paul. *Ethiek en gezondheidszorg.* 4th ed. Baarn: Amboboeken, 1979.

Sporken, C. Paul. "Ethische reflexies: Experimenten met de mens." *Katholieke Gezondheidszorg* 37 (1968): 190–94.

Sporken, C. Paul. "Katholieke moraal en abortus." *Medisch Contact* 22 (1967): 385–89.

Sporken, C. Paul. "Medisch-ethische vragen in verband met anesthesie." *Medisch Contact* 25 (1970): 669–73.

Sporken, C. Paul. "Medische ethiek als cultuurkritiek: Naar aanleiding van revalidatie, levensverlenging en euthanasia." *Medisch Contact* 24 (1969): 1431–34.

Sporken, C. Paul. "Vijftig jaar medische ethiek in het Katholiek Artsenblad." *Metamedica* 49 (1970): 395–411.

Sporken, C. Paul. *Voorlopige diagnose: inleiding tot een medische ethiek.* Utrecht: Ambo, 1969.

Spreeuwenberg, C. "Een handboek tegen xenofobie." *Medisch Contact* 46 (1991): 423.

Spreeuwenberg, C. "Staan patiëntenwetten de gezondheid in de weg?" *Medisch Contact* 46 (1991): 1019.

Staatscourant. "Voorschriften omtrent onderzoek voor wetenschappelijke doeleinden ten aanzien van hen die rechtens vrijheidsbeneming ondergaan." June 9, 1980.

Stam, F. C. "Prof. Dr. L. van der Horst 50 jaar arts." *Nederlands Tijdschrift voor Geneeskunde* 114 (1970): 785–86.

Stark, Laura J. M. *Behind Closed Doors: IRBs and the Making of Ethical Research.* Chicago: University of Chicago Press, 2012.

Stark, Laura J. M. "Morality in Science: How Research is Evaluated in the Age of Human Subjects Regulation." PhD diss., Princeton University, 2006.

Sterrenberg, L. "Ethisch aspectenonderzoek: dans met beleid." In *Beleid en ethiek,* edited by Frans W. A. Brom, B. J. van den Bergh, and A. K. Huibers, 26–33. Assen: Van Gorcum, 1993.

"Stervensbegeleiding: Medisch-ethische plicht? Door Dr. C.P. Sporken, ethicus, directeur van het Mgr. Bekkers Centrum, Katholieke Universiteit Nijmegen." *Medisch Contact* 25 (1970): 418–24.

Stevens, M. L. Tina. *Bioethics in America: Origins and Cultural Politics.* Baltimore, MD: Johns Hopkins University Press, 2000.

Stewart, Larry. "Pneumatic Chemistry, Self-Experimentation and the Burden of Revolution, 1780–1805." In *The Uses of Humans in Experiment: Perspectives from the 17th to the 20th Century,* edited by Erika Dyck and Larry Stewart, 139–69. Leiden: Brill Rodopi, 2016.

Strathern, Marilyn, ed. *Audit Cultures: Anthropological Studies in Accountability, Ethics and the Academy.* London: Routledge, 2000.

"Streptomycin Treatment of Pulmonary Tuberculosis: A Medical Research Council Investigation." *British Medical Journal* 2, 4582 (1948): 769–82.

Swart, J., R. Tramper, and M. Jonker, eds. *Afwegen, hoe doe je dat?* Budel: Damon, 2009.

Swellengrebel, N. H. "Levensbericht C.D. de Langen." In *Jaarboek KNAW 1966–1967,* 353–57. Amsterdam: KNAW, 1967.

Swierstra, Tsjalling. "De commissie Biotechnologie bij Dieren: toets of glijmiddel?" In *Afwegen, hoe doe je dat?,* edited by J. Swart, R. Tramper, and M. Jonker, 154–64. Budel: Damon, 2009.

Tamboer, K. "Groningse zenuwarts R.H. van den Hoofdakker: 'Artsenstandsleepanker dat vooruitgang afremt.'" *Het Vrije Volk,* August 30, 1969: 5.

Taylor, Telford. "Opening Statement of the Prosecution: December 9, 1946." Reprinted in *The Nazi Doctors and the Nuremberg Code: Human Rights in Human Experimentation*, edited by George J. Annas and Michael A. Grodin, 67–93. Oxford: Oxford University Press, 1992.

Teijgeler, C. A., ed. *Het College ter Beoordeling van Geneesmiddelen: Een Registratie.* Bloemendaal, 1988.

Temin, Peter. "Government Actions in Times of Crisis: Lessons from the History of Drug Regulation." *Journal of Social History* 18 (1985): 433–38.

Temin, Peter. *Taking Your Medicine: Drug Regulation in the United States.* Cambridge, MA: Harvard University Press, 1980.

Terborgh-Dupuis, H. *Medische ethiek in perspectief: Een onderzoek naar normen en argumentaties in de (medische) ethiek.* Leiden: Stafleu, 1976.

Terburgh, H. S. "Groeiende mondigheid patiënt door overheid weer afgenomen?" *NRC Handelsblad*, October 4, 1975: 4.

Theling, J. J. "Vijftien jaren van strijd tegen de vivisectie." *Meededeelingen Lustrum-Nummer* 15 (1946): 3–4.

Timmermans, H., and D. D. Breimer. "Levensbericht Everhardus Jacobus Ariëns." In KNAW, *Levensberichten en Herdenkingen 2007*, 6–17. Amsterdam: Koninklijke Nederlandse Akademie van Wetenschappen, 2007.

Tongeren, Paul van. "De ethicus versus de ingenieur." In *Beleid en ethiek*, edited by Frans W. A. Brom, B. J. van den Bergh, and A. K. Huibers, 205–11. Assen: Van Gorcum, 1993.

Tongeren, Paul van. "De smalle moraal: pluralisme of uniformiteit?" *Algemeen Nederlands Tijdschrift voor de Wijsbegeerte* 80 (1988): 92–102.

Tongeren, Paul van. "Ethiek en Praktijk." *Filosofie en Praktijk* 9 (1988): 113–27.

Tonkens, E. H. *Het zelfontplooiingsregime: De actualiteit van Dennendal en de jaren zestig.* Amsterdam: Bakker, 1999.

Toth, B. "Clinical Trials in British Medicine 1858–1948, with special reference to the development of the randomised controlled trial." PhD diss., University of Bristol, 1998.

Toulmin, Stephen. "How Medicine Saved the Life of Ethics." *Perspectives in Biology and Medicine* 25 (1982): 736–50.

Treub, Hector. *Medische fatsoensleer: Drie colleges.* Amsterdam: Scheltema & Holkema, 1903.

Tröhler, Ulrich. "The Long Road of Moral Concern: Doctors' Ethos and Statute Law Relating to Human Research in Europe." In *History and Theory of Human Experimentation*, edited by Andreas Frewer and Ulf Schmidt, 27–54. Frankfurt: Steiner, 2007.

Tröhler, Ulrich. "'To Improve the Evidence of Medicine': Arithmetic Observation in Clinical Medicine in the Eighteenth and Early Nineteenth Centuries." *History and Philosophy of the Life Sciences* 10, supplement (1988): 31–40.

Tröhler, Ulrich, and Stella Reiter-Theil, eds. *Ethics Codes in Medicine: Foundations and Achievements of Codification since 1947*. Aldershot: Ashgate, 1998.

Trouw. "Ik roep walging op: Interview met Theo van Willigenburg." October 11, 2014.

Tsuchiya, Takashi. "The Imperial Japanese Experiments in China." In *The Oxford Textbook of Clinical Research Ethics*, edited by Ezekiel J. Emanuel et al., 31–45. Oxford: Oxford University Press, 2008.

Vandenbroucke, J. P. "De opkomst van medische statistiek en epidemiologie in het klinisch wetenschappelijk onderzoek van de afgelopen eeuw." *Nederlands Tijdschrift Voor Geneeskunde* 143 (1999): 2625–28.

Vandenbroucke, J. P. "Het Centraal Bureau voor de Statistiek: de begraafplaats van onze doodsoorzaken." *Nederlands Tijdschrift voor Geneeskunde* 133 (1989): 2112–14.

Vandenbroucke, J. P. "Medische ethiek en gezondheidsrecht: hinderpalen voor de verdere toename van kennis in de geneeskunde?" *Nederlands Tijdschrift voor Geneeskunde* 134 (1990): 5–6.

Vandenbroucke, J. P. "Reactie." *Nederlands Tijdschrift voor Geneeskunde* 124 (1990): 928.

Vandendriessche, Joris, Evert Peeters, and Kaat Wils. *Scientists' Expertise as Performance: Between State and Society, 1860–1960*. London: Pickering & Chatto, 2015.

"Varia." *Medisch Contact* 20 (1965): 278.

"Varia: Het dogma in de medische ethiek." *Medisch Contact* 22 (1967): 1163.

Veatch, Robert M. "The Birth of Bioethics: Autobiographical Reflections of a Patient Person." *Cambridge Quarterly of Health Ethics* 11 (2002): 344–52.

Veen, E.-B. van. "Het betrekken van incompetenten bij experimenten." *Tijdschrift voor Gezondheidsrecht* 14 (1990): 33–35.

Veen, E.-B. van. "Het betrekken van incompetenten in experimenten–een commentaar op enige commentaren." *Tijdschrift voor Gezondheidsrecht* 13 (1989): 536–51.

"Veiligheid van Nieuwe Geneesmiddelen." *Medisch Contact* 18 (1963): 359–61.

Vereniging voor Gezondheidsrecht, ed. *Oratiebundel gezondheidsrecht: Verzamelde redes 1971–2011*. The Hague: SDU Uitgevers, 2012.

Verkerk, M., ed. *Filosofie, ethiek en praktijk: Liber amicorum voor Koo van der Wal*. Rotterdam: Erasmus Universiteit Rotterdam, Faculteit der Wijsbegeerte, 2000.

Verkerk, M. "Zorgethiek: naar een geografie van verantwoordelijkheid." In *In gesprek over goede zorg*, edited by H. M. Manschot and H. van Dartel, 177–84. Meppel: Boom, 2005.

Vermij, R. H. *David de Wied: Toponderzoeker in polderland*. Utrecht: Universiteit van Utrecht, 2008.

Vicedo, Marga. "Introduction: The Secret Lives of Textbooks." *Isis* 103 (2012): 83–87.

Visser, M. B. H. "Ethische aspecten van medische experimenten op de mens (I) & (II)." *Medisch Contact* 34 (1979): 1351–58, 1386–90.

Visser, M. B. H. "Medische experimenten: Van experimenten op mensen naar experimenten met mensen." Medisch Contact 37 (1982): 711–13.

Visser, M. B. H. "Nieuwe richtlijnen voor biomedisch onderzoek." *Medisch Contact* 36 (1981): 23–24.

Vogel, Morris J., and Charles E. Rosenberg, eds. *The Therapeutic Revolution: Essays in the Social History of American Medicine*. Philadelphia: University of Pennsylvania Press, 1979.

"Voordrachten: Dr. H. Hamminga, onderwerp 'Enige medisch-ethische problemen.'" *Medisch Contact* 22 (1967): 469.

"Voordrachten: internist C.L.C. Nieuwenhuizen, onderwerp 'De ethische consequenties van de moderne ontwikkeling in de geneeskunde en biologie.'" *Medisch Contact* 22 (1967): 377.

Vorstenbosch, Jan. "Dierethiek in Nederland." In *Ethiek in Nederland*, edited by Bert Musschenga et al., 251–76. Budel: Damon, 2010.

Vosman, Frans, and Carlo Leget. "Rooms-katholieke moraaltheologie in Nederland." In *Ethiek in Nederland*, edited by Bert Musschenga et al., 13–40. Budel: Damon, 2010.

Vries, Gerard H. de. *Gerede Twijfel: Over de rol van de medische ethiek in Nederland*. Amsterdam: De Balie, 1993.

Vries, Gerard H. de. "Medische technologie en morele twijfel." In *Redes gehouden op de 16e Dies Natalis van de Rijksuniversiteit Limburg, 10 januari 1992*, edited by M. J. Cohen and Gerard H. de Vries, 5–13. Maastricht: Rijksuniversiteit Limburg, 1992.

Vries, Gerard H. de, and Sara van Epenhuysen. "Niet de handelingen maar het stuk: ethiek en het experimenten met mensen." *De Gids* 154 (1991): 861–70.

Vries, Jouke de. *Paars en de managementstaat: Het eerste kabinet-Kok (1994–1998)*. Apeldoorn: Garant, 2002.

Wachter, M. A. M. de. "Toestemming van proefpersonen." *Medisch Contact* 33 (1978): 925–28.

Warner, John Harley. *Against the Spirit of System: The French Impulse in Nineteenth-Century American Medicine*. Princeton, NJ: Princeton University Press, 1998.

Warner, John Harley. "Ideals of Science and Their Discontents in Late Nineteenth-Century American Medicine." *Isis* 82 (1991): 454–78.

Warner, John Harley. *The Therapeutic Perspective: Medical Practice, Knowledge, and Identity in America, 1820–1885*. Princeton, NJ: Princeton University Press, 1997.

Waterman, Alan T. "Introduction." In Vannevar Bush, *Science: The Endless Frontier*, reprint ed., xi-xii. Washington, DC: National Science Foundation, 1960 [1945]. https://archive.org/stream/scienceendlessfr00unit#page/n15/mode/2up.

Wear, Andrew. "The Discourses of Practitioners in Sixteenth- and Seventeenth Century Europe." In *The Cambridge World History of Medical Ethics*, edited by Robert B. Baker and Laurence B. McCullough, 379–90. Cambridge: Cambridge University Press, 2009.

Weatherall, Miles. *In Search of a Cure: A History of Pharmaceutical Discovery*. Oxford: Oxford University Press, 1990.

Webster, Charles. *The National Health Service: A Political History (New Edition)*. Oxford: Oxford University Press, 1998.

Weindling, Paul J. "The Nazi Medical Experiments." In *The Oxford Textbook of Clinical Research Ethics*, edited by Ezekiel J. Emanuel et al., 18–30. Oxford: Oxford University Press, 2008.

Weindling, Paul J. "The Origins of Informed Consent: The International Scientific Commission on Medical War Crimes, and the Nuremberg Code." *Bulletin of the History of Medicine* 75 (2001): 37–71.

Wennen-Van der Mey, C. "Medische ethiek ter discussie." *De Groene Amsterdammer*, October 4, 1969: 10.

Westendorp Boerma, F. "Prof. Dr. A. Pondman 70 jaar." *Nederlands Tijdschrift voor Geneeskunde* 104 (1960): 1008–10.

Wet regelende de uitoefening der artsenijbereidkunst, 1 Junij 1865.

Wet van 28 juli 1958, houdende nieuwe regelen nopens de geneesmiddelenvoorziening en de uitoefening der artsenijbereidkunst (Wet op de geneesmiddelenvoorziening). https://wetten.overheid.nl/BWBR0002290/2006-03-01.

Wet van 24 oktober 1997, houdende regels betreffende bijzondere verrichtingen op het gebied van de gezondheidszorg (Wet op bijzondere medische verrichtingen). https://wetten.overheid.nl/BWBR0008974/2021-07-01.

Wet van 26 februari 1998, houdende regelen inzake medisch-wetenschappelijk onderzoek met mensen (Wet medisch-wetenschappelijk onderzoek met mensen). https://wetten.overheid.nl/BWBR0009408/2021-07-01.

Wet van 12 april 2001, houdende toetsing van levensbeëindiging op verzoek en hulp bij zelfdoding en wijziging van het Wetboek van Strafrecht en van de Wet op de lijkbezorging (Wet toetsing levensbeëdiging op verzoek en hulp bij zelfdoding). https://wetten.overheid.nl/BWBR0012410/2020-03-19.

Weyers, H. *Euthanasie: Het proces van rechtsverandering*. Amsterdam: Amsterdam University Press, 2004.

Wibaut, F. "Notulen vergadering 5 februari 1949." *Medisch Contact* 4 (1949): 22–27.

Wibaut, F. "Reorganisatie der Maatschappij, betekenis der te stichten secties." *Medisch Contact* 2 (1947): 1–4.

Wied, D. de. "Erik Noach: collega en vriend." In *Geneeskunde en ethiek in harmonie*, edited by F. A. Wolff, 11–18. The Hague: Pasmans Offset Drukkerij BV, 2001.

"Wie had de Nobelprijs moeten krijgen?" *Nederlands Tijdschrift voor Geneeskunde* 151 (2007): 73–77.

Wielenga, Friso. *Nederland in de twintigste eeuw*. Amsterdam: Boom, 2009.

Wiese, K. "Buikhuisen volhardt in gevaarlijke denkfouten." *Nieuwsblad van het Noorden*, October 10, 1978: 4.

Willigenburg, Theo van. "Ik ben een ethisch ingenieur!" In *Beleid en ethiek*, edited by Frans W. A. Brom, B. J. van den Bergh, and A. K. Huibers, 189–204. Assen: Van Gorcum, 1993.

Willigenburg, Theo van. "Inleiding." In *Beleid en ethiek,* edited by Frans W. A. Brom, B. J. van den Bergh, and A. K. Huibers, 187–88. Assen: Van Gorcum, 1993.

Willigenburg, Theo van. *Inside the Ethical Expert: Problem Solving in Applied Ethics.* Kampen: Kok Pharos Publishing House, 1991.

Wilson, Duncan. *The Making of British Bioethics.* Manchester: Manchester University Press, 2014.

Wilson, Duncan. "What Can History Do for Bioethics?" *Bioethics* 27 (2013): 215–23.

Wolff, F. A., ed. *Geneeskunde en ethiek in harmonie: Liber amicorum voor Prof.Dr E.L. Noach bij diens 8oste verjaardag op 21 November 2001.* The Hague: Pasmans Offset Drukkerij BV, 2001.

Wolters, W. H. G. *Medische experimenten met mensen: Mogelijkheden en grenzen.* Utrecht: Bohn, Scheltema & Holkema, 1980.

World Health Organization. "Principles for the Clinical Evaluation of Drugs." *World Health Organization Technical Report Series* 403 (Geneva, 1968): 6.

Yoshioka, Alan. "Use of Randomisation in the Medical Research Council's Clinical Trial of Streptomycin in Pulmonary Tuberculosis in the 1940s." *British Medical Journal* 317 (1998): 1120–223.

Zwart, Hub. *Boude Bewoordingen: De historische fenomenologie ("metabletica") van Jan Hendrik van den Berg.* Kampen: Uitgeverij Klement, 2002.

Zwart, Hub. "De Intolerantie van een Pluralistische Ethiek: De Engelhardt/Callahan-controverse." *Filosofie en Praktijk* 12 (1991): 113–24.

Zwart, Hub. *Ethische consensus in een pluralistische samenleving: De gezondheidsethiek als casus.* Amsterdam: Thesis Publishers, 1993.

INDEX

INDEX

Dutch Hospital Council, 155

Dutch Journal of Medicine, 32; ethics of medicine, 33, 78–79; human experimentation, 35–36, 109; Nazi experiments, 35

Dutch Medical Association. *See* KNMG (Royal Dutch Medical Association)

Dutch Patient-Consumer Federation, 159

Dutch Society for Bioethics, 134

Dutch Society for Health Law, 93

Dutch Society for Medical Ethics Review Committees, 155

Dutch Society for the Advancement of Medicine. *See* KNMG (Royal Dutch Medical Association)

Dutch Society for Voluntary Euthanasia, 135

Dutch Society of Ethicists, 132

Dyck, Erika, 29

EMA (European Medicines Agency), 2

embryo research, 3, 19, 147, 149, 156–57, 167

Engelhardt, H. Tristram, 134

epistemic filter, 16, 66, 69–70, 117, 179–80, 181

Erasistratus, 2

ethical engineer, 137, 144–45

ethical expertise, 134, 143, 146, 162, 169–71, 178

ethics booklets, (K)NMG, 34, 78–80, 82, 84

etiquette, 32, 79, 82

European Economic Community, 153

European Medicines Agency, 2

euthanasia and physician-assisted suicide: Dutch ethical debate, 79, 84, 87, 89, 104, 134–35; Dutch legislation and policy, 15, 156–57, 161–63, 171

Evans, John, 10, 164

expert-reviewer, 155

external control, 18; concept, 11–12; growing call for, 77; human experi-

mentation, 98, 109; research ethics committees as tools of, 99, 114

FDA (Food and Drug Administration), 2, 55, 151, 153

fetal research, 7–8, 149, 156–57

Food and Drug Administration, 2, 55, 151, 153

Fortuyn, Pim, 166

Foucault, Michel, 137

Gaarenstroom, Johan, 59–60

Geneva Declaration. *See* Declaration of Geneva

Georgetown mantra, 136, 138

germ theory of disease, 27, 30

Gilded Age of clinical research, 55

golden rule, 29

Good Clinical Practice for Trials of Medicinal Products in the European Community, 153

Graaf, Johannes de, 80–81

Groningen University, 152, 155

Gusfield, Joseph, 12

Hahnemann, teachings of, 42

Halpern, Sydney, 29–30

Hamburger, Roel, 39–40, 46

Have, Henk ten, 137, 139–40, 143, 171

Health Council, 42; Committee for Clinical Drug Research, 64–70; Committee for Clinical Pharmacology, 71–72; Committee for Medical Ethics, 88–94, 133; Committee for Tests upon Human Beings, 25, 37, 42, 46–50; Committee on Animal Vivisection, 42, 45; Committee on Vivisection-Free Medicine, 42–43, 48; Standing Committee for Health Ethics, 133, 156, 166

health ethics, 125–46; contemporary reflections, 171–72; political function, 164–69. *See also* Institute for Health Ethics; Standing Committee for Health Ethics, Health Council health law, 93–94. *See also* Leenen, Henk

Hedgecoe, Adam, 4–5, 11–12, 126

Heering, Herman, 65, 84–85, 89, 93, 131–32, 133

Hellegers, André, 134

Helsinki Declaration. *See* Declaration of Helsinki

Heringa, Gerard, 36, 40, 44

hermeneutic perspective on ethics, 136, 145, 170–71

Herophilus, 2

Heymans, Gerardus, 129

Hippocratic Oath, 9, 25, 39, 48, 127

Hoofdakker, Rudi van den, 77, 88, 92

horizontal relations of consultation and participation, 78, 94, 97, 114, 117

Huize Assisië, 107–9

Hurlbut, Benjamin, 163

Illich, Ivan, 137

incapacitated individuals, research with, 3, 149, 156–58, 162, 182

Independent Review Board Foundation, 154

informed consent. *See* consent

Institute for Health Ethics, 133–34, 155

Institute of Radio Pathology and Radiation Protection, 151

institutional isomorphism, 21, 194n69

institutional review board, 2, 4, 9–12, 111, 153

internal control, 12, 17, 25–73; *artsenstand*, 32–33, 40; criticism of, 109; Dutch medical ethics, 78; Health Council Committee for Tests upon Human Beings, 47, 51; therapeutic reform movement, 58

International Covenant on Civil and Political Rights, 149

Introduction to the Study of Experimental Medicine, 27

IRB (institutional review board), 2, 4, 9–12, 111, 153

Jacobs, Frans, 140–41

Jasanoff, Sheila, 20

Jewish Chronic Disease Hospital study, 100–101, 104

Jongh, Samuel de, 46, 57–58, 59, 60, 64

Jonsen, Albert, 9

Journal of the American Medical Association, 40

Juliana, Queen, 7

KEMO (Core Committee for Ethics and Medical Research), 156, 157

Kennedy Center for Bioethics, 134

Kluveld, Amanda, 31

KNMG (Royal Dutch Medical Association): *artsenstand*, 28–29, 33–34, 36–40, 41, 44–45, 50; creation of and Royal prefix, 28, 38–39; Dutch crisis of medical ethics, 4, 78–82, 84–88; ethics booklets, 34, 78–80, 82, 84; health ethics, 131, 132; international historiography, 15, 135; research ethics committees, 155

Kok, Wim, 157, 169–70

Kopland, Rutger. *See* Hoofdakker, Rudi van den

Krop, Henri, 130

Kuhn, Thomas, 6

Kuitert, Harry, 136

Kuyper, Abraham, 31

Labor Party (Dutch). *See* PvdA (Dutch Labor Party)

Langen, Cornelis Douwe de, 46, 47, 48

Lansink, Ad, 147

Laqueur, Ernst, 57, 205n18

Large Advisory Committee on Illegality, 36–37

Latour, Bruno, 21

Lederer, Susan, 15, 31

Leenen, Henk, 93–96, 104–5, 111–12, 120–21, 133

Leeuwen-Schut, Dian van, 167, 168–69

Leiden University, 1, 46, 57, 64, 105, 150

Lévy-Bruhl, Lucien, 129
liberal democracy, 7, 19, 164, 169–70,
181–82
liberal ethics, 139, 140
Lindeboom, Gerrit Arie, 79–80
Loghem, Joghem van, 35
logic of lesser harms, 29
Lombroso, Cesare, 105
Louis, Pierre, 27, 53
Lubbers, Ruud, 148–49

Marks, Harry, 53–55
Marlet, Jan, 83; and brothers, 83
MEB (Medicines Evaluation Board), 62,
69, 104, 207n47
medical ethics: *artsenstand*, 33, 40, 78–
86; clinical trials, 55–56, 59, 65–70;
Dutch crisis of, 78–86, 103; Dutch
political dealings with, 86–97, 163–
73; historiography, 8–15; KNMG, 39,
78–86; human experimentation, 103–
4, 119–21; medical tests upon human
beings, 34, 45–51; modern medicine,
25, 45–51; modern society, 77–97; new
authorities on, 126–35. *See also* bioethics; Committee for Medical Ethics,
Health Council; health ethics
Medical Ethics Review Committee, 3
medical insiders, 8–13, 16, 65, 167. See
also *artsenstand*
medical outsiders: call for, 102; danger
of, 178; dismissal and neglect, 33, 46,
84; health ethics, 128; historiography,
8–13, 78; KNMG, 84, 86, 92; movement of, 51, 128; overbearing concerns
of, 110, 115; participation of, 111
Medical Research Involving Human
Subjects Act. *See* WMO
Medicines Evaluation Board, 62, 69, 104,
207n47
Medicines Supply Act (Dutch), 62–63
Medisch Contact, 20, 36; antivivisectionists, 44; Borst, 156; Brutel de la
Rivière, 36–37; Dutch crisis of medi-

cal ethics, 78–83, 85; health ethics, 132;
letter of Leiden surgeon, 1, 3, 4; medical tests upon human beings, 35, 36,
40; research ethics committees, 150,
152, 153; Visser, 98, 109, 112, 114, 120
Medisch Contact: resistance group,
36–37
Medische ethiek en gedragsleer, 78–80, 82,
84
Medische macht en medische ethiek, 87
METC (Medical Ethics Review Committee), 3
Mijn, Wim van der, 95–96, 97, 105, 120–21
minimum morality, 138, 140
mondig: assertive citizens, 93–94; assertive patients, 83, 86, 94, 96, 98, 128, 156,
211n36; *mondigheid* as ethical principle, 133, 137
moral engineering, 137, 139, 144–45
moral lingua franca, 134, 136–37, 164, 173,
178
moral obligation, 27
Musschenga, Bert, 130

Nagel, Thomas, 178
National Institutes of Health, 4–5, 10, 54
National Research Act (United States),
101
Nelemans, Frans, 58–61, 63–64, 65, 67–
68, 180
neoliberalism, 18, 126, 148–49, 181
Netherlands Organization of Applied
Scientific Research. *See* TNO
new Marxism, 174
NIH (National Institutes of Health),
4–5, 10, 54
Nijmegen school of ethics, 145
NMG (Dutch Medical Association). *See*
KNMG (Royal Dutch Medical Asso-
ciation)
Noach, Erik, 8, 64; Central Council
for Public Health, 73, 99, 111, 113–20;
Health Council Committee for Clin-
ical Drug Research, 64–70; Health

Noach, Erik (*continued*)
  Council Committee for Clinical Pharmacology, 71–72; Leiden Committee for Medical Ethics, 151–52; Leiden postgraduate course, 155, 156; objectivity, 176
numerical method, 27
Nuremberg Code, 14, 15, 55
NVMETC (Dutch Society for Medical Ethics Review Committees), 155

objectivity in ethics review, 175–78
object lessons, 5
obligatory passage points, 2
Office of Scientific Research and Development, 54
Organon, 57, 205n18
Orthodox Protestant Party. *See* SGP (Staatkundig Gereformeerde Partij)
Ortt, Felix, 30–31
OSRD (Office of Scientific Research and Development), 54

Pannekoek, Job, 25, 46, 48
Pappworth, Maurice, 14, 101–2, 103
participatory decision-making, 18, 96, 126, 177
patient law, 93, 94, 112
patient material, 27, 28–29, 41, 60
patients' consent. *See* consent
patients' rights, 10, 13; Dutch codification of, 72, 95–97; Dutch movement and frame, 33, 78, 88–94; language of, 55; relation to human experimentation, 98–102, 104–5, 111, 118, 120, 179–80
Pernick, Martin, 29–30
"Peter and the Commissar" (Sherman), 174
PHS (United States Public Health Service), 5, 11, 101, 151
physicians' oath, Dutch response, 39
pillarization, 37, 82, 167, 169
Plate, Willem Paul, 46
pluralistic perspectives, 86, 97

pluralistic society, 19, 89; ethicists' discussion of, 134–36, 138–40; and objective decision-making, 177–80; and public governance, 147–48, 161–66
polder model, 119, 169–70
Porter, Dorothy, 127
Porter, Roy, 127
Porter, Theodore, 182
Principles for Those in Research and Experimentation, 40
procedural approach to ethics, 138–39
public accountability, 18–19; contemporary function of Dutch ethics review, 177–78; democratic control, 6, 112, 126; neoliberalism, 164
Purple Coalitions, 157, 166, 169–70
PvdA (Dutch Labor Party), 64, 86, 94, 107, 157, 159, 167

Querido, Arie, 90, 103

Rang, Jaap, 84, 93–94, 104, 112
rational therapeutics, ideals of, 54, 58, 60, 179
RCT (randomized controlled trial), 5, 17, 54–56, 58, 61–64, 71
research ethics committees: call for uniform procedures, 154–56; Central Council Committee for the Rights of the Patient, 97, 99, 110–18; Dutch parliamentary debates, 155–56, 162–63; Dutch rise of, 150–54; epistemic filters, 16, 64–70, 117; Health Council Committee for Clinical Drug Research, 61, 68–70; Health Council Committee for Clinical Pharmacology, 71; Health Council Committee for Tests upon Human Beings, 50; health ethics, 126, 136, 139, 143, 171–73; historiography, 4–5, 8–15; importance of historical research, 5–7; instruments of social control, 18, 73, 77–78, 110–14; obligatory passage points, 2–3; WMO, 170–71

Research School of Ethics (Dutch), 130, 145
Research School of Philosophy (Dutch), 130, 145
Rockefeller Institute, 57
Rothman, David, 8–9, 11–13, 55, 99–101
Rouvoet, André, 161
Royal Dutch Medical Association. *See* KNMG (Royal Dutch Medical Association)
Rümke, Chris, 58–60

Schiebinger, Londa, 26
School for Theology and Religion (Dutch), 130
Schrag, Zachary, 5, 12, 21
Schuyt, Kees, 105–6
SGP (Staatkundig Gereformeerde Partij), 42–43, 159, 165
Sherman, Allan, 174
Simmel, Georg, 129
Slob, Arie, 157
social-liberal party (Dutch). *See* D66 (Dutch social-liberal party)
Societas Ethica, 132
society representatives, 18, 99, 113, 117, 120, 156–60
Sporken, C. Paul, 85–86, 87, 89, 91, 93, 131–34
Standing Committee for Health Ethics, Health Council, 133, 156, 166
Stark, Laura, 3, 4, 10–12, 16, 126
State University of Limburg (Maastricht University), 133
Stevens, M. L. Tina, 10
Stewart, Larry, 29
Structure of Scientific Revolutions, The, 6

ten Have, Henk. *See* Have, Henk ten
Thatcher, Margaret, 148
therapeutic reform: concept and history, 53–56; crisis of modern medicine, 179–81; Dutch attempts at, 56–61; Health Council Commit-

tee for Clinical Drug Research, 66–70; narrative of egalitarian decision-making, 99; Noach and Van Bekkum, 115, 118
Third Way politics, 19, 170
Tilanus, Arnold, 86–88, 91
TNO (Netherlands Organization of Applied Scientific Research), 59; Committee for Clinical Drug Research, 60, 62–63, 65; Gaarenstroom's memo, 59; Radiobiological Institute and Van Bekkum, 110–11; State's Defense Force, 57; survey on research ethics committees, 152
Tongeren, Paul van, 136, 138–40, 144–45, 167, 171
Toulmin, Stephen, 126–27, 130
Tuskegee syphilis study, 5, 14, 101, 103

United States Department of Health, Education, and Welfare, 151, 153
United States Public Health Service, 5, 11, 101, 151
Utrecht Center for Bioethics and Health Law, 134, 140
Utrecht school of ethics, 145

van Bekkum, Dirk. *See* Bekkum, Dirk van
van den Berg, Jan Hendrik. *See* Berg, Jan Hendrik van den
van den Berg, Joop. *See* Berg, Joop van den
van den Hoofdakker, Rudi. *See* Hoofdakker, Rudi van den
van der Mijn, Wim. *See* Mijn, Wim van der
van der Wal, Koo. *See* Wal, Koo van der
van Leeuwen-Schut, Dian. *See* Leeuwen-Schut, Dian van
van Loghem, Joghem. *See* Loghem, Joghem van
van Tongeren, Paul. *See* Tongeren, Paul van

van Willigenburg, Theo. *See* Willigenburg, Theo van

Veatch, Robert, 9, 127

vertical relations of dependence and subordination, 78, 94, 96–97, 117

Visser, Matthijs, 98, 109–10, 112–14, 118, 120

vivisection-free medicine, 41–45

Vonhoff, Henk, 61–64, 71, 219n34

Vreeze, Jan de, 92

Vries, Gerard de, 139–40, 145, 164, 167, 171–72

VVD (Dutch conservative-liberal party), 61, 94, 106, 157, 159, 165, 166, 167

Wal, Koo van der, 130

Weber, Max, 139

Wilhelmina, Queen, 36

Willigenburg, Theo van, 142–45, 168, 171

Willowbrook State School study, 100–101

Wilson, Duncan, 11, 13, 14, 102, 127–28, 163–64

WHO (World Health Organization), 66, 90

WMA (World Medical Association), 14, 15, 39–40, 46

WMO (Medical Research Involving Human Subjects Act), 3, 147; debates in parliament, 156–63

World Federation of Doctors Who Respect Human Life, 7

World Health Organization, 66, 90

World Medical Association, 14, 15, 39–40, 46

yellow-fever experiments: US army, 5

Zwart, Hub, 138–39

Milton Keynes UK
Ingram Content Group UK Ltd.
UKHW011818140923
428699UK00004B/245